Clinical Nursing: A Process Approach

Clinical Nursing: A Process Approach

Editor: Jim Carrey

hayle medical
New York

Hayle Medical,
750 Third Avenue, 9th Floor,
New York, NY 10017, USA

Visit us on the World Wide Web at:
www.haylemedical.com

ISBN 978-1-64647-581-0 (Hardback)

Cataloging-in-Publication Data

Clinical nursing : a process approach / edited by Jim Carrey.
p. cm.
Includes bibliographical references and index.
ISBN 978-1-64647-581-0
1. Nursing. 2. Nurses. 3. Care of the sick. 4. Nursing services. 5. Medical care. I. Carrey, Jim.
RT42 .C55 2023
610.73--dc23

Contents

Preface

Clinical nursing is an advanced nursing practice that involves providing advice related to specific conditions or treatment pathways. It specializes in evidence-based nursing practice in a particular specialization of medicine. It is involved in designing, implementing and evaluating both population-based and patient-specific programs of care. There are five principal steps involved in the process of nursing, which include assessment, diagnosis, outcomes, implementation and planning. The process of assessment is concerned with analyzing a patient on the basis of in-depth physiological, economic, social and lifestyle factors. The diagnosis involves a thorough and careful examination of a patient's physical symptoms and behavior. Following this, realistic goals are set for the recovery of patients based on prior experience. It is followed by an implementation of the care plan and recording the progress of a patient. Evaluation is the final step that seeks to investigate the effectiveness of the care plan and examine the response of a patient. This book provides comprehensive insights into the field of clinical nursing. It consists of contributions made by international experts. Researchers and students in this field will be assisted by this book.

This book is a comprehensive compilation of works of different researchers from varied parts of the world. It includes valuable experiences of the researchers with the sole objective of providing the readers (learners) with a proper knowledge of the concerned field. This book will be beneficial in evoking inspiration and enhancing the knowledge of the interested readers.

In the end, I would like to extend my heartiest thanks to the authors who worked with great determination on their chapters. I also appreciate the publisher's support in the course of the book. I would also like to deeply acknowledge my family who stood by me as a source of inspiration during the project.

Editor

1

The Effect of a Nurse-Led Cognitive Behavioral Protocol on Depressive Symptoms and Coping Strategies of Dementia Caregivers

Yuqin PAN[1]* • Ruyi CHEN[2]

ABSTRACT

Background: Family caregivers of patients with dementia (PWD) often experience depressive symptoms and use poor coping strategies. Cognitive behavioral interventions may enhance positive appraisals of caregiving-related issues and the utilization of active coping strategies among caregivers, which may help prevent caregiver depression. However, there is a shortage of primary, community-based mental health services in China, and little research has been conducted on the effect of nurse-led mental health programs in this population.

Purpose: This study explored the effect of a nurse-led cognitive behavioral intervention on depressive symptoms and coping strategies among family caregivers of PWD in China.

Methods: This randomized controlled trial used data from a sample of 112 caregivers screened from 276 potential participants in a city in southeastern China. The sample was randomly assigned to an intervention group ($n = 56$) and a control group ($n = 56$). The intervention group received five monthly in-home, nurse-led cognitive behavioral sessions and telephone consultations after each session. The control group received five monthly, short, general conversations with nurse interventionists at the participants' homes, in the hospital, or via telephone. Depressive symptoms, coping strategies, and the demographics of caregiving dyads were collected at Time 1 (baseline), Time 2 (the end of the 5-month intervention), and Time 3 (2-month follow-up). IBM SPSS Statistics Version 19.0 was used for data analysis.

Results: Eighty-two participants (intervention group: $n = 47$, control group: $n = 35$) completed the three evaluations. No significant group differences were found in baseline characteristics between the two groups. The general linear model repeated-measures analysis of variance indicated a significant difference in depressive symptoms and active coping between groups over time, with $p < .001$ for the interaction between depressive symptoms and groups and $p < .01$ for the interaction between active coping and groups. A similar result did not occur for passive coping. The *t* tests further supported a significant interventional effect on participants' depressive symptoms and active coping.

Conclusions/Implications for Practice: This nurse-led cognitive behavioral intervention was effective in decreasing depressive symptoms and improving active coping among study participants. The findings suggest the improvement of mental health services and social policies in China to support family caregivers of PWD.

KEY WORDS:
randomized controlled trial, cognitive behavioral intervention, family caregivers, patients with dementia, China.

Introduction

Caregiver Depression and Coping

The number of patients with dementia (PWD) is increasing rapidly worldwide, and family caregiving to PWD is stressful as patient's cognitive and functional ability declines, accompanied by behavioral symptoms (Alzheimer's Disease International, 2016). The prevalence of depression in family caregivers of PWD has been reported as between 14.9% and 80% globally (Alfakhri et al., 2018; Hashimoto et al., 2013; Schoenmakers, Buntinx, & Delepeleire, 2010). In China, the prevalence was 22.4%, but family caregiving may be more challenging than in Western countries (Liang et al., 2016). It has been estimated that China accounts for 20% of PWD worldwide. In China, there are expectations of family care because of the cultural value of filial piety, legal requirements, and disparity between care needs and service provisions in the community (Wu & Lam, 2016). Coupled with social stigma about dementia and a lack of mental health services in primary care, family caregivers may face difficulties in coping with PWD care needs and thus face a higher risk of depression.

Coping, an important concept in Lazarus and Folkman's (1984) stress and coping theory, refers to "constantly changing cognitive and behavioral efforts to manage specific external or internal demands that are appraised as taxing or exceeding the resources." Coping strategies are frequently categorized as active versus passive, problem-focused versus emotion-focused, or approach-based versus avoidance-based/dysfunctional

[1]PhD, RN, Associate Professor, Faculty of Jinhua Polytechnic, Zhejiang Province, China • [2]MS, RN, Intermediate Laboratory Instructor, Faculty of Jinhua Polytechnic, Zhejiang Province, China.

(Lazarus & Folkman, 1984; Pearlin & Schooler, 1978; Xie, 1998). Overlaps exist among these categories. For example, active confrontation, seeking helpful resources, and positive appraisals are strategies of active coping that combine elements of problem-focused coping, approach-based coping, and emotion-focused coping, whereas acceptance and avoidance are strategies of passive coping that overlap with emotion-focused coping and avoidance-based/dysfunctional coping (Rodríguez-Pérez, Abreu-Sánchez, Rojas-Ocaña, & del-Pino-Casado, 2017; Snyder et al., 2015). Different coping strategies may affect the mental health outcomes of caregivers differently. For example, utilization of active coping has been reported to reduce depressive symptoms, and passive coping has been correlated with more depressive symptoms among caregivers (Gilhooly et al., 2016; Lu, Liu, Wang, & Lou, 2017; Roche, Croot, MacCann, Cramer, & Diehl-Schmid, 2015). Thus, mental health services that focus on coping strategies may help to prevent caregiver depression.

The Nature and Effectiveness of Cognitive Behavioral Therapy

Cognitive behavioral therapy (CBT), a psychosocial intervention, has been widely used to manage depression and coping among caregivers. The cognitive aspect of CBT helps caregivers through the use of positive reappraisals (Lazarus & Folkman, 1984). Identifying benefits is a powerful element of active and positive cognitive restructuring in which caregivers reflect on caregiving-related benefits, rewards, and positive changes. The intent is to help caregivers develop active coping skills such as problem-solving skills, promoting emotional closeness with PWD, using relaxation techniques, and balancing daily life to maintain their health. CBT, often conducted by psychologists, psychiatrists, or psychological therapists, has employed online communications, face-to-face meetings, and telephone consultations (Scott et al., 2016; Wilz & Soellner, 2016).

The evidence for the effects of face-to-face CBT on depressive symptoms and coping strategies among family caregivers of PWD is inconclusive. Although systematic reviews and meta-analyses indicate that CBT may decrease depressive symptoms, the format in which CBT is delivered must be explored further (Hopkinson, Reavell, Lane, & Mallikarjun, 2018). Prior studies have shown that CBT facilitates an adaptive coping response among caregivers (Kinnear, 2012), increases positive coping along with an increase in dysfunctional coping (Li, Cooper, Austin, & Livingston, 2013), or may reduce dysfunctional thoughts only (Kwon, Ahn, Kim, & Park, 2017). Despite these different findings, very few of the studies that were included in these systematic reviews or meta-analyses were performed in Asian countries.

Individual studies from Italy (Passoni et al., 2014) and Brazil (Aboulafia-Brakha, Suchecki, Gouveia-Paulino, Nitrini, & Ptak, 2014; Fialho, Köenig, dos Santos, Barbosa, & Caramelli, 2012) reported no significant changes in depressive symptoms of PWD caregivers after CBT, whereas other studies from Colombia (Arango-Lasprilla et al., 2014) and Spain (Vázquez et al., 2016) found a significant effect for CBT. Similarly, Fialho et al. (2012) found that family caregivers of PWD in Brazil were more optimistic and more focused on solving problems post-CBT. Moreover, Losada et al. (2015) revealed that CBT selectively affected the coping strategies of caregivers in Spain, resulting in a decrease in their dysfunctional thoughts but without a decrease in the use of avoidance.

These inconsistent findings may be caused by the limited rigor of the study designs. For example, Passoni et al. (2014) used no treatment control group for family caregivers of PWD, whereas Cheng et al. (2017) used a psychoeducation lecture group for comparison. Moreover, the focus of an intervention and its means of delivery may also be influential. An individual CBT program that focused on identifying benefits and a culturally sensitive group CBT program achieved positive effects in Chinese and Latino caregivers, respectively (Gonyea, López, & Velásquez, 2016). In contrast, a general group CBT program with education, sharing feelings, and pleasant activities was found to be ineffective (Aboulafia-Brakha et al., 2014). Finally, treatment intensity may not affect efficacy. Although duration of CBT varied between four and eight weekly or biweekly sessions, longer durations of CBT were not definitively associated with a better effect (Hopkinson et al., 2018; Vázquez et al., 2016).

Few studies by nurses have employed individual CBT among community-living family caregivers in China. Systematic reviews of relevant topics in the domestic literature have shown that coping-driven interventions increase active coping and decrease passive coping among caregivers, with their depressive symptoms relieved by multicomponent interventions. However, most studies have used group interventions in hospital settings. Studies that have used interventions similar to this study reported an effect on the depressive symptoms of Chinese family caregivers, but they were not conducted by nurses and were conducted in Australia and Hong Kong (Cheng et al., 2017; Leone et al., 2014).

Summary and Purpose of This Study

Community-based mental health nursing is urgently needed for the large number of family caregivers of PWD because of the shortage of primary mental health practitioners in China. As previously discussed, the effects of CBT on the depressive symptoms and coping strategies of caregivers are currently unclear, and little research has focused on nurse-led, individual-based cognitive behavioral interventions for community-living family caregivers in China. Thus, the purpose of this study is to explore the effect of a nurse-led cognitive behavioral intervention on depressive symptoms and coping strategies of family caregivers of PWD in China.

Methods

Study Design and Sample

This randomized controlled trial was approved by the Science and Technology Bureau (including the review of human subjects protections) in the city in which the data were collected (Project no. 2016-4-017). A convenience sample of 112 family caregivers of PWD was recruited from community health centers and an 880-bed tertiary hospital (discharge lists of neurological units) in a city in southeastern China. Inclusion criteria for caregivers were as follows: (a) being 20 years old or above, (b) serving as a primary caregiver of a family member diagnosed with Alzheimer's disease or vascular dementia or having a Mini Mental Status Examination (MMSE) score of less than 17, (c) living in the target city or its metropolitan area, (d) having a depressive symptom score of 10 or greater but less than 20, and (e) being able to understand and speak Mandarin. Individuals who showed signs of suicidal tendencies, history or evidence of a psychotic disorder, or intellectual deficits or were being treated at a mental health clinic were excluded.

Procedure

The researcher telephoned the administrators of the community health centers and the hospital to explain the study and obtain entry permission. The study was announced using flyers and word of mouth to the health staff and community residents. The researcher contacted potential participants to confirm eligibility and obtain verbal consent. Research assistants administered the anonymous surveys by appointment at three time points, namely, Time 1 (baseline), Time 2 (the end of the 5-month intervention), and Time 3 (2-month follow-up), at either the participants' homes or in hospital units during medical visits. Caregivers completed the questionnaires within 15–20 minutes, either independently according to instructions or with the help of research assistants, who also evaluated the cognitive status of PWD. A 5-month intervention period was adopted based on the duration of 2–7 months reported in previous studies and a minimum recommended intervention period of 3–4 months for an observable effect (Kwon et al., 2017). To maximize the effective time of intervention and minimize the possibility of dropouts, a 2-month follow-up was used.

After the initial assessment, participants were assigned to one of the five nurse interventionists based on area of residence. Nurses were trained in the intervention protocol and the relevant psychosocial skills and were instructed to follow the protocol. A Wechat group (Tencent, Shenzen, China) allowed the nurse interventionists to discuss procedural issues as a way to maintain intervention consistency. Participants were reminded at the initial session to keep each appointment; an additional appointment was amended over the subsequent few days if one was missed. Collected data were kept in a secure location. The data file was encrypted and stored in the researcher's personal computer.

Sample Size Calculation

G*power (Heinrich Heine Universitat, Dusseldorf, Germany) was used to calculate the sample size for this study. An *F* test, with three repeated measurements for two independent groups, a default effect size of 0.25, $\alpha = .05$, power = .85, and an expected $r = .5$ between measurements, yielded a sample size of 98. Considering a possible attrition rate of 10%–15%, the final sample size was set to 112.

Randomization and Masking

After oral consent was obtained from the participants, a computerized random number was generated at a ratio of 1:1 for the intervention-to-control group, with 56 participants in each. Group assignments were delivered to each participant in a sealed envelope. The participants and data collectors were blinded to the assignments. The data processing staff did not know the participants who were being studied. However, masking was not possible for the nurse interventionists when the treatment was initiated.

Cognitive Behavioral Intervention and Control

Intervention group

The cognitive behavioral intervention consisted of five monthly 60-minute, face-to-face, individual sessions with a 20- to 30-minute telephone consultation after each session. The face-to-face sessions were conducted by nurse interventionists early in the month. This five-module intervention (Table 1) was constructed based on the CBT strategy recommendations of Aboulafia-Brakha et al. (2014), Cheng et al. (2017), and Schinköthe and Wilz (2014). Details were flexible and tailored to the culture of family caregivers of PWD. Telephone consultations were conducted to obtain participant feedback, reinforce strategies, and answer questions.

Control group

Participants in the control group received five monthly, short, general conversations from nurse interventionists early in the month at participants' homes, in the hospital units during medical visits, or via telephone contact. The conversation was a 5- to 10-minute casual chat about daily life and health. The interventionists responded naturally by showing concern but with no in-depth instructions. Participants did not receive any additional interventions, with the possible exception of regularly scheduled medical visits.

Measures

Depression

The 10-item Center for Epidemiological Studies Depression Scale (CES-D 10) was used to assess the frequency of caregiver's depressive symptoms during the past week. An example of a CES-D 10 item is "My sleep is restless." All items are rated on a 4-point scale that ranges from 0 (*rarely or none of the time*) to 3 (*most of the time or all of the time*). The scale score is the sum of item scores, with 10 or greater indicating the presence of clinical depression. The Chinese version of CES-D 10 has been applied among caregivers in China, with a Cronbach's α of .82 (Pan, 2014).

TABLE 1.
The Nurse-Led Cognitive Behavioral Intervention Protocol

Module/Purpose	Description of Session Content
1. Assessing/ Familiarize with caregivers' situations and their perceptions	(1) Caregivers are encouraged to share their caregiving background such as personal data, family network and socioeconomic status, history of acquiring the caregiver role, patients' condition, caregiving demands, support, and daily routine. (2) Caregivers are encouraged to describe their perceptions of the caregiver role, caregiving dyadic relationship, family relationship related to caregiving, dementia, patients' behavioral symptoms, and the support resources available. (3) Caregivers are then invited to discuss issues related to dementia care such as social stigma and role demands, which may concern them the most.
2. Diagnosing/ Clarify caregivers' stressors, appraisals, and coping strategies	(1) Caregivers are encouraged to list a number of difficult caregiving scenarios and their previous management. (2) Caregivers are helped to reflect on these scenarios to identify caregiving stressors, appraisals, coping strategies, and the consequences. (3) Caregivers are then made aware of positive appraisals and active coping strategies that may facilitate stress reduction and promote problem-solving skills, along with negative appraisals and passive coping strategies that may increase stress and depressive symptoms.
3. Cognitive training/ Elicit positive appraisals and avoid negative appraisals	(1) Caregivers are further encouraged to explore caregiving scenarios that are considered as successful or difficult and specifically discuss the positive or negative appraisals utilized. (2) Caregivers are taught how to identify benefits, such as looking at the positive sides of caregiving, caregiver role, caregiving relationship, and the PWD, and identify the benefits or gains experienced during caregiving. (3) Caregivers are encouraged to rehearse by identifying benefits in difficult caregiving scenarios and avoid negative appraisals, thoughts, or emotions.
4. Coping behavioral training/ Reinforce active coping strategies and avoid passive coping strategies	(1) Caregivers are further encouraged to explore caregiving scenarios that are considered as successful or difficult and to discuss the active or passive coping strategies utilized. (2) Caregivers are guided to utilize active coping strategies in specific caregiving situations, such as building support, venting anxiety, seeking help to solve problems, and nurturing a good caregiver–care receiver relationship or a friendly caregiving environment. (3) Caregivers are reinforced with these active coping strategies in examples of specific challenging caregiving scenarios and also trained to avoid passive coping strategies.
5. Relaxation and self-maintenance skill training/ Stress reduction and self-care	(1) Caregivers are taught with relaxation skills such as deep breathing, diary writing, music listening, exercising, and throwing soft pillows and allowed time to practice these skills. (2) More behavioral changes focused on personal health maintenance such as improving time management, assuming pleasant activities or hobbies, balancing nutrients, and employing sleeping tips. (3) Caregivers are encouraged to develop other personal skills beneficial to their health.
Session	**Procedures and Approximate Timing**
1. Five 60-minute, face-to-face monthly sessions conducted early in the month	(1) Building rapport (3–5 minutes) (2) Conducting the session by reviewing of previous session content and making transient to new session. Following the list of session content and taking notes for each session (45–50 minutes) (3) Summarizing, assigning homework, and terminating (5–10 minutes)
2. Five 20- to 30-min monthly telephone consultations in the middle of the month	(1) Building rapport (2–3 minutes) (2) Conducting the consultation by reviewing the previous session according to the session content list. Asking for feedbacks, reinforcing knowledge, positive appraisals or active coping skills, and taking notes for each consultation (15–20 minutes) (3) Summarizing, assigning homework, and terminating (3–5 minutes)

Coping

The 20-item simplified coping scale (Xie, 1998) was developed with Chinese adults and used to measure caregiver coping strategies. Cronbach's α was .90 for the full scale, .89 for the 12-item subscale of active coping, and .78 for the eight-item subscale of passive coping. Examples of scale items are "Try to identify several solutions to solve the problem" and "Try to forget the whole thing." All items are rated on a 4-point scale that ranges from 0 (*never used*) to 3 (*often used*). The subscale scores are averages of the respective items. Higher scores for active coping are associated with better coping ability, whereas higher scores for passive coping are associated with poorer coping ability.

Care receivers' self-maintainance ability

The 14-item Activities of Daily Living Scale measures both basic and more complicated self-maintenance activities for PWD. One example of a scale item is "Are you having difficulty bathing?" All items are scored on a 4-point scale that ranges from 1 (*perform without difficulty*) to 4 (*unable to perform*). The scale score is the sum of item scores. Higher scores indicate lower functional ability. The Chinese version of this scale has been used in studies of disabled older adults in China, with a Cronbach's α of .97 (Pan, 2014).

Care receivers' cognitive function

The cognitive function of PWD was assessed using the Chinese version of the MMSE, which has been widely tested with satisfactory psychometrics and used with older adults in China (Yu, Li, & Huang, 2012). The MMSE consists of 10 cognitive function domains such as orientation, memory, and calculation with a maximum score of 30 points. Higher scores indicate better cognitive function. The cutoff point for diagnosing cognitive impairment is 16–19 for those with less than primary education. Therefore, a recruitment criterion of 17 points was adopted.

Demographic and caregiving characteristics

A researcher-designed questionnaire was used to collect demographic data for participants and PWD, with caregiving characteristics listed in Table 2.

Data Analysis

Data were analyzed using IBM SPSS Statistics Version 19.0 (IBM, Armonk, NY, USA). Descriptive data were evaluated with frequencies and measures of central tendency. Group differences in the characteristics of caregiving dyads were analyzed using an independent-samples t test for continuous variables that met the assumptions of normality and homogeneity and the Mann–Whitney U test for variables that did not. The chi-square test was used for all categorical data.

The differences in depressive symptoms, active coping, and passive coping between the two groups over time (Time 1, Time 2, and Time 3) were evaluated, respectively, using general linear model repeated-measures analysis of variance (GLM repeated-measures ANOVA) with one within-subject factor (one of the three main variables studied) and one between-subject factor (groups) as the assumptions of normality, homogeneity, and sphericity were met. The differences in the study variables between groups were analyzed using independent-samples t tests, and the pre-differences and post-differences for the study variables in the same group were analyzed using paired t tests. Intention-to-treat analysis was not conducted because of the relatively large attrition rate.

Results

This study continued from mid-May 2016 to mid-March 2017. A sample comprising 112 family caregivers of PWD was enrolled after 276 potential participants were screened. This sample was randomly assigned to either the intervention group (n = 56) or the control group (n = 56). Eighty-two participants (intervention group: n = 47, control group: n = 35) completed all three evaluations (Figure 1). Demographic characteristics are shown in Table 2. No significant group differences were found in the characteristics of the caregiving dyads.

The GLM repeated-measures ANOVA, with one within-subject factor (depressive symptoms, active coping, or passive coping) and one between-subject factor (groups), indicated significant differences, respectively, in depressive symptoms and active coping between groups over time (Table 3). The p value for the interaction between depressive symptoms and groups was < .001. The related mean plot showed a small difference in depressive symptoms between groups at Time 1, which became much larger at Time 2 and Time 3 (Figure 2). Active coping reflected a similar change, except that it increased at Time 2, and the p value for the interaction between active coping and the groups was < .01 (Table 3, Figure 2). Conversely, no significance was found for the interaction between passive coping and groups ($p > .05$ for the interaction).

Table 3 shows no significant group differences in the study variables at Time 1. However, the independent-samples t tests showed significant group differences in depressive symptoms ($t = -3.53$, $p < .01$) and active coping ($t = 4.20$, $p < .001$) at Time 2, with improvements in the intervention group, and the significance persisted at Time 3. However, similar changes did not occur in passive coping. The paired t tests revealed significant decreases in depressive symptoms ($t = 10.12$, $p < .001$) and passive coping ($t = 2.29$, $p < .05$) and a significant increase in active coping ($t = -7.50$, $p < .001$) between Time 1 and Time 2 in the intervention group, with significance sustained between Time 1 and Time 3. In addition, significant changes were noted in depressive symptoms and passive coping in the control group at different times.

Discussion

Effect of the Intervention on Depressive Symptoms

This study found the nurse-led cognitive behavioral intervention to be effective in reducing depressive symptoms among

TABLE 2.

Sample Characteristics at Baseline (N = 112)

Variable	Total (*N* = 112)		Intervention Group (*n* = 56)		Control Group (*n* = 56)		$t/\chi^2/Z$	*p*
	n	%	*n*	%	*n*	%		
Caregivers								
Age (*M* ± *SD*)	62.7	10.9	63.3	11.2	62.1	10.6	$t = 0.57$	.57
Gender							$\chi^2 = 2.44$	.12
Male	42	37.5	25	44.6	17	30.4		
Female	70	62.5	31	55.4	39	69.6		
Relationships							$\chi^2 = 0.14$	.71
Spouse	54	48.2	28	50.0	26	46.4		
Other family members	58	51.8	28	50.0	30	53.6		
Education							$\chi^2 = 0.001$	.99
Junior, middle school, and below	100	89.3	50	89.3	50	89.3		
High school and above	12	10.7	6	10.7	6	10.7		
Monthly income (RMB)							$\chi^2 = 2.19$	.14
≤ 3,000	92	82.1	43	76.8	49	87.5		
> 3,000	20	17.9	13	23.2	7	12.5		
Number of CD (*M* ± *SD*)	1.1	1.1	1.3	1.3	0.9	0.9	$Z = -1.89$	.07
Living status							$\chi^2 = 0.49$	.48
Co-resident	89	79.5	46	82.1	43	76.8		
Resides separately	23	20.5	10	17.9	13	23.2		
Duration of care (months; *M* ± *SD*)	67.3	75.6	71.2	85.6	63.3	64.6	$Z = -0.52$	.60
Hours of care per day (*M* ± *SD*)	17.0	8.8	17.7	8.5	16.4	9.1	$t = 0.79$	.43
Burden							$\chi^2 = 0.69$	.40
No or infrequent	15	13.4	6	10.7	9	16.1		
Frequent or very frequent	97	86.6	50	89.3	47	83.9		
Care receivers								
Age (*M* ± *SD*)	79.5	9.5	79.0	9.4	80.0	9.8	$t = -0.53$	.60
Gender							$\chi^2 = 3.12$	.08
Male	41	36.6	16	28.6	25	44.6		
Female	71	63.4	40	71.4	31	55.4		
MMSE (*M* ± *SD*)	6.5	5.9	6.5	5.9	6.6	5.9	$t = -0.18$	.86
ADLs (*M* ± *SD*)	43.9	10.5	42.9	10.7	44.9	10.4	$t = -0.98$	.33
Psychobehavioral symptoms							$\chi^2 = 0.54$	.46
Yes	39	35.0	21	37.5	17	30.3		
No	73	65.0	35	62.5	39	69.7		
History of hospitalization							$\chi^2 = 0.04$	.84
Yes	75	67.0	37	66.1	38	67.9		
No	37	33.0	19	33.9	18	32.1		

Note. MMSE = Mini Mental Status Examination; ADLs = activities of daily living; CD = chronic diseases; *Z* = *Z* score from the Mann–Whitney *U* test.

participants, as the mean differences in depressive symptoms differed significantly between groups over time (Table 3, Figure 2). This finding agrees with those reported by Arango-Lasprilla et al. (2014), Kwon et al. (2017), and Vázquez et al. (2016) but contradicts the findings of Passoni et al. (2014). The diversity of research designs in terms of number of subgroups, conditions of intervention or control, and means of delivery used in these studies may be largely responsible for these inconsistencies.

Several potential explanations exist for the decrease in depressive symptoms after the cognitive behavioral intervention. First, participants in the intervention group may have developed coping skills for problem solving and stress reduction. This explanation is supported by the work of Gallagher-Thompson, Gray, Dupart, Jimenez, and Thompson (2008), who reported that the use of coping skills and perceived helpfulness helped reduce depressive symptoms in caregivers after they had received CBT. Second, caregiving in China is a family responsibility with insufficient support and no pay, which may cause resentment among caregivers. The strategies of cognitive reappraisal used in the intervention group helped caregivers consider the benefits and rewards of caregiving, which may have enhanced their perceptions of the meaning of caregiving and self-worth. Third, family caregivers are often homebound, socially isolated, and neglected. Participants in the intervention

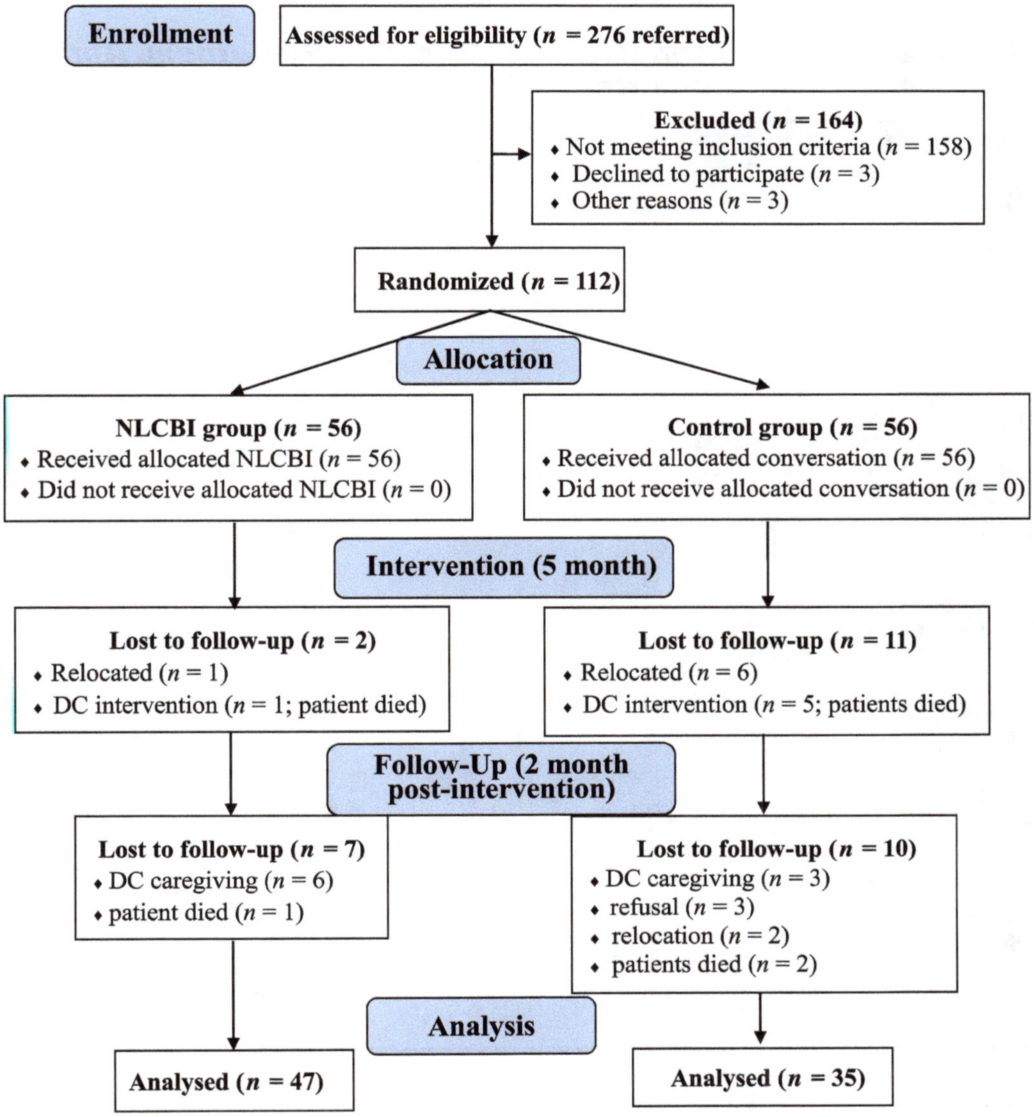

Figure 1. Research process. NLCBI = nurse-led cognitive behavioral intervention; DC = discontinue.

group had a greater opportunity to privately express concerns regarding caregiving demands and to experience being the focus of others' concern. Hence, they received more social support than their peers in the control group (Pan, 2014). Thus, mental health nursing services, such as the cognitive behavioral intervention reported in this article, are an important source of support for the family caregivers of PWD.

Although the group differences in depressive symptoms at both Time 2 and Time 3 were significant (Table 3, independent-samples *t* test), confirming the effectiveness of this cognitive behavioral intervention, depressive symptom scores dropped steeply at Time 2 but rose again at Time 3 (Figure 2). This trend is similar to the findings of Arango-Lasprilla et al. (2014) at a 3-month follow-up and contrary to the findings of Vázquez et al. (2016), who found a 12-month effect of CBT. Because of the varied length of follow-up periods among the different studies, it is difficult to conclude whether the rise in depressive symptoms at Time 3 represented a fluctuation in an overall downward progression or indicated an upward trend. Therefore, further investigation is necessary to determine the long-term effect of this intervention.

Furthermore, as caregiving situations are often complicated, multiple social factors such as the repeated hospitalizations of PWD may exacerbate caregiver depression and confound the interventional effect. Additional analysis using GLM repeated-measures ANOVA found a slight change in the significance levels of the interactions when the data were stratified by repeated PWD hospitalizations (yes/no). However, the work of Kuo et al. (2017) tended to support the idea that caregiver depression should remain stable despite the disruption of repeated hospitalizations, because depression is deeply rooted in the caregiving process. The intensity of the cognitive behavioral intervention provided in this study may be inadequate to

TABLE 3.
Within- or Between-Group Differences in Depressive Symptoms, Active Coping, Passive Coping, and Their Interactions With Group

Variable/Time/Group	*n*	*M*	*SD*	Independent *t*	Paired *t*	*p*[a]
Depressive symptoms						$p = .0001$
Time 1	112			1.15		
Intervention group	56	13.9	3.5			Depression × Groups
Control group	56	13.2	3.1			$p = .0001$
Time 2	99			−3.53**	Time 1 vs. Time 2	
Intervention group	54	9.4	3.5		10.12***	
Control group	45	12.0	3.8		2.80*	
Time 3	82			−2.30*	Time 1 vs. Time 3	
Intervention group	47	10.2	3.0		7.09***	
Control group	35	12.1	5.0		0.75	
Active coping						$p = .0001$
Time 1	112			−0.37		
Intervention group	56	1.2	0.4			Active Coping × Groups
Control group	56	1.2	0.4			$p = .002$
Time 2	99			4.20***	Time 1 vs. Time 2	
Intervention group	54	1.6	0.5		−7.50***	
Control group	45	1.3	0.4		−1.50	
Time 3	82			2.13*	Time 1 vs. Time 3	
Intervention group	47	1.5	0.5		−4.50***	
Control group	35	1.2	0.4		−1.93	
Passive coping						$p = .001$
Time 1	112			−0.21		
Intervention group	56	1.4	0.4			Passive Coping × Groups
Control group	56	1.4	0.4			$p = .690$
Time 2	99			−0.44	Time 1 vs. Time 2	
Intervention group	54	1.2	0.4		2.29*	
Control group	45	1.3	0.4		1.63	
Time 3	82			0.52	Time 1 vs. Time 3	
Intervention group	47	1.1	0.4		2.21*	
Control group	35	1.1	0.4		3.47**	

Note. Time 1 = baseline; Time 2 = end of the 5-month intervention; Time 3 = 2-month follow-up; I = intervention group; C = control group.
[a]Within-subject effects (sphericity assumed).
*$p < .05$. ** $p < .01$. *** $p < .001$.

eradicate depression. Instead, the intervention should occur regularly to effectively alleviate the depressive symptoms of caregivers over the long term and be subject to longer follow-ups to further confirm the effect.

Finally, depressive symptoms in the control group also decreased significantly at Time 2, although not as significantly as in the intervention group (Table 3, independent-samples *t* test). There are several potential explanations for this finding. Depressed caregivers may be more responsive to interventions than those who are not (Ho, 2017; Otero et al., 2015). The participants in this study had moderate depression, whereas most previous studies included both depressed and nondepressed caregivers. Another potential explanation is that, similar to Chang (1999), an unexpected placebo effect may have occurred. Furthermore, this phenomenon may illustrate that mental health services for caregivers of PWD in China are sufficiently meager so that even short general conversations have a measurable impact, implying that family caregivers are in great need of mental health nursing care.

Effect of the Intervention on Active Coping

The nurse-led cognitive behavioral intervention in this study significantly improved active coping skills among participants; there was a significant difference in active coping scores between the groups over time (Table 3, Figure 2). This finding is similar to Li et al. (2013) and Fialho et al. (2012). As Chinese caregivers are inclined not to ask for help even in difficult situations (Au, Shardlow, Teng, Tsien, & Chan, 2013), this nurse-led cognitive behavioral intervention aimed not only to increase participants' positive appraisals and improve their ability to deal with emotions but also to encourage the use of strategies to solve caregiving-related problems. For example, after the intervention, participants may have felt less stigmatized

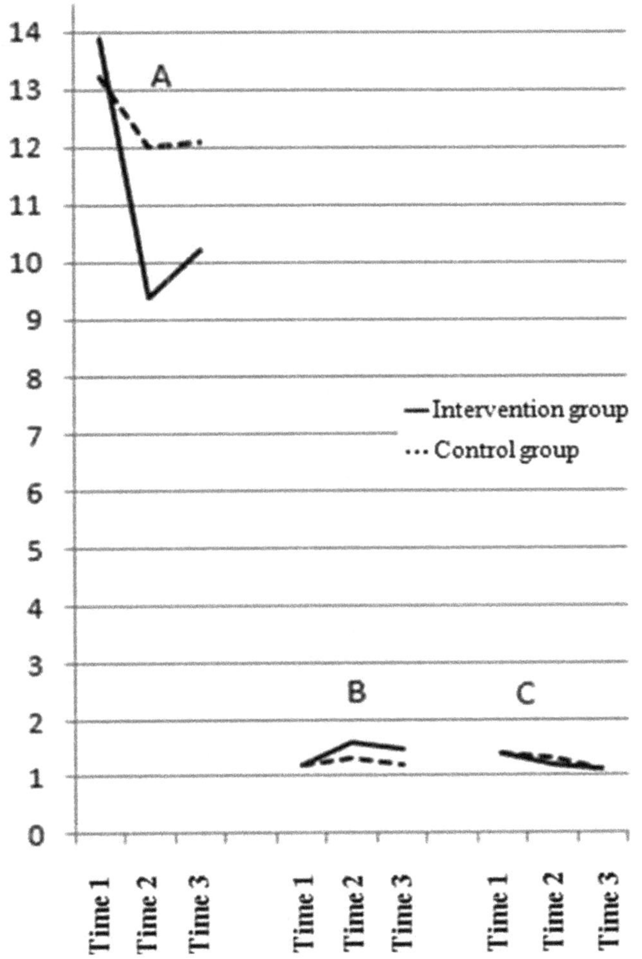

Figure 2. Changes in the means of depressive symptoms (A), active coping (B), and passive coping (C) between groups over three time points.

as a caregiver of a PWD, viewed their caregiving experience and relationships with PWD more positively, sought help and support, and developed caregiving and self-care skills. These findings support the stress and coping theory tenets (Lazarus & Folkman, 1984) that positive appraisals lead to active coping and better health outcomes. Therefore, this intervention was effective in improving the active coping strategies of participants, which may benefit family caregivers of PWD in China.

Effect of the Intervention on Passive Coping

This study did not reveal a significant interventional effect on passive coping, as indicated by the results of GLM repeated-measures ANOVA (Table 3, Figure 2). Nevertheless, passive coping in both groups declined significantly from Time 1 to Time 3 (paired *t* tests). This finding is inconsistent with the work of Li et al. (2013), in which CBT increased passive coping such as dysfunctional coping in caregivers, and partly in line with the work of Losada et al. (2015), in which CBT selectively decreased dysfunctional thoughts in caregivers. Reasons for these differences are not clear but may be related to the research design of each study and the different control conditions, coping scales, sample characteristics, and sample ethnicities used. Furthermore, this may indicate that Chinese caregivers in both groups gradually accepted the fact that dementia is not curable and that some PWD were moving toward the end of life as the disease progressed. More investigations must be conducted to clarify the effect of this intervention on passive coping as well as its mechanisms and potential influencing factors.

Limitations, Future Directions, and Implications

This study investigated the effect of a nurse-led cognitive behavioral intervention on the depressive symptoms and coping strategies of family caregivers in China. Several limitations should be considered when interpreting the findings.

First, the relatively high attrition rate may have decreased the power of this study. The response rate was 84.0% (47 from 56) in the intervention group and 62.5% (35 from 56) in the control group (Figure 1). This may be because of participant relocating, seeking alternative care, or losing interest in this study or of patient death. Future recruitment plans should exclude caregivers with a high risk of withdrawal and patients with severe conditions.

Second, the PWD in this study were older (M = 79.5 years old) with chronic conditions. Most (67.0%) were hospitalized during the intervention period (Table 2). This may have interfered with the emotional experience of participants, as both the stress and the support received in the hospital environment, in transition, and at home vary. Therefore, future recruitment efforts should focus on caregivers of PWD who are typical and stable.

Third, although the nurse interventionists were trained in relevant skills, participant adherence and treatment fidelity were not studied. Moreover, the effect of the intervention may be subject to participant trust in nurses, learning capacity, and adherence to the intervention as well as the nurses' communication skills. Future studies should set goals for caregivers and nurses in each session to maintain the quality of the intervention.

This study has important implications for nursing practice. The intervention may be helpful in training family caregivers to develop active coping strategies that reduce their depressive symptoms. Countries like China, which has an increasing number of PWD but few primary mental health practitioners, are well positioned to benefit from related nursing interventions. Early detection, continuous monitoring, and support through nurse-led community service programs are essential to sustain the mental health of family caregivers.

Various ways to deliver this intervention are available, and face-to-face cognitive behavioral sessions with telephone consultations may be a feasible approach for homebound family caregivers. The caregiver-oriented nursing interaction was based on cognitive behavioral training and developed a trusting relationship that gave nurses access to participant homes, which may have facilitated the positive results.

To confirm these results, future research on nurse-led cognitive behavioral interventions should recruit larger samples and/or adopt strategies to minimize dropouts, attempt to maintain treatment fidelity and caregiver adherence, lengthen the time frame because the effect of this intervention may be evident over a longer term, confirm the effect of this intervention on active and passive coping, and study the mechanisms that reduce depressive symptoms in caregivers.

This research has implications for social policy in China. As formal support is sparse, this study recommends that family caregivers of PWD be eligible for financial subsidies and regular mental health services. Strategies such as consultations, psychoeducation, cognitive behavioral interventions, and other supportive services should be developed for family caregivers in the community. Optimizing the health of family caregivers will have substantial social and economic benefits by decreasing the need to institutionalize PWD, which would not only honor the general preference of older adults to age in their homes but also greatly reduce the nationwide burden.

Conclusions

This nurse-led cognitive behavioral intervention was shown to be effective in reducing depressive symptoms and increasing active coping strategies in a sample of family caregivers of PWD in China. It is suggested that an appropriate mental health nursing program be initiated in the community and combined with social support for family caregivers who are at risk of depression as one strategy, to ameliorate the growing crisis in dementia care in China.

Acknowledgments

This research was supported by grant (No. 2016-4-017) from Jin Hua Science and Technology Bureau.

References

Aboulafia-Brakha, T., Suchecki, D., Gouveia-Paulino, F., Nitrini, R., & Ptak, R. (2014). Cognitive–behavioural group therapy improves a psychophysiological marker of stress in caregivers of patients with Alzheimer's disease. *Aging & Mental Health, 18*(6), 801–808. https://doi.org/10.1080/13607863.2014.880406

Alfakhri, A. S., Alshudukhi, A. W., Alqahtani, A. A., Alhumaid, A. M., Alhathlol, O. A., Almojali, A. I., ... Alaqeel, M. K. (2018). Depression among caregivers of patients with dementia. *INQUIRY: The Journal of Medical Care Organization Provision & Financing, 55*(9), 551–556. https://doi.org/10.1177/0046958017750432

Alzheimer's Disease International. (2016). *World Alzheimer Report 2016: Improving healthcare for people living with dementia.* Retrieved from https://www.alz.co.uk/research/worldalzheimerreport2016sheet.pdf

Arango-Lasprilla, J. C., Panyavin, I., Merchán, E. J. H., Perrin, P. B., Arroyo-Anlló, E. M., Snipes, D. J., & Arabia, J. (2014). Evaluation of a group cognitive–behavioral dementia caregiver intervention in Latin America. *American Journal of Alzheimer's Disease & Other Dementias, 29*(6), 548–555. https://doi.org/10.1177/1533317514523668

Au, A., Shardlow, S. M., Teng, Y., Tsien, T., & Chan, C. (2013). Coping strategies and social support-seeking behaviour among Chinese caring for older people with dementia. *Ageing & Society, 33*(8), 1422–1441. https://doi.org/10.1017/S0144686X12000724

Chang, B. L. (1999). Cognitive–behavioral intervention for homebound caregivers of persons with dementia. *Nursing Research, 48*(3), 173–182. https://doi.org/10.1097/00006199-199905000-00007

Cheng, S. T., Mak, E. P. M., Fung, H. H., Kwok, T., Lee, D. T. F., & Lam, L. C. W. (2017). Benefit-finding and effect on caregiver depression: A double-blind randomized controlled trial. *Journal of Consulting & Clinical Psychology, 85*(5), 521–529. https://doi.org/10.1037/ccp0000176

Fialho, P. P., Köenig, A. M., dos Santos, M. D. L., Barbosa, M. T., & Caramelli, P. (2012). Positive effects of a cognitive–behavioral intervention program for family caregivers of demented elderly. *Arquivos de Neuro-Psiquiatria, 70*(10), 786–792. https://doi.org/10.1590/S0004-282X2012001000007

Gallagher-Thompson, D., Gray, H. L., Dupart, T., Jimenez, D., & Thompson, L. W. (2008). Effectiveness of cognitive/behavioral small group intervention for reduction of depression and stress in non-Hispanic white and Hispanic/Latino women dementia family caregivers: Outcomes and mediators of change. *Journal of Rational-Emotive & Cognitive-Behavior Therapy, 26*(4), 286–303. https://doi.org/10.1007/s10942-008-0087-4

Gilhooly, K. J., Gilhooly, M. L., Sullivan, M. P., McIntyre, A., Wilson, L., Harding, E., ... Crutch, S. (2016). A meta-review of stress, coping and interventions in dementia and dementia caregiving. *BMC Geriatrics, 16*(1), 106. https://doi.org/10.1186/s12877-016-0280-8

Gonyea, J. G., López, L. M., & Velásquez, E. H. (2016). The effectiveness of a culturally sensitive cognitive behavioral group intervention for Latino Alzheimer's caregivers. *The Gerontologist, 56*(2), 292–302. https://doi.org/10.1093/geront/gnu045

Hashimoto, E., Washio, M., Arai, Y., Sasaki, R., Mori, M., & Saito, T. (2013). Depression among family caregivers of patients with dementia attending to a psychiatric dispensary in northern Japan. *International Medical Journal, 20*(1), 9–12. Retrieved from https://www.researchgate.net/publication/289436414

Ho, J. S. (2017). *Mediators and moderators of dementia caregiver depression and CVD risk outcomes in the pleasant events program* (Unpublished doctoral dissertation). University of California at San Diego, San Diego State University. Retrieved from http://hdl.handle.net/10211.3/174575

Hopkinson, M. D., Reavell, J., Lane, D. A., & Mallikarjun, P. (2018). Cognitive behavioral therapy for depression, anxiety, and stress in caregivers of dementia patients: A systematic review and meta-analysis. *The Gerontologist*, gnx217. https://doi.org/10.1093/geront/gnx217

Kinnear, V. (2012). *Systematic review and meta-analysis of psychological interventions for informal dementia caregivers* (Unpublished doctoral dissertation). University of Edinburgh, UK. Retrieved from https://www.researchgate.net/publication/292450154

Kuo, L. M., Huang, H. L., Liang, J., Kwok, Y. T., Hsu, W. C., Su, P. L., & Shyu, Y. L. (2017). A randomized controlled trial of a home-based training programme to decrease depression in family caregivers of persons with dementia. *Journal of Advanced Nursing, 73*(3), 585–598. https://doi.org/10.1111/jan.13157

Kwon, O. Y., Ahn, H. S., Kim, H. J., & Park, K. W. (2017). Effectiveness of cognitive behavioral therapy for caregivers of people with dementia: A systematic review and meta-analysis. *Journal of Clinical Neurology, 13*(4), 394–404. https://doi.org/10.3988/jcn.2017.13.4.394

Lazarus, R. S., & Folkman, S. (1984). *Stress, appraisal, and coping.* New York, NY: Springer.

Leone, D., Carragher, N., Santalucia, Y., Draper, B., Thompson, L. W., Shanley, C., ... Thompson, D. G. (2014). A pilot of an intervention delivered to Chinese- and Spanish-speaking carers of people with dementia in Australia. *American Journal of Alzheimer's Disease & Other Dementias, 29*(1), 32–37. https://doi.org/10.1177/1533317513505130

Li, R., Cooper, C., Austin, A., & Livingston, G. (2013). Do changes in coping style explain the effectiveness of interventions for psychological morbidity in family carers of people with dementia? A systematic review and meta-analysis. *International Psychogeriatrics, 25*(2), 204–214. https://doi.org/10.1017/S1041610212001755

Liang, X., Guo, Q., Luo, J., Li, F., Ding, D., Zhao, Q., & Hong, Z. (2016). Anxiety and depression symptoms among caregivers of care-recipients with subjective cognitive decline and cognitive impairment. *BMC Neurology, 16*(1), 191–199. https://doi.org/10.1186/s12883-016-0712-2

Losada, A., Márquez González, M., Romero Moreno, R., Mausbach, B. T., López, J., Fernández Fernández, V., & Nogales-Gonzalez, C. (2015). Cognitive–behavioral therapy (CBT) versus acceptance and commitment therapy (ACT) for dementia family caregivers with significant depressive symptoms: Results of a randomized clinical trial. *Journal of Consulting & Clinical Psychology, 83*(4), 760–772. https://doi.org/10.1037/ccp0000028

Lu, N., Liu, J., Wang, F., & Lou, V. W. (2017). Caring for disabled older adults with musculoskeletal conditions: A transactional model of caregiver burden, coping strategies, and depressive symptoms. *Archives of Gerontology and Geriatrics, 69*, 1–7. https://doi.org/10.1016/j.archger.2016.11.001

Otero, P., Smit, F., Cuijpers, P., DeRubeis, R. J., Torres, Á., & Vázquez, F. L. (2015). Differential response to depression prevention among a sample of informal caregivers: Moderator analysis of longer-term follow-up trial data. *Psychiatry Research, 230*(2), 271–278. https://doi.org/org/10.1016/j.psychres.2015.09.005

Pan, Y. (2014). *Predictors of health in adult child caregivers of parent stroke survivors in China* (Doctoral dissertation, Loma Linda University). Retrieved from http://scholarsrepository.llu.edu/etd/170/

Passoni, S., Moroni, L., Toraldo, A., Mazzà, M. T., Bertolotti, G., Vanacore, N., & Bottini, G. (2014). Cognitive behavioral group intervention for Alzheimer caregivers. *Alzheimer Disease & Associated Disorders, 28*(3), 275–282. https://doi.org/10.1097/WAD.0000000000000033

Pearlin, L. I., & Schooler, C. (1978). The structure of coping. *Journal of Health and Social Behavior, 19*(1), 2–21. https://doi.org/10.2307/2136319

Roche, L., Croot, K., MacCann, C., Cramer, B., & Diehl-Schmid, J. (2015). The role of coping strategies in psychological outcomes for frontotemporal dementia caregivers. *Journal of Geriatric Psychiatry and Neurology, 28*(3), 218–228. https://doi.org/10.1177/0891988715588830

Rodríguez-Pérez, M., Abreu-Sánchez, A., Rojas-Ocaña, M. J., & del-Pino-Casado, R. (2017). Coping strategies and quality of life in caregivers of dependent elderly relatives. *Health and Quality of Life Outcomes, 15*, 71. https://doi.org/10.1186/s12955-017-0634-8

Schinköthe, D., & Wilz, G. (2014). The assessment of treatment integrity in a cognitive behavioral telephone intervention study with dementia caregivers. *Clinical Gerontologist, 37*(3), 211–234. https://doi.org/10.1080/07317115.2014.886653

Schoenmakers, B., Buntinx, F., & Delepeleire, J. (2010). Factors determining the impact of care-giving on caregivers of elderly patients with dementia: A systematic literature review. *Maturitas, 66*(2), 191–200. https://doi.org/10.1016/j.maturitas.2010.02.009

Scott, J. L., Dawkins, S., Quinn, M. G., Sanderson, K., Elliott, K. E., Stirling, C., ... Robinson, A. (2016). Caring for the carer: A systematic review of pure technology-based cognitive behavioral therapy (TB-CBT) interventions for dementia carers. *Aging & Mental Health, 20*(8), 793–803. https://doi.org/10.1080/13607863.2015.1040724

Snyder, C. M., Fauth, E., Wanzek, J., Piercy, K. W., Norton, M. C., Corcoran, C., ... Tschanz, J. T. (2015). Dementia caregivers' coping strategies and their relationship to health and well-being: The cache county study. *Aging & Mental Health, 19*(5), 390–399. https://doi.org/10.1080/13607863.2014.939610

Vázquez, F. L., Torres, Á., Blanco, V., Otero, P., Díaz, O., & Ferraces, M. J. (2016). Long-term follow-up of a randomized clinical trial assessing the efficacy of a brief cognitive–behavioral depression prevention intervention for caregivers with elevated depressive symptoms. *American Journal of Geriatric Psychiatry, 24*(6), 421–432. https://doi.org/10.1016/j.jagp.2016.02.050

Wilz, G., & Soellner, R. (2016). Evaluation of a short-term telephone-based cognitive behavioral intervention for dementia family caregivers. *Clinical Gerontologist, 39*(1), 25–47. https://doi.org/10.1080/07317115.2015.1101631

Wu, D., & Lam, T. P. (2016). Underuse of primary care in China: The scale, causes, and solutions. *Journal of the American Board of Family Medicine, 29*(2), 240–247. https://doi.org/10.3122/jabfm.2016.02.150159

Xie, Y. (1998). Reliability and validity of the simplified Coping Style Questionnaire. *Chinese Journal of Clinical Psychology, 6*(2), 114–115.

Yu, J., Li, J., & Huang, X. (2012). The Beijing version of the Montreal cognitive assessment as a brief screening tool for mild cognitive impairment: A community-based study. *BMC Psychiatry, 12*(1), 156. https://doi.org/10.1186/1471-244X-12-156

2

Using a Text Mining Approach to Explore the Recording Quality of a Nursing Record System

Hsiu-Mei CHANG[1] • Ean-Weng HUANG[2] • I-Ching HOU[3] • Hsiu-Yun LIU[4] • Fang-Shan LI[5] • Shwu-Fen CHIOU[6]*

ABSTRACT

Background: Most nursing records in Taiwan have been computerized, resulting in a large amount of unstructured text data. The quality of these records has rarely been discussed.

Purpose: This study used a text mining method to analyze the quality of a nursing record system to establish an auditing model and associated tools for nursing records, with the ultimate objective of improving the quality of electronic nursing records.

Methods: This study utilized a retrospective method to collect the electronic nursing records of 6,277 patients who had been discharged from the internal medicine departments of a medical center in northern Taiwan from January to June 2014. SAS Enterprise Guide Version 6.1 and SAS Text Miner Version 13.2 software were used to perform text mining. Nursing experts were invited to examine the electronic nursing records. The text mining results were compared against a benchmark that was developed by the experts, and the efficiency of SAS Text Miner was examined using the criteria of specificity, sensitivity, and accuracy.

Results: In this study, 27,356 nurse-formulated events were used in the analysis. The results of the nurse-formulated events showed an 8.08% similar error with system-formulated events, 29.72% were identified as necessary and appropriate names, 17.53% were retained, 10.15% involved error event names, and 34.52% were not classified. In this study, the sensitivity of SAS text mining in the training (testing) data set was 96% (95%), and the specificity and accuracy were both 99% (99%).

Conclusions: The results of this study show that text mining is an effective approach to auditing the quality of electronic nursing records. SAS Text Miner software was shown to identify inappropriate nursing record content quickly and efficiently. Furthermore, the results of this study may be included in in-service education teaching materials to promote the writing of better nursing records to improve the quality of electronic nursing records.

KEY WORDS:
nursing record, record quality, text mining.

Introduction

The computerization of medical information is a global trend. Increasingly, governments are facilitating the integration of information technology in healthcare and related settings. Using information systems allows patient information to be collected, retrieved, stored, and managed rapidly and accurately, and delivered instantly and correctly. It also effectively enhances team communication and enables patient-centered care. Nursing records are an important component of computerization and include information about patient physiological and psychological changes that nurses record in patient medical records after providing nursing care. These records are also critical legal documents representing the process of nursing care. Moreover, they are a crucial reference for clinical decision making (Almasalha et al., 2013; Feng, Tseng, Yan, Huang, & Chang, 2013; Paans, Sermeus, Nieweg, & Van Der Schans, 2010).

Nursing record computerization enhances the quality of medical records, reduces recording time, facilitates information sharing, and establishes standard nursing care guidelines, thus improving the efficacy of nursing work. Most medical institutions computerize nursing records using "nursing care plans" or "Focus Charting" record methods. In addition, a minority of institutions adopt an integrated approach that includes descriptive nursing records. Regardless of how the records are compiled, the content of nursing records should be objective, concise, clear, specific, immediate, organized, and accurate (Chang, Lee, & Lin, 2013; Hung, Han, & Lai, 2010; Wang, Yang, Sung, Liou, & Chen, 2011).

Information technology has been increasingly integrated into healthcare. Various research methods such as surveys of user attitudes toward the computerization of healthcare and nurse perceptions toward using computers in clinical settings have been used to evaluate nursing information systems. The results indicate that when recording templates or the interface design of the nursing information system does not

[1]MSN, RN, Department of Nursing, National Taiwan University Hospital, Taiwan, ROC • [2]PhD, Professor, Department of Information Management, National Taipei University of Nursing and Health Sciences, Taiwan, ROC • [3]PhD, RN, Assistant Professor, Department of Nursing, National Yang Ming University, Taiwan, ROC • [4]MSN, RN, Supervisor, Department of Nursing, National Taiwan University Hospital, Taiwan, ROC • [5]MSN, RN, Director, Department of Nursing, National Taiwan University Hospital Hsin-Chu Branch, Taiwan, ROC • [6]PhD, RN, Adjunct Associate Professor, School of Nursing, National Taipei University of Nursing and Health Sciences, Taiwan, ROC.

meet user needs, user intention to use the system as well as the quality of information in the system may be affected (DeLone & McLean, 1992; Han, Kamber, & Pei, 2011; Yee et al., 2012).

In recent years, studies have applied data mining to select correct and useful information from large stores of data in electronic medical records. Information quality has been used as a criterion for nursing record management to improve the quality of medical care (Almasalha et al., 2013; Hunt, Sproat, & Kitzmiller, 2010; Lee, Lin, Mills, & Kuo, 2012). Text mining, a data mining approach, is used to search information to identify useful text fragments and further establish data analysis models, trends, or rules that may serve as the basis for monitoring information quality. For example, Kushima, Araki, Suzuki, Araki, and Nikama (2011) adopted a text mining approach to analyze the medical records of patients with chronic hepatitis. Relevant information was investigated by analyzing appropriate terms and feature words in nursing records to improve patient care quality (Byrne & Lang, 2013; Fayyad, Piatetsky-Shapiro, & Smyth, 1996; Park, Cho, & Chung, 2011).

Electronic nursing records may contain massive numbers of words. Record quality may be examined using a number of methods. For example, von Krogh, Nåden, and Aasland (2012) examined the record quality of a nursing information system based on the completeness, comprehensiveness, and coherence of the record content. Paans et al. (2010) applied the Delphi method to develop a D-Catch instrument, which they used to evaluate the quality of nursing records. Therefore, database quality management, which is the process of auditing and managing a large amount of electronic medical records, is a crucial topic in clinical nursing settings.

Recent studies on electronic nursing records have focused mostly on the evaluation of the developed system or on the degree of user satisfaction (Chang et al., 2013; Liao, Chu, & Chu, 2014; Wang et al., 2011). Few studies have investigated the quality of computerized nursing records. Therefore, this study used the text mining method to analyze the degree of accuracy with which the content of electronic nursing records complied with relevant hospital regulations, to determine the quality of these nursing records, and to propose a generally applicable model and set of tools to audit nursing records in order to facilitate improvements in recording quality.

Methods

Study Design

A retrospective method was used to collect the electronic nursing records of 6,277 patients discharged from the internal medicine departments of a medical center in northern Taiwan from January to June 2014. The records of patients younger than 20 years old and patients positive for human immunodeficiency virus were excluded from the research samples. SAS Enterprise Guide Version 6.1 and SAS Text Miner Version 13.2 (SAS, Cary, NC, USA) software were used to perform text mining. The following sections describe data processing and data mining, and Figure 1 illustrates the related steps.

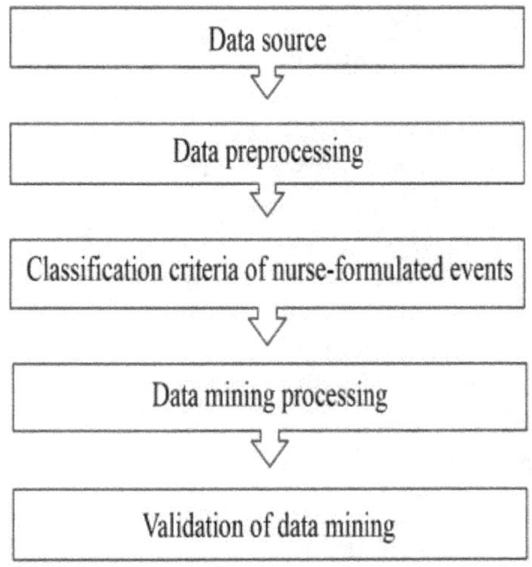

Figure 1. Flow chart of data processing and data mining.

Data Source

In this study, the basic patient demographic data set and diagnosis data set were obtained from the hospital information system, and data were obtained from the electronic nursing records of the nursing information system. Collected data included patient age, gender, diagnosis, and number of hospitalization days as well as subspecialty and nursing record. The electronic nursing record included the names of system-formulated events (SFEs), the nurse-formulated events (NFEs), and other event information with regard to nursing assessments, interventions, and outcomes.

The medical center targeted in this study identified health problems and events during the process of patient care and input this information into the electronic nursing record system to form electronic nursing records, which comprised the SFEs and NFEs that were chosen by the nurses. The process used to develop the nursing recording system was based on the principles or guidelines proposed in *On Call Principles and Protocols* edited by Marshall and Ruedy (2011). In this process, nursing staff of various wards were asked to provide lists of common health problems, which were then sorted systematically and used to build a system for the event. The nursing recording system was categorized into three record columns, including event name, nursing assessment and intervention, and evaluation/outcomes.

The SFEs comprised 93 types of events, which were categorized according to event classifications, including biological systems, nerves/muscles/bones, cardiovascular system, respiratory system, gastrointestinal system, skin, sensory perception, urinary system, psychological and social events, cancer treatment, obstetrics and pediatrics, value anomalies, patient tendencies, and common events. The nursing record system provided phrases regarding the nursing assessment, nursing intervention, and nursing outcomes related to a specific event, allowing nurses to select the appropriate phrases to write and edit in the record.

If no appropriate SFEs are available, nurses may add new events in blank fields based on patient conditions and edit the content of the events, which constitute the NFEs. As with the SFE, NFE content includes event name, nursing assessment and intervention, and evaluation/outcomes. The NFE comprises unstructured records and further includes a free-text column, in which nurses may edit any word.

Data Preprocessing

Patient demographic and diagnosis information, as well as the electronic nursing record data file provided by the research hospital, were imported into a Microsoft Access database (Microsoft, Redmond, WA, USA). The data were transformed into a consistent format to build the data column required for research. Structured query language (SQL) was used to combine data files and process missing values. The data were then categorized, recoded, and input into SAS Enterprise Guide 6.1 and SAS Text Miner 13.2 for data mining and text mining.

The original data were collected from 235,798 electronic nursing records, of which 208,442 (88.40%) contained SFEs, indicating that a high proportion of nurses used the SFEs. In this study, 27,356 NFEs were used, accounting for 11.60% of the original data. This study analyzed the quality of the 27,356 NFEs using a text mining method.

Classification Criteria for Nurse-Formulated Events

Three nursing experts were invited to examine the electronic nursing records and establish the classification criteria for the review of the NFEs in a meeting that discussed the hospital's nursing record writing regulations and guidelines and related literature. These nursing experts each had 10 years of working experience in cardiovascular, gastroenterology, endocrine, and hematology and oncology nursing, respectively and were responsible for nursing quality management and medical record reviews at the participating hospital.

The review of nursing records for the NFEs was divided into two stages. Figure 2 shows the NFE data analysis process. In the first stage of the review, the experts determined whether an NFE was similar to any SFE. "Similar SFE" meant that different names were used to describe a very similar/same event in the SFE and NFE. In these cases, nurses should use SFE names rather than creating a new name. Therefore, this situation was classified as "Category A: Set error event name." For example, when a nurse set a name in the NFE as "hyperthermia" and the event was similar to the "fever" event of SFE, this was regarded as an error of event similarity and was not reviewed again in the second stage.

When names of events differed from the SFE, the experts examined whether the event name was appropriate in the second stage. If the nurses described a new event name that had no equivalent SFE and was correct in terms of name and content, this event was classified as "Category B1: Add to SFE." For example, the event names "discharge nursing care" and "examination and treatment" were considered appropriate to add to the system. Infrequent events that were not SFEs, but did not need to be included in the SFEs of the nursing record information systems, were classified as "Category B2: Retain as NFE." An example of this would be when a nurse sets the name "changes renal tissue perfusion" to an event.

When nurses create an inappropriate NFE name, the experts analyzed the relevance of the event name to the content. If the NFE name was related to the content but the event could not be classified, it was categorized as "Category B3: Not classified event." For example, nurses described a "summary" event that had an NFE name related to the content, but this summary was used as a substitute on the three shift nursing records. Finally, when NFE names or contents are irrelevant or provided with an incorrect event name, they are classified as "Category B4: Event name error." For example, nurses created an "on dopamine" event name that was identified through expert review of the nursing record content and discussion; it was considered suitable to select the "shock and hypotension" of SFEs. In cases such as this, the nurse should use the SFE correctly and should not set an error event name.

Following these classification criteria helps determine the quality of nursing records. Categories B1 and B2 were considered "good quality" nursing records, and Categories A, B3, and B4 were considered "poor quality" nursing records. Nurses should try to use the SFE name to avoid using inappropriate names for events. These criteria were thus used as the data mining rules and algorithm.

Data Mining Processing

This study performed text mining on 27,356 NFEs using SAS Text Miner 13.2 software. A random month was selected, and the data in that month were used as the training set. The data from all of the other months constituted the testing set. SAS Enterprise Guide 6.1 software was used to convert the data of 27,356 NFEs into SAS files, which were input in SAS Text Miner to establish a data source.

The text mining rules and algorithm were based on the expert review classification criteria (Figure 2), and text mining was conducted on the data of the training set and testing set using SAS Text Miner. The text mining results were compared with the benchmark, which is considered the gold standard of event classification. Our benchmark was developed by nursing experts, and the efficiency of SAS Text Miner was examined using criteria for specificity, sensitivity, and accuracy.

Validation of Data Mining

The quality of the NFEs was evaluated based on expert review of nursing records. The three experts reviewed the training set separately and spent 8 weeks reviewing the nursing records of the training set as the gold standard for

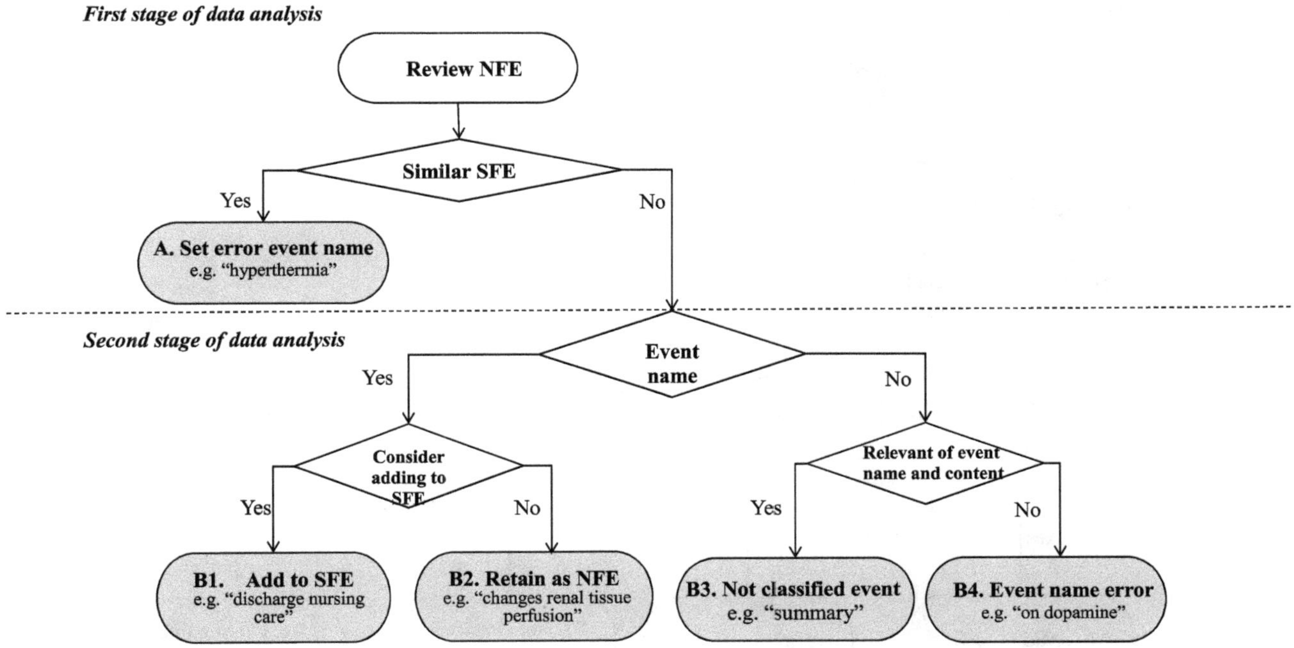

Figure 2. Nurse-formulated event (NFE) data analysis process. SFE = system-formulated event.

verifying training set data. However, because of limited time and manpower, only one nursing expert conducted the nursing record review for the testing set. The kappa statistic method was used to measure nursing expert interrater reliability, and these examination results were applied as the gold standard for verifying the results of SAS Text Miner.

The results of the two-stage review given by Experts 1 and 2 were identical, with each stage kappa value of 1.0. The results of Expert 3 and those of the other two experts were highly consistent, with the combined kappa values for the two stages of 0.98 and 0.99, respectively. The three experts discussed the items in 29 sets of data again to reach a consensus that served as the standard in the subsequent review of the testing set.

Ethical Considerations

The requested data resource was retrieved from the database of the hospital's information center after personal information had been de-identified. This study was approved by the institutional review board of the target institution (no. 201408056RINC). The medical records were recoded through link removal. Only the data related to this study were selected for overall analysis, and no distinguishable personal information was present.

Results

Analysis of the Quality of Electronic Nursing Records

Nursing records should be objective, clear, timely, organized, and accurate. Electronic nursing records are clearer and more organized than traditional, handwritten records. In this study, the electronic nursing record quality was evaluated using a text mining method that includes the use of accurate event names and correlation between the event name and content.

The nursing records in the target hospital comprised SFEs and NFEs. In this study, 27,356 NFEs were used, accounting for 11.60% of the original data. The name and content of the NFEs were diverse and the terms used were varied. For example, the events for inserting an intravenous catheter were written as "ON CATH," "ON CATHETER," "ON IV CATH," "inserting catheter," "inserting intravenous catheter," "catheter placement," "placing catheter," "placing intravenous catheter," and "inserting tube." Therefore, before data mining, it was necessary to clean, recode, and classify the NFEs to gain an accurate picture of the actual situation. As with the catheter example above, a large number of the NFEs were actually the same event but identified with disparate names.

Figure 3 shows the results of the NFE distribution. The analysis of the quality of the NFEs found that the recording quality for Categories B1 and B2 were good, whereas the event names and contents of Categories A, B3, and B4 were poor and must be improved. The expert review revealed that 8.08% of the NFEs were errors due to their similarity with the SFEs (Category A), 29.72% could be added as new SFEs because the event names were associated with the content and the terms were correctly used (Category B1), and 17.53% could be retained as NFEs (Category B2) because in part of prior noninclusion in the system's list of SFEs.

Finally, 34.52% of the events were identified as having inappropriate names or as not classifiable (Category B3), and 10.15% had names that were irrelevant to the content or used incorrect names (Category B4). Overall, the results show

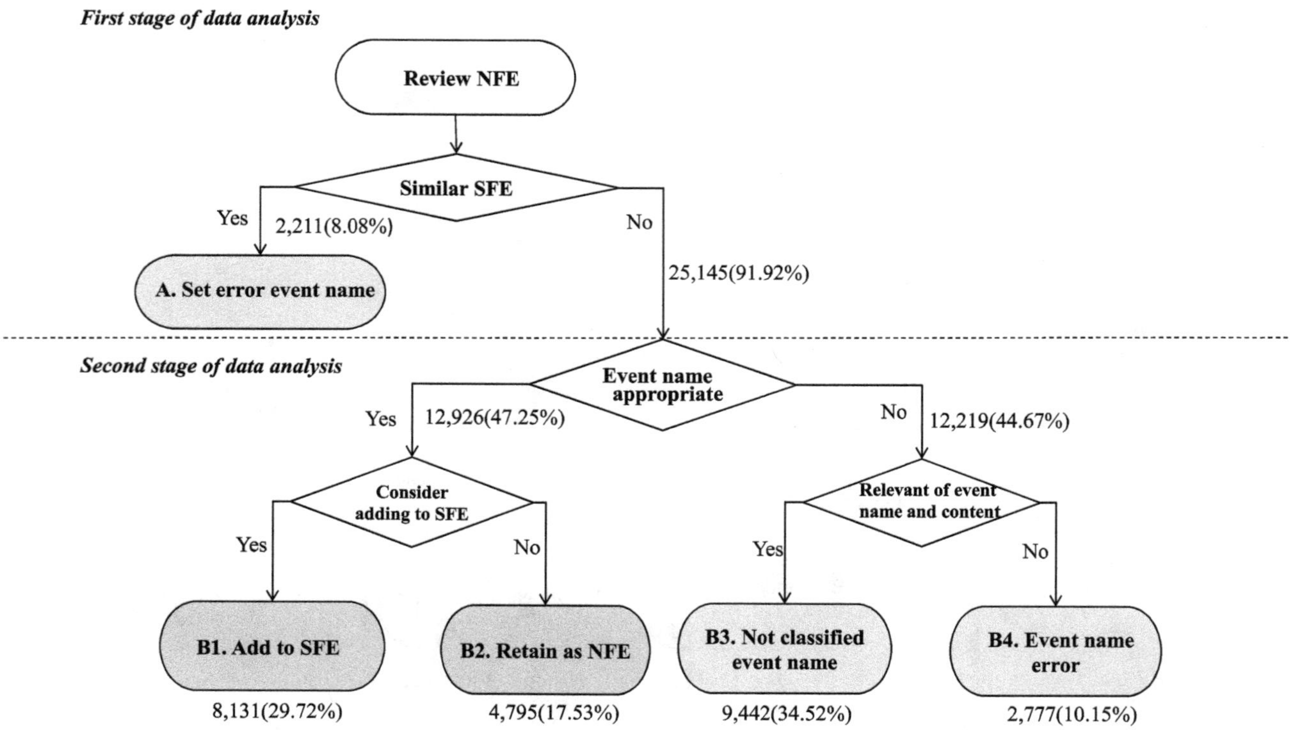

Figure 3. The results of the expert review of the nurse-formulated event (NFE). SFE = system-formulated event.

that 47.25% of the NFE records were accurate (Categories B1 and B2); these NFE records were assessed as having good recording quality. Approximately 52.75% of the NFE records were assessed as having poor recording quality and contained Categories A, B3, and B4.

Analysis of the Efficiency of SAS Text Miner

The experts established the rules for the text mining of the 3,800 NFEs in the training set. In the first stage, SAS Text Miner analyzed the level of similarity between the NFEs and the SFEs. The "event name" column was set as a variable, and the terms in the NFEs that were similar to the system-formulated terms were identified and set as the keywords for text mining. SAS Text Miner selected 463 NFEs that were similar to the SFEs. The analysis results found that the number of data analyzed correctly and incorrectly by the software was 441 and 27 events, respectively. Therefore, the sensitivity of SAS Text Miner was 96%, and the specificity and accuracy were both 99%.

The same text mining rules were applied to the 23,556 NFEs in the testing set. The SAS Text Miner selected 1,783 NFEs that were similar to the SFEs. The selected 1,783 events were compared with the 1,743 benchmark events identified by the experts, and the results showed that SAS Text Miner analyzed 1,649 events correctly and 134 events incorrectly. The sensitivity, specificity, and accuracy of SAS Text Miner for the training and testing sets are shown in Table 1, indicating that SAS Text Miner had high efficiency in analyzing the similarity between NFEs and SFEs. The testing set sensitivity of the software was 95%, and the specificity and accuracy were both 99%.

If the NFEs differed from the SFEs, SAS Text Miner should determine in the second stage whether the event names were related to the content and accuracy of the terms used. The software is only able to search entire files using keywords, whereas using the "text filter snippet" mining function can filter related keywords and terms to select files related to the keywords. The content of these mining results must be examined by experts to determine the accuracy of terms and the level of association between the event names and the content. Therefore, the analysis conducted by SAS Text Miner in the second stage should be used only as a supplementary tool for audits of nursing record quality.

Discussion

Quality of Electronic Nursing Record

Of the electronic nursing records examined in this study, 88.40% used SFEs. Using a customized nursing record information system enhanced the association between nursing record content and the completeness and clarity of the records. Overall, the

TABLE 1.

Sensitivity, Specificity, and Accuracy in the SAS Text Miner

Data Set	Sensitivity (%)	Specificity (%)	Accuracy (%)
Training set	96	99	99
Testing set	95	99	99

quality of nursing records improved. Approximately 11.60% of the NFEs were created by nurses because they did not find appropriate SFEs for use in the nursing record.

According to the results, 29.72% of the NFEs may be added directly into groups of SFEs with the correct use of event names. It is recommended that the hospital use common NFEs as SFEs with consistent terms to prevent nurses from using inconsistent terms or inappropriate abbreviations for the same NFE. Examples of this include "wound care," "discharge nursing care," "invasive examination and treatment," and "drug dosage adjustment."

This study analyzed the quality of NFEs and found that 17.53% of the events were appropriate for retention in their current nurse-formulated form—a result that is consistent with Lee (2006) and Yee et al. (2012). When an event could not be recorded using standardized nursing language, nurses adapted accordingly, indicating that a nursing record system that provides NFEs promotes the flexibility and convenience needed for nurses to compose nursing records.

However, if the NFE is similar to the SFE, the data in the nursing recording system database may be inconsistent, which will affect future data analysis. In this study, 8.08% of the NFEs were classified as the error event name being similar to SFEs. For example, NFEs that included terms such as "respiratory wheezing," "wheezing," "wheezing during activity," and "gasping for breath" were actually describing the same event as the SFE "shortness of breath." In addition, 10.15% of the NFEs were categorized into error event name categories. For example, nurses should not create NFE of "on dopamine," because it belongs to event category of the cardiovascular system "hypotension and shock" in the SFE.

This study performed only data mining and did not investigate the real experience of nurses using the nursing record system. Therefore, the reasons proposed for our results are only suggested as being the same as those for not using the recording templates of nursing record system in Wang et al. (2011); that is, the nurses felt that making their own records was faster and more convenient than using record templates provided in the system.

The nursing record system used in the target hospital was unable to identify errors of similarity between NFEs and SFEs. According to the results, as shown in Figure 3, poor-quality nursing records, including Categories A, B3, and B4, accounted for approximately 52.75% of the NFEs. Thus, hospitals should provide these inadequate record examples for in-service nursing education and train nurses to understand how to use SFEs correctly to reduce errors and promote clarity in nursing records.

In addition, the nursing department should establish a standard for regular audits of electronic nursing records to ensure compliance and improve the quality of electronic nursing records. Moreover, when performing system updates, the hospital should either add a function to search for synonyms of system-formulated terms or provide experts with the function of automatic assessment to reduce errors of event similarity and data inconsistency.

In this study, nursing staff of different divisions used a variety of terms to record the same nursing care activity. For example, "abdominal tapping" was also termed "abd tapping," "paracentesis," and "abdominal paracentesis drainage." This result is consistent with that of Wu, Chen, and Chen (2009) and Yee et al. (2012), who indicated the difficulty with use of standardizing nursing language. This study analyzed NFEs and found that content used Chinese, English, uppercase and lowercase English letters, and various medical terminologies intermittently.

The original data were examined manually to determine whether the same nursing activities and terms could be collated, reclassified, and coded for subsequent data interpretation. In other words, data processing entailed a significant amount of time and energy. Therefore, as suggested by Feng et al. (2013), structured and coherent languages and methods comprise a critical base and foundation for establishing medical information systems.

Text Mining Software-Facilitated Auditing of the Quality of Nursing Records

Paans et al. (2010) adopted the D-Catch instrument as a tool to assess nursing records. However, their process of assessment was complex and time consuming. Text mining provides information search, association, prediction, analysis, management, and decision-making support for a rapid and accurate analysis of unstructured text (Han et al., 2011; Liao et al., 2014; SAS Resource Center, 2014). This study employed SAS Text Miner to conduct text mining on electronic nursing records, identified the information hidden in the NFEs, and determined a method for auditing the quality of electronic nursing records. The results were consistent with those of Kushima et al. (2011), which suggested that text mining may be used as a basis for improving medical care quality.

In addition, this study used SAS Text Miner to analyze the quality of electronic nursing records and found the software to have high sensitivity, specificity, and accuracy in both the training and testing data sets. SAS Text Miner efficiently and accurately analyzed the NFEs that were similar to SFEs. Moreover, its "text filter snippet" mining function permitted the selection of words with high association coefficients and identified related documents.

In this study, 34.52% of the NFEs were identified as having inappropriate event names. For example, "summary" was used to refer to the nursing records of three shifts. Nursing expert analysis of the events described by "summary" found a diverse range of contents. SAS Text Miner performed text mining on the 9,442 events of "summary" and identified the events related only to SFEs within a few minutes.

The results of this study indicated that SAS Text Miner has a fast and effective text mining tool and supported text mining as a strategy to reduce the amount of time spent on manually examining electronic nursing records. Therefore, this software package can be used as an auxiliary tool for auditing electronic nursing records.

Conclusions

This study analyzed the association between the NFEs and the SFEs and found that 8.08% of the NFEs had an error of being similar to SFEs. Among the NFEs, 29.72% of the terms could be added as new SFEs because their content was correct, and 17.53% should be retained as NFEs. This result may be referenced by professionals who design and implement updates of nursing record systems. In addition, 10.15% of the NFEs were classified as the error category of "incorrect event name," and 34.52% of the event names could not be adequately classified. This result may serve as a teaching material reference for in-service education related to nursing records in nursing record systems.

This study conducted text mining on NFEs using SAS Text Miner. The sensitivity, specificity, and accuracy of SAS Text Miner for the training set were 96%, 99%, and 99%, respectively, whereas those for the testing set were 95%, 99%, and 99%, respectively. These results indicate that SAS Text Miner is an excellent audit tool for electronic nursing records.

Implications for Nursing Practice

The recommended applications of the findings of this study in future clinical nursing include the following:

1. By evaluating the nursing recording system and the text mining model of NFEs, it is possible to identify NFEs that are commonly used by nurses as well as those that should be added as SFEs. In addition, the nursing recording system should enhance the search function and set the list of common SFE names for various units to improve nursing record consistency and accuracy.

2. In-service education on electronic nursing records should be provided for nursing staff. Nursing documentation teaching materials should discuss the SFE terms that are typically incorrectly chosen (resulting in NFE names that are similar to SFEs), NFEs that are difficult or currently impossible to classify, and event names that are selected incorrectly. In-service education should promote the correct use of structured SFE names to enhance the consistency and accuracy of nursing records and the regular audit of nursing records to improve the quality of nursing records.

3. SAS Text Miner software is able to quickly identify relevant items from a large number of documents, reducing the time and cost involved in manual reviews of medical records. It is suggested that SAS Text Miner be used as a tool for nursing record quality management.

4. In the future, the text mining model proposed in this study may be applied to the unstructured text forms of data files of medical institutions and used as a way to audit the quality of electronic medical records.

Limitations

This study targeted only the nursing records of patients in the internal medicine wards of one medical center in northern Taiwan because of limitations in time, manpower, and material resources. Moreover, as electronic nursing record system designs vary from hospital to hospital, further verification is necessary to determine whether this research method can be used in other hospitals. In this study, a retrospective electronic data analysis was conducted to evaluate the quality of nursing records in terms of accuracy, association, and completeness of content, but the timeliness of the records could not be evaluated. Although SAS Text Miner was used in this study, other data mining software such as IBM DB2 Intelligent Miner and PolyAnalyst are available. Therefore, future studies may also investigate the efficiency of other text mining software.

Acknowledgments

The research was supported by the National Taiwan University Hospital. The authors are grateful to the Information Technology Office for providing the data and for assistance with data processing as well as to the Supervisor of Nursing Information for providing administrative assistance and support.

References

Almasalha, F., Xu, D., Keenan, G. M., Khokhar, A., Yao, Y., Chen, Y. C., ... Wilkie, D. J. (2013). Data mining nursing care plans of end-of-life patients: A study to improve healthcare decision making. *International Journal of Nursing Knowledge, 24*(1), 15–24. https://doi.org/10.1111/j.2047-3095.2012.01217.x

Byrne, M. D., & Lang, N. (2013). Examination of nursing data elements from evidence-based recommendations for clinical decision support. *CIN: Computers, Informatics, Nursing, 31*(12), 605–614. https://doi.org/10.1097/CIN.0000000000000013

Chang, F. M., Lee, T. T., & Lin, K. C. (2013). Exploring nurse, usage effectiveness of mobile nursing station. *The Journal of Nursing, 60*(2), 32–40. https://doi.org/10.6224/JN.60.2.32 (Original work published in Chinese)

DeLone, W. H., & McLean, E. R. (1992). Information systems success: The quest for the dependent variable. *Information Systems Research, 3*(1), 60–95. https://doi.org/10.1287/isre.3.1.60

Fayyad, U., Piatetsky-Shapiro, G., & Smyth, P. (1996). From data mining to knowledge discovery in databases. *AI Magazine, 17*(3), 37–54. https://doi.org/10.1609/aimag.v17i3.1230

Feng, R. C., Tseng, K. J., Yan, H. F., Huang, H. Y., & Chang, P. (2013). A preliminary study on the use of clinical care classification in nursing documentation data sets. *Computer Methods and Programs in Biomedicine, 112*(3), 713–719. https://doi.org/10.1016/j.cmpb.2013.07.019

Han, J., Kamber M., & Pei, J. (2011). *Data mining: Concepts and techniques* (3rd ed.). Burlington, NJ: Morgan Kaufmann Elsevier.

Hung, L. C., Han, C. H., & Lai, W. W. (2010). The exploration of satisfaction about clinical information system application in the intensive care unit of a medical center. *The Journal of Taiwan Association for Medical Informatics, 19*(3), 35–46. https://doi.org/10.29829/TJTAMI.201009.0003 (Original work published in Chinese)

Hunt, E. C., Sproat, S. B., & Kitzmiller, R. R. (2010). *The nursing informatics implementation guide.* New York, NY: Springer.

Kushima, M., Araki, K., Suzuki, M., Araki, S., & Nikama, T. (2011). Text data mining of in-patient nursing records within electronic medical records using KeyGraph. *IAENG International Journal of Computer Science, 38*(3), 215–224.

Lee, T. T. (2006). Nurses' perceptions of their documentation experiences in a computerized nursing care planning system. *Journal of Clinical Nursing, 15*(11), 1376–1382. https://doi.org/10.1111/j.1365-2702.2006.01480.x

Lee, T. T., Lin, K. C., Mills, M. E., & Kuo, Y. H. (2012). Factors related to the prevention and management of pressure ulcers. *CIN: Computers, Informatics, Nursing, 30*(9), 489–495. https://doi.org/10.1097/NXN.0b013e3182573aec

Liao, P. H., Chu, W., & Chu, W. C. (2014). Evaluation of the mining techniques in constructing a traditional Chinese-language nursing recording system. *CIN: Computers, Informatics, Nursing, 32*(5), 223–231. https://doi.org/10.1097/CIN.0000000000000051

Marshall, S. A., & Ruedy, J. (2011). *On call principles and protocols* (5th ed.). St. Louis, MO: Saunders Elsevier.

Paans, W., Sermeus, W., Nieweg, R. M. B., & Van Der Schans, C. P. (2010). D-Catch instrument: Development and psychometric testing of a measurement instrument for nursing documentation in hospitals. *Journal of Advanced Nursing, 66*(6), 1388–1400. https://doi.org/10.1111/j.1365-2648.2010.05302.x

Park, H. A., Cho, I., & Chung, E. (2011). Exploring use of a clinical data repository containing international classification for nursing practice-based nursing practice data. *CIN: Computers, Informatics, Nursing, 29*(7), 419–426. https://doi.org/10.1097/NCN.0b013e3181f9dc6e

SAS Resource Center. (2014). *SAS Text Miner makes it easy to use text mining to find out important information!*. Retrieved from http://www.sasresource.com/artical285.html (Original work published in Chinese)

von Krogh, G., Nåden, D., & Aasland, O. G. (2012). Testing a nursing- specific model of electronic patient record documentation with regard to information completeness, comprehensiveness and consistency. *Journal of Clinical Nursing, 21*(19–20), 2930–2939. https://doi.org/10.1111/j.1365-2702.2012.04185.x

Wang, M. T., Yang, S. H., Sung, C. Y., Liou, S. F., & Chen, B. L. (2011). The influential factors of nurses using the standardized nursing record. *VGH Nursing, 28*(3), 241–248. https://doi.org/10.6142/VGHN.28.3.241 (Original work published in Chinese)

Wu, W. R., Chen, J. Y., & Chen, C. H. (2009). Standardized nursing language: The bedrock of computerized nursing records. *The Journal of Nursing, 56*(5), 75–79. https://doi.org/10.6224/JN.56.5.75 (Original work published in Chinese)

Yee, T., Needleman, J., Pearson, M., Parkerton, P., Parkerton, M., & Wolstein, J. (2012). The influence of integrated electronic medical records and computerized nursing notes on nurses' time spent in documentation. *CIN: Computers, Informatics, Nursing, 30*(6), 287–292. https://doi.org/10.1097/NXN.0b013e31824af835

3

Effectiveness of a Nurse-Delivered Intervention on Illness Perceptions and Quality of Life in Patients with Injury

Wen-Chih FANN[1] • Chang-Chiao HUNG[2] • Wendy CHABOYER[3] • Bih-O LEE[4]*

ABSTRACT

Background: Research has shown that nursing interventions are able to affect short-term outcomes in patients with injury. However, evidence based on a comprehensive nurse-led intervention may be beneficial for trauma care.

Purpose: This study was designed to assess the effect of a nursing intervention on the illness perceptions and quality of life of patients with injury.

Methods: A two-group experimental design and a follow-up period of 12 months were used. Ninety-four patients were randomly assigned to either the experimental group or the control group. A nurse-led cognitive behavioral therapy intervention was used to improve outcomes.

Results: The illness perception variables of "personal control" and "treatment control" were found to be significantly improved in the experimental group at 3 months after discharge, whereas "emotional perception" was significantly improved at 6 months after discharge. The intervention was also shown to improve "social quality of life" at 6 and 12 months after injury.

Conclusions: This study adds new knowledge related to nursing interventions for patients with injury in terms of the intervention achieving longer-term effects than the interventions examined in previous studies. The results highlight the importance of providing interprofessional collaborative care. However, the intervention protocol should be tested further in future studies.

Key Words:
illness perceptions, nurse-delivered intervention, patients with injury, quality of life.

Introduction

Injury is the leading cause of death among people aged 45 years and younger in many countries, including the United States (Centers for Disease Control and Prevention, 2016), the United Kingdom (Kanani & Hartshorn, 2016), and Taiwan (Ministry of Health and Welfare, National Health Insurance Administration, Taiwan, ROC, 2019). Annual medical costs related to mortal injuries total 21.4 billion USD in the United States (Centers for Disease Control and Prevention, 2016). In Taiwan, medical costs associated with injury-related hospitalizations exceed 470 million USD annually (Ministry of Health and Welfare, National Health Insurance Administration, Taiwan, ROC, 2019). Survivors of injury may experience permanent disabilities associated with alarmingly high medication and rehabilitation costs (Kanani & Hartshorn, 2016). Although healthcare professionals have traditionally focused on physical disabilities (Chaboyer et al., 2010), the need to understand and treat cognitive, behavioral, and other disabilities is being increasingly recognized to maximize health outcomes such as quality of life (Baker et al., 2018). Patients with injury may experience short- and longer-term physical and psychological disabilities (Schneiderman et al., 2013). Physical and psychological problems are found in patients with injury and correlate with quality of life (Chaboyer et al., 2010; Schneiderman et al., 2013). For example, a longitudinal study of Swedish patients with trauma found that patients experienced physical functioning declines 3 months after an injury incident (Ringdal et al., 2010). According to Chaboyer et al. (2010), over 50% of patients experienced psychological and functional disabilities 6 months after an injury incident. More recently, some cohort studies have followed patients with injury for up to 1 year. For example, one study performed follow-up assessments of patients at 3 months and 1 year after injury, reporting that patients with visible injuries may have poor psychological health and posttraumatic stress disorder (PTSD) at 12 months after injury (Baecher et al., 2018). Another retrospective study found that the long-term physical functioning and quality of life

[1]*MSc, MD, Attending Physician, Department of Emergency Medicine, Chia-Yi Chang Gung Memorial Hospital, Taiwan* • [2]*PhD, RN, Associate Professor, Department of Nursing, Chang Gung University of Science and Technology, and Associate Research Fellow, Department of Nursing, Chia-Yi Chang Gung Memorial Hospital, Taiwan* • [3]*PhD, RN, Professor, School of Nursing and Midwifery, Menzies Health Institute Queensland, Griffith University, Queensland, Australia* • [4]*PhD, RN, Professor, College of Nursing, Kaohsiung Medical University, Taiwan, and Adjunct Professor, Faculty of Nursing, Universitas Airlangga, Indonesia.*

of patients with severe injury were poorer than those of the general population (Banierink et al., 2019).

The concept of illness perception has been commonly applied in patients with injury as well as in other patient groups. Illness perceptions are the organized, cognitive, and emotional perceptions that individuals experience when facing an illness or health-threatening condition (Leventhal et al., 2016; Willemse et al., 2019). Illness perception was originally modeled to address the five components of consequences, timeline, control, identity, and causes, with each component reflecting different perceptions or internal beliefs toward an illness (Leventhal et al., 2016; Willemse et al., 2019). Moss-Morris et al. (2002) used different patient populations to reconceptualize the components of illness perception, with two components added: illness coherence and emotional representations. Timeline is divided into two subscales, timeline-acute/chronic and timeline cyclical, whereas control is divided into personal control and treatment control (Moss-Morris et al., 2002).

Illness perceptions, related to several health outcomes, have been studied in various patient populations (Sawyer et al., 2019). For example, the relationship between illness perceptions and quality of life has been studied in patients with irritable bowel syndrome (Knowles et al., 2017) and patients with injury (Lee et al., 2008). In previous studies, patients with injury were found to have relatively poor quality of life (Bayo et al., 2019; Van Son et al., 2017) and to have developed negative illness perceptions at 3 months after their injury (Lee et al., 2010). In another study of Taiwanese patients, three components of illness perception, including identity, consequences, and timeline, were identified as significant predictors of the physical quality of life of patients with injury at 3 months after injury (Lee et al., 2008). Moreover, Chaboyer et al. (2010) found that the three components of identity, emotional perceptions, and timeline were found to be predictors of the physical and mental health quality of life of patients with injury at 6 months after injury.

Background

Research has shown that nursing interventions can affect illness perceptions and other health outcomes in different patient groups. For example, in one study, an educational intervention was used on patients with pacemaker implantations. Rakhshan et al. (2013) found that all of the components of illness perception, with the exception of treatment control, were positively changed in patients with pacemakers by an intervention. Vranceanu et al. (2015) conducted a study that examined the implementation of a mind–body, skills-based intervention in patients with injury over a period of 1–2 months. The results showed that overall disability and pain were improved, although no change in coping strategies or emotional status was observed. In addition, Zatzick et al. (2013) conducted a study that involved patients who developed severe PTSD after experiencing injuries. Patients in the experimental group were subjected to a stepped intervention that included combined care management, psychopharmacology, and cognitive behavioral psychotherapy. These patients exhibited significantly reduced PTSD symptoms compared with their control group peers. Furthermore, the patients in the intervention group achieved significant improvements in physical function over the 1-year posttest period.

Cognitive behavioral therapy (CBT) has emerged as one of the most effective, evidence-based adjunctive treatments for illnesses (Halford & Brown, 2009). In Siemonsma et al. (2013), a CBT intervention was found to reduce the consequences and to increase personal control in people with chronic low back pain within 4.5 months. In another study using nursing interventions combined with skills learned via CBT, injury-related physical symptoms and perceptions of controllability were found to be positively affected 3 months after injury because of a nursing intervention (Lee et al., 2015). A recent systematic review suggested that the effectiveness of different patterns of intervention on outcomes in patients with injury remains inconclusive (Shepherd-Banigan et al., 2018). Thus, the authors of this research speculated that there may be an opportunity to add new knowledge related to nursing research and nursing practice by conducting a study to examine the effects over 1 year of a nursing intervention on illness perceptions and quality of life in patients with injury.

Methods

This study was designed to examine the effect of a nurse-delivered intervention on the illness perceptions and quality of life of patients with injury. The Transparent Reporting of Evaluations with Nonrandomized Designs statement checklist was adopted to enhance reporting quality. The Transparent Reporting of Evaluations with Nonrandomized Designs statement is a 22-item checklist that helps validate the use of nonrandomized and quasi-experimental designs to evaluate interventions (Des Jarlais et al., 2004).

Design

A two-group experimental design was used, and the participants were followed up for 12 months.

Participants

Adults aged 20–65 years who had experienced a moderate-to-severe injury were eligible to participate in this study. An Injury Severity Score (ISS) of 9–15 was adopted to indicate moderate injury, and an ISS of 16 or greater was adopted to indicate severe injury (Sluys et al., 2016). To be included in the study, participants were required to have had an ISS ≥ 9, and their injury must have resulted from an accident. Patients with severe head injuries, spinal cord injuries, or burns were excluded. Two participants were matched in terms of ISS scores and gender by artificial selection from the hospital computer by a nurse practitioner (NP) and then randomly assigned to either the experimental or control group. The participants and their carers were blinded to study group assignment. Participants were recruited from one teaching hospital with 2,450 beds. The hospital is one of 14 medical centers in Taiwan that treats more than 2,000 patients with injury each year. Data collection was conducted in five ward units in which patients with injury are treated.

Previous data were used to calculate the correlations between Time 1 and Time 2 and between Time 2 and Time 3 (Lee et al., 2010). The results showed that the correlation coefficients were .45 and .50, respectively. On the basis of the suggestions of Diggle et al. (2013), using a medium effect size of $d = 0.5$, a power of 0.80, an alpha of .05, a correlation of outcomes between Time 1 and Time 2 of .45, and the number of time intervals set as 4, the required minimum sample size for each group was determined to be 37. Using an anticipated attrition rate of 20%, the target number of participants in each group was set at 45.

The Intervention

CBT is a psychotherapeutic modality, with plentiful evidence of efficacy across multiple morbidities (Dekker et al., 2012). Training nurses in CBT can expand the pool of therapists available to promote patient health outcomes (Halford & Brown, 2009). The intervention NP attended a CBT training program held by the Chinese Association of Group Psychotherapy. The program included basic and advanced courses.

The nurse-delivered CBT intervention was provided to patients in three sessions. The first and second sessions were parts of an in-hospital intervention that was modified from a previous study (Lee et al., 2015) and that was focused on depicting the existing feelings or perceptions regarding the injury based on the dimension of the illness perceptions (Broadbent et al., 2006). The objective of the first session was to establish rapport with the participant, to help the participant understand the meaning of illness perceptions, and to guide the participant in discussing all of the components of injury-related illness perceptions. The second session, held 24 hours after the first session based on the participant's condition and convenience, was designed to clarify and discuss useful information related to injury recovery.

The third session extended the in-hospital intervention using a method described by Lee et al. (2015) and subsequently tailored for this study. This third session includes a follow-up telephone interview early after hospital discharge and focuses on helping patients adapt to the postinjury transitional period. The extension strategies added to the intervention in this study made this intervention somewhat different from that in Lee et al. (2015). These included a follow-up telephone call made at 10–14 days after hospital

Table 1
Demographic and Clinical Data for the Experimental and Control Groups

Variable	Experimental Group (n = 47)		Control Group (n = 47)		p
	n	%	n	%	
Gender					1.000
Male	31	66.0	31	66.0	
Female	16	34.0	16	34.0	
Age (years; M and SD)	32.4	10.3	32.6	10.2	.904
Marital status					.249
Single	37	78.7	31	66.0	
With spouse	10	21.3	16	34.0	
Education (years)					.435
< 12	2	4.3	5	10.6	
≥ 12	45	95.7	42	89.4	
Employment					.386
Yes	38	80.9	42	89.4	
No	9	19.1	5	10.6	
Injury mechanism					1.000
Vehicle accident	37	78.7	38	80.9	
Fall or other	10	21.3	9	19.1	
Injury severity score (M and SD)	11.6	4.7	11.3	3.5	.711
Injury severity					1.000
9–15	39	83.0	40	85.1	
16–25	8	17.0	7	14.9	
Length of hospital stay (days; M and SD)	10.4	5.3	9.4	5.9	.392

Note. Data are expressed as mean (standard deviation) for continuous variables and frequency (percentage) for categorical variables.

Table 2
Descriptive Statistics of Brief IPQ and WHOQOL-BREF Across the Follow-Ups in the Experimental and Control Groups

Scale/Domain	Experimental Group								Control Group							
	Baseline (*n* = 47)		3 Month (*n* = 37)		6 Month (*n* = 34)		12 Month (*n* = 32)		Baseline (*n* = 47)		3 Month (*n* = 40)		6 Month (*n* = 39)		12 Month (*n* = 32)	
	B	*p*	*B*	*p*	*B*	*p*	*B*	*p*	*B*	*p*	*B*	*p*	*B*	*p*	*B*	*p*
Brief IPQ																
Personal control [a]	6.5	1.6	7.9	1.9	7.4	1.9	7.4	1.6	6.2	1.8	6.3	1.6	7.1	1.8	6.8	2.2
Treatment control [a]	7.7	1.7	8.3	1.7	7.7	1.7	7.5	2.1	7.7	1.7	6.7	1.9	7.5	2.1	7.5	2.0
Consequences [b]	7.8	2.0	5.8	1.9	4.6	2.0	4.4	2.6	8.1	2.1	6.7	2.0	5.8	2.3	5.2	2.5
Timeline [b]	5.4	2.0	4.8	1.7	4.8	2.0	4.8	1.8	5.7	1.8	5.5	2.0	5.6	2.6	5.6	2.4
Identity [b]	5.8	2.6	4.0	1.6	4.4	1.8	4.4	1.9	6.1	2.1	5.5	1.7	5.1	2.2	4.8	2.0
Illness concern [b]	8.7	1.7	9.0	1.5	7.2	1.6	7.8	2.2	9.3	1.3	9.0	2.0	8.5	2.0	8.0	2.1
Coherence [a]	7.8	1.9	8.4	1.5	8.6	1.7	8.1	1.9	8.0	1.9	8.1	1.7	7.9	1.8	8.4	1.8
Emotional representation [b]	5.1	2.9	6.0	2.5	3.9	2.3	5.0	2.5	4.9	2.9	6.4	2.2	6.3	2.1	5.0	2.7
Overall score [b]	5.1	0.9	4.4	0.7	3.9	1.0	4.2	1.0	5.3	1.0	5.2	1.2	4.8	1.3	4.5	1.2
WHOQOL-BREF																
Physical health	14.6	3.2	13.6	1.9	13.9	1.9	14.7	2.4	15.6	2.8	13.1	2.7	14.0	3.1	14.3	2.8
Psychological health	14.8	2.0	14.4	2.4	14.6	2.5	15.3	2.2	14.5	2.2	14.2	2.4	14.5	2.6	13.8	2.7
Social relationships	14.8	1.8	14.6	2.5	15.3	2.6	15.0	2.7	15.3	2.4	14.3	2.5	14.4	2.4	14.5	2.5
Environment	14.9	2.1	15.1	2.3	15.7	2.0	15.9	1.9	14.8	2.4	14.0	2.0	15.0	2.5	14.8	2.6

Note. IPQ = Illness Perception Questionnaire; WHOQOL-BREF = World Health Organization Quality of Life Questionnaire.
[a] 1 = *worst* to 10 = *best.* [b] 1 = *best* to 10 = *worst.*

discharge and the use of a common-thinking-errors sheet and an evidence-for-and-against useful thoughts sheet based on CBT (Cohen & Mannarino, 2008).

An NP who was not involved in recruitment or data collection delivered the intervention. The intervention NP had been working with patients with injury for more than 15 years, was trained in CBT techniques by a practicing psychologist for 16 hours, and was CBT certified.

Data Collection

A senior NP who held national NP certification was in charge of collecting preintervention data, following up with the participants, and assessing the outcomes. This NP was blinded to the study group assignment. Demographic and clinical data and the Brief Illness Perception Questionnaire (the Brief IPQ) were collected before hospital discharge. Follow-up data on the two groups were collected at 3, 6, and 12 months after hospital

Table 3
GEE Analysis of Intervention Effect on Brief IPQ

Variable	Consequences		Timeline		Personal Control		Treatment Control	
Intercept	7.76***	< .001	4.53***	< .001	4.47***	< .001	8.14***	< .001
Treatment								
Experimental vs. control	−0.35	.400	−0.40	.308	0.21	.545	−0.07	.841
Time								
3 months vs. baseline	−1.41***	< .001	−0.31	.408	0.08	.838	−0.95**	.008
6 months vs. baseline	−2.26***	< .001	−0.19	.697	0.79*	.028	−0.17	.585
12 months vs. baseline	−2.91***	< .001	−0.29	.524	0.59	.195	−0.13	.780
Interaction term								
3 months vs. baseline	−0.49	.326	−0.25	.636	1.26*	.021	1.50**	.002
6 months vs. baseline	−0.95	.081	−0.54	.393	0.09	.861	0.23	.613
12 months vs. baseline	−0.62	.306	−0.21	.726	0.35	.535	−0.02	.968

Note. GEE = generalized estimating equation; IPQ = Illness Perception Questionnaire.
**p* < .05. ***p* < .01. ****p* < .001.

discharge using the Brief IPQ and the World Health Organization Quality of Life Questionnaire (the WHOQOL-BREF). The recruiting NP and the researchers were blinded to group allocation. The allocation concealment ended when a given pair of two patients was discharged from the hospital. Data were collected from January 2013 to December 2015.

Measures

The Brief IPQ is a nine-item scale that provides a rapid assessment of an individual's perceptions of illness (Broadbent et al., 2006; Woodhouse et al., 2018). Each item in this scale is designed to assess one dimension of illness perception. The ninth item, that is, the item addressing the cause of injury, was excluded because the indicated reasons for injury did not apply to the patients in this study (Chaboyer et al., 2010). Thus, the eight items used in the Brief IPQ addressed the following dimensions: consequences, timeline, personal control, treatment control, identity, illness concern, coherence, and emotional representation. Three items, namely, personal control, treatment control, and coherence, are scored from 1 (*worst*) to 10 (*best*), whereas the remaining five items are scored from 1 (*best*) to 10 (*worst*). The overall score ranges from a best possible score of 1 to a worst possible score of 10. The Chinese version of the Brief IPQ was translated by Lin and Xue (The Illness Perception Questionnaire, 2020). The coefficients of test–retest reliability for the Brief IPQ ranged from .69 to .73, and the Cronbach's α of the subscales ranged from .70 to .84.

The WHOQOL-BREF is a 28-item scale used to measure four domains, including physical, psychological, social relationship, and environment. This scale has been tested transculturally in clinical settings (Yao, 2000). Scores range from 1 to 5, with higher scores indicating better quality of life (Yao, 2000). The reliability and validity of the Chinese WHOQOL-BREF have been tested in several clinical settings, including on caregivers of patients with injury (Wu et al., 2014). In this study, the Cronbach's α of the subscales for the WHOQOL-BREF ranged from .86 to .89, and the overall Cronbach's α of the scale was .90.

Ethical Considerations

Institutional review board approval (IRB No. 10202-013) was received from the board of the study hospital. The purposes of the study were explained to the participants. The participants received both written and oral information about the study before they provided informed consent.

Statistical Analyses

Descriptive statistics were used to summarize the sample and the scores on the Brief IPQ and the WHOQOL-BREF. Group differences in sample characteristics were assessed using independent-sample *t* tests for continuous variables and Fisher's exact tests for categorical variables. Generalized estimating equation (GEE) analysis was used to evaluate the intervention effects on the Brief IPQ and the WHOQOL-BREF across the follow-ups. Each GEE model included the main effects of time (baseline as the reference category) and intervention effect (control group as the reference category), the two-way interaction effects of Time × Intervention, and the main effects of control variables (patient characteristics). The differences between the two groups in terms of the change from baseline to the later follow-ups were warranted when the interaction effects were significant, suggesting the intervention effect was supported. Patient characteristics (Table 1) were treated as the control variables in the GEE model. Robust standard errors were selected to calculate significance of parameter estimates, and the exchangeable working correlation matrix was used to adjust for the time effect (Liang & Zeger, 1986). All of the analyses were performed using SPSS Version 22 (IBM, Inc., Armonk, NY, USA).

Table 3

GEE Analysis of Intervention Effect on Brief IPQ, Continued

Identity		Illness Concern		Coherence		Emotional Representation		Overall Score	
5.97***	< .001	9.73***	< .001	8.79***	< .001	4.03**	.005	5.03***	< .001
−0.45	.345	−0.48	.134	−0.15	.691	0.17	.764	−0.19	.344
−0.57	.143	−0.26	.414	0.23	.479	1.37*	.012	−0.07	.672
−0.94*	.011	−0.77**	.009	−0.02	.953	1.42**	.005	−0.42*	.016
−1.45***	<.001	−1.25***	<.001	0.50	.176	0.05	.930	−0.88***	<.001
−1.10	.059	0.50	.254	0.32	.454	−0.55	.467	−0.60*	.011
−0.59	.308	−0.73	.111	0.82	.096	−2.59***	< .001	−0.82***	.001
0.10	.866	0.40	.462	−0.15	.763	−0.15	.842	−0.05	.846

Results

Ninety-four patients with injury were recruited and randomized into the experimental and control groups. The participants in both groups had an average age in the early 30s. A substantial majority in both groups were employed before injury, injured in vehicular accidents, and classified as having a moderate injury (ISS = 9–15). A minority in both groups were classified as having a severe injury (ISS > 16). The mean lengths of hospital stay in the experimental and control groups were 10.4 ($SD = 5.3$) and 9.4 ($SD = 5.9$) days, respectively (Table 1). No significant differences in gender, age, marital status, educational level, employment status, injury mechanism, ISS, injury severity, or length of hospital stay were found between the two groups (Table 1).

The descriptive statistics of the Brief IPQ across the follow-ups in both groups are shown in Table 2, and the summary statistics of the GEE models for each domain and the overall score of the Brief IPQ are shown in Table 3. The results show that the interaction effect of the intervention over time was significant at 3 months in the personal control domain ($B = 1.26, p < .05$) and the treatment control domain ($B = 1.50, p < .01$), indicating that improvement from baseline to 3 months was greater in the experimental group than in the control group. The interaction effect of the intervention over time was significant at 6 months in the emotional representation domain ($B = -2.59, p < .001$), indicating the positive effect of the intervention at 6 months. Noticeably, the intervention effect on the Brief IPQ overall score was supported at 3 months ($B = -0.60, p < .05$) and 6 months ($B = -0.82, p < .001$). However, no evidence for an intervention effect was found for any domains of the Brief IPQ at 12 months (see Figure 1).

The descriptive statistics of the WHOQOL-BREF across follow-ups in both groups are presented in Table 2, and the summary statistics of the GEE models for each WHOQOL domain are presented in Table 4. The results of the GEE indicate that the interaction effects of the intervention at 6 months ($B = 1.38$, $p < .01$) and 12 months ($B = 1.06, p < .05$) were significant in the social relationships domain, revealing that the improvements from baseline to 6 months and to 12 months were greater in the experimental group than in the control group. However, no

Figure 1

Observed Mean Values of (A) Personal Control, (B) Treatment Control, (C) Emotional Representation, and (D) Total Score of the IPQ in the Experimental and Control Groups Across Follow-Ups

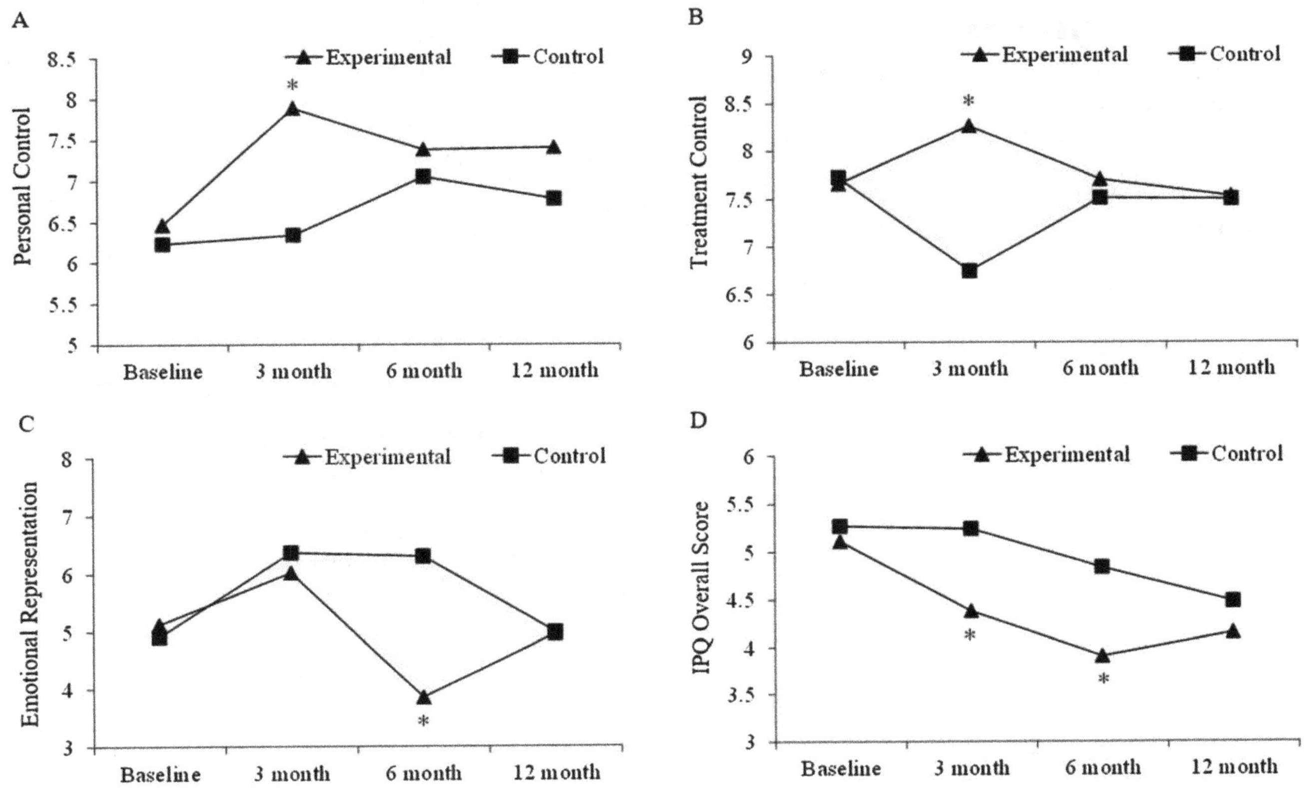

Note. IPQ = Illness Perception Questionnaire. * indicates the change in mean values between baseline and the later time point differed significantly between the two groups.

Table 4
GEE Analysis of Intervention Effect on WHOQOL-BREF

Variable	Physical Health		Psychological Health		Social Relationships		Environment	
	B	*p*	*B*	*p*	*B*	*p*	*B*	*p*
Intercept	14.35***	< .001	14.22***	< .001	15.32***	< .001	14.51***	< .001
Treatment Experimental vs. control	−0.96	.123	0.29	.502	−0.45	.298	0.06	.902
Time								
3 months vs. baseline	−2.34***	< .001	−0.27	.497	−0.96*	.015	−0.73	.051
6 months vs. baseline	−1.61**	.002	−0.08	.839	−0.80*	.025	0.18	.638
12 months vs. baseline	−1.05*	.047	−0.67	.137	−0.97*	.012	0.02	.962
Interaction term								
3 months vs. baseline	1.37	.074	−0.08	.887	0.87	.098	0.86	.087
6 months vs. baseline	1.02	.213	−0.08	.891	1.38**	.008	0.56	.277
12 months vs. baseline	1.09	.170	1.04	.071	1.06*	.044	0.87	.121

Note. GEE = generalized estimating equation; WHOQOL-BREF = World Health Organization Quality of Life Questionnaire.
*$p < .05$. **$p < .01$. ***$p < .001$.

evidence for an intervention effect was found at 3 months or at all for the other domains of the WHOQOL-BREF. The changes in the "social relationships domain" across the follow-ups in each group are presented in Figure 2.

Discussion

The effects of a nurse-delivered intervention over a 12-month follow-up period were examined in this study. The outcomes showed that the intervention had positive effects on the cognitive illness perceptions, emotional perceptions, and quality of life of the participants in the experimental group at 3, 6, and 12 months after hospital discharge.

Figure 2
Observed Mean Values of the Social Relationships Domain of the World Health Organization Quality of Life Questionnaire in the Experimental and Control Groups Across Follow-Ups

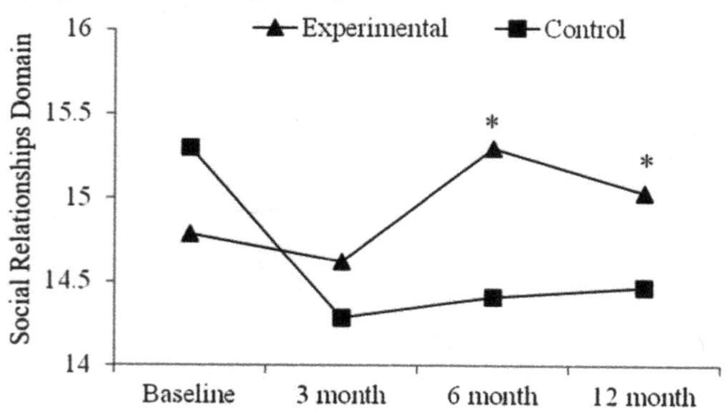

Note. * indicates the change in mean values between baseline and a later time point differed significantly between the two groups.

Moreover, these participants registered significant improvements in personal control and treatment control at 3 months after injury, suggesting that the intervention helped promote confidence in recovery and greater adherence to postinjury treatment. These findings are consistent with those in the study by Lee et al. (2015), which showed that in-hospital interventions help patients improve their perceptions and increase their confidence in their ability to control their postinjury conditions at 3 months after injury.

These findings do make sense for patients with injury because the time around 3 months after an injury is typically a transitional period for patients from the subacute stage to the rehabilitation stage. However, different from Lee et al.'s (2015) study, this study did not detect significant decreases in injury-related physical symptoms. This may be attributable to the average age of the patients in this study being lower than the average ages of the patients in Lee et al. (2015) and Chaboyer et al. (2010), which may have led to the participants in this study to self-perceive a relatively fast physical recovery and a lower intervention effect on this dimension.

Although previous studies have reported many physical symptoms in patients with injury at 3 months after injury (Chaboyer et al., 2010; Lee et al., 2008), no intervention effect on physical outcomes at 3 months after injury was found in this study. Importantly, positive changes in 3-month overall illness perceptions in the experimental group were found in this study. General illness perceptions include the physical symptoms domain. These findings may not contradict with previous findings, as positive perceptions may fluctuate in patients with injury who experience physical or psychological disabilities.

The intervention changed the emotional perceptions of participants at 6 months after injury. As standardized care for patients with injury is not provided across hospitals in Taiwan, the participants in this study appeared to have emotional problems that require greater focus in terms of treatment. This result is quite important because previous studies found that patients with injury experience emotional problems at 6 months after hospital discharge (Chaboyer et al., 2010; Schneiderman et al., 2013). This new evidence indicates that it is crucial for clinicians to provide mental support during the first 6 months after injury.

Findings from this study indicate that the overall score for illness perceptions was positively changed by the intervention at 3 and 6 months after injury. These results are similar to Rakhshan et al. (2013), although the intervention effects in this study persisted significantly longer. These results may be attributable to the combined effect of the nursing intervention and CBT skills helping patients change their perceptions.

No evidence of intervention effects on illness perceptions was found at 12 months after hospital discharge. Therefore, the intervention may not provide an effect that extends beyond 6 months after injury. This may be because the patients have almost completely recovered from their injury or have already acclimated to their postinjury status. Although research has shown that up to 40% of patients with severe injury experience psychological problems at 12 months after injury (Vles et al., 2005), this study did not indicate that the intervention had any effect on 12-month health outcomes. We speculate that over 80% of the participants in this study had moderate rather than major injuries. Thus, the extent of long-term disability may be significantly less in this study than in Vles et al. (2005).

The intervention resulted in better "social relationships" in terms of quality of life at 6 and 12 months after injury. These participants had better social relationships with others, indicating that the intervention improved connections with their social networks. We speculate that the patients were influenced in terms of their cognitive perceptions at 3 months and emotional perceptions at 6 months after injury and thus may have had better social skills at 6–12 months after injury. No prior research evidence is available to compare with these results. To retest the intervention effects, future research may adopt the intervention protocol and follow-up time points used in this study to investigate patients with major injuries or specific types of injuries (e.g., injuries to extremities).

In summary, this study aimed to explore whether the developed nurse-driven intervention has short- and long-term impacts on outcomes in patients with injury, including illness perceptions and quality of life. The nurse intervention was found to partially improve patients' short- and long-term outcomes. Most importantly, this study provides a new and unique finding that the investigated nurse intervention may affect 1-year outcomes in patients with injury. The study results are of significant value for patients, clinicians, and the government. With regard to patients, their postinjury expectations should be regularly assessed to identify the critical barriers to recovery. Meanwhile, clinicians, including nurses, physicians, rehabilitation therapists, and social workers, should be made better aware of patient outcomes after injury. By receiving treatment consisting of interdisciplinary interventions, patients may obtain better quality-of-life-related health outcomes, which may ultimately reduce national medical costs.

Relevance to Clinical Practice

The findings of this study suggest that case management may be necessary to improve outcomes in patients with injury and that the core concept of case management should include injury-related interventions, even when a hospital does not have a standard care management protocol for these patients. Under a care management model, nurses and other clinicians such as physicians, rehabilitation therapists, and social workers may be made better aware of the illness perceptions and care needs of patients by visiting these patients on a daily basis to review progress, ensure optimal care is given, and schedule regular postdischarge follow-up visits.

Hospitals may incorporate illness perceptions as a foundation for assessment. It is important to implement early identification of expectations to highlight the needs of patients with injury and to assist them to reshape their illness perceptions. For example, the Brief IPQ (Broadbent et al., 2006) may be used to quickly assess patient expectations regarding an injury at hospital discharge and at 3 and 6 months after discharge. After these assessments, multidisciplinary professional services may be deployed to help patients reduce inconsistencies between these expectations and reality.

With regard to rehabilitation efforts, providing comprehensive care to patients with injury to help them adapt to postinjury recovery rather than providing acute care, nurses and clinicians may combine rehabilitation practice and test the effects on the illness perceptions of these patients. In rehabilitation units or during outpatient department visits, regular assessments of each patient's expectations and barriers to recover may be necessary to improve the quality of life of patients with injury.

Limitations

The data were collected in only one hospital, which may limit the external validity of this study. Another limitation was the complicated nature of injury mechanisms, which may limit the applicability of findings to patients in other injury categories. Finally, only a minority of the patients included in the study were classified with a severe injury. This may be attributable to the exclusion of patients with severe head, spinal cord, or burn injuries.

Conclusions

The findings showed that the nurse-delivered CBT intervention had long-term effects and positively changed patients' illness perceptions and quality of life. This study adds some new evidence that may facilitate the recovery of patients with injury, especially in the 6- to 12-month postinjury period. Moreover, the findings of this study suggest that nurses and other clinicians should be involved in the intervention to provide interprofessional care at different periods for patients. In addition, regular assessment of the illness perceptions and self-care abilities of patients with injury may be helpful to their successful recovery and rehabilitation. Although some components of illness perceptions and quality of life were not changed by the intervention, further research may be used to test the applicability of the intervention.

Acknowledgments

The authors would like to thank National Science Council (grant number: NSC 101-2314-B-255-005-MY3) and Kaohsiung Medical University Neuroscience (grant number: KMU-TC109B03) for providing the research grants for this study.

Authors Contributions

Study conception and design: BOL
Data collection: BOL
Data analysis and interpretation: BOL, CCH
Drafting of the article: WCF, BOL
Critical revision of the article: BOL, WCF, WC

References

Baecher, K., Kangas, M., Taylor, A., O'Donnell, M. L., Bryant, R. A., Silove, D., McFarlane, A. C., & Wade, D. (2018). The role of site and severity of injury as predictors of mental health outcomes following traumatic injury. *Stress and Health, 34*(4), 545–551. https://doi.org/10.1002/smi.2815

Baker, E., Xyrichis, A., Norton, C., Hopkins, P., & Lee, G. (2018). The long-term outcomes and health-related quality of life of patients following blunt thoracic injury: A narrative literature review. *Scandinavian Journal of Trauma, Resuscitation and Emergency Medicine, 26*(1), Article No. 67. https://doi.org/10.1186/s13049-018-0535-9

Banierink, H., Reininga, I. H. F., Heineman, E., Wendt, K. W., ten Duis, K., & IJpma, F. F. A. (2019). Long-term physical functioning and quality of life after pelvic ring injuries. *Archives of Orthopaedic and Trauma Surgery, 139*(9), 1225–1233. https://doi.org/10.1007/s00402-019-03170-2

Bayo, H. L., Montmany, S., Rebasa, P., Secanella, M., Alberich, M., & Navarro, S. (2019). Analysis of quality of life after major trauma: A Spanish follow-up cohort study. *European Journal of Trauma and Emergency Surgery, 45*(2), 289–297. https://doi.org/10.1007/s00068-018-0920-0

Broadbent, E., Petrie, K. J., Main, J., & Weinman, J. (2006). The brief illness perception questionnaire. *Journal of Psychosomatic Research, 60*(6), 631–637. https://doi.org/10.1016/j.jpsychores.2005.10.020

Centers for Disease Control and Prevention. (2016). *Cost of injuries and violence in the United States.* http://medbox.iiab.me/modules/en-cdc/www.cdc.gov/injury/wisqars/overview/cost_of_injury.html

Chaboyer, W., Lee, B. O, Wallis, M., Gillespie, B., & Jones, C. (2010). Illness representations predict health-related quality of life 6 months after hospital discharge in individuals with injury: A predictive survey. *Journal of Advanced Nursing, 66*(12), 2743–2750. https://doi.org/10.1111/j.1365-2648.2010.05431.x

Cohen, J. A., & Mannarino, A. P. (2008). Trauma-focused cognitive behavioural therapy for children and parents. *Child and Adolescent Mental Health, 13*(4), 158–162. https://doi.org/10.1111/j.1475-3588.2008.00502.x

Dekker, R. L., Moser, D. K., Peden, A. R., & Lennie, T. A. (2012). Cognitive therapy improves three-month outcomes in hospitalized patients with heart failure. *Journal of Cardiac Failure, 18*(1), 10–20. https://doi.org/10.1016/j.cardfail.2011.09.008

Des Jarlais, D. C., Lyles, C., Crepaz, N., & the TREND Group. (2004). Improving the reporting quality of nonrandomized evaluations of behavioral and public health interventions: The TREND statement. *American Journal of Public Health, 94*(3), 361–366. https://doi.org/10.2105/ajph.94.3.361

Diggle, P. J., Heagerty, P. J., Liang, K.-Y., & Zeger, S. L. (2013). *Analysis of longitudinal data* (2nd ed.). Oxford University Press.

Halford, J., & Brown, T. (2009). Cognitive-behavioural therapy as an adjunctive treatment in chronic physical illness. *Advances in Psychiatric Treatment, 15*(4), 306–317. https://doi.org/10.1192/apt.bp.107.003731

Kanani, A. N., & Hartshorn, S. (2016). *NICE clinical guideline NG39: Major trauma: Assessment and initial management. ADC Education & Practice, 102*(1), 20–23. https://doi.org/10.1136/archdischild-2016-310869

Knowles, S. R., Austin, D. W., Sivanesan, S., Tye-Din, J., Leung, C., Wilson, J., Castle, D., Kamm, M. A., Macrae, F., & Hebbard, G. (2017). Relations between symptom severity, illness perceptions, visceral sensitivity, coping strategies and well-being in irritable bowel syndrome guided by the common sense model of illness. *Psychology, Health & Medicine, 22*(5), 524–534. https://doi.org/10.1080/13548506.2016.1168932

Lee, B. O, Chaboyer, W., & Wallis, M. (2008). Predictors of health-related quality of life 3 months after traumatic injury. *Journal of Nursing Scholarship, 40*(1), 83–90. https://doi.org/10.1111/j.1547-5069.2008.00210.x

Lee, B. O, Chaboyer, W., & Wallis, M. (2010). Illness representations in patients with traumatic injury: A longitudinal study. *Journal of Clinical Nursing, 19*(3–4), 556–563. https://doi.org/10.1111/j.1365-2702.2009.02972.x

Lee, B. O, Chien, C. S., Hung, C. C., & Chou, P. L. (2015). Effects of an in-hospital nursing intervention on changing illness perceptions in patients with injury. *Journal of Advanced Nursing, 71*(11), 2540–2550. https://doi.org/10.1111/jan.12716

Leventhal, H., Phillips, L. A., & Burns, E. (2016). The common-sense model of self-regulation (CSM): A dynamic framework for understanding illness self-management. *Journal of Behavioral Medicine, 39*(6), 935–946. https://doi.org/10.1007/s10865-016-9782-2

Liang, K.-Y., & Zeger, S. L. (1986). Longitudinal data analysis using generalized linear models. *Biometrika, 73*(1), 13–22. https://doi.org/10.1093/biomet/73.1.13

Ministry of Health and Welfare, National Health Insurance Administration, Taiwan, ROC. (2019). *Statistical annual reports: The national health insurance statistics, 2018.* https://www.nhi.gov.tw/ english/Content_ List.aspx?n= D8ECF7F6C9D80FC1&topn=616B97F8DF2C3614

Moss-Morris, R., Weinman, J., Petrie, K., Horne, R., Cameron, L., & Buick, D. (2002). The revised illness perception questionnaire (IPQ-R). *Psychology and Health, 17*(1), 1–16. https://doi.org/10.1080/08870440290001494

Rakhshan, M., Hassani, P., Ashktorab, T., & Majd, H. A. (2013). The nature and course of illness perception following cardiac pacemaker implantation: A self-regulatory approach. *International*

Journal of Nursing Practice, 19(3), 318–325. https://doi.org/10.1111/ijn.12073

Ringdal, M., Plos, K., Örtenwall, P., & Bergbom, I. (2010). Memories and health-related quality of life after intensive care: A follow-up study. *Critical Care Medicine, 38*(1), 38–44. https://doi.org/10.1097/ccm.0b013e3181b42909

Sawyer, A. T., Harris, S. L., & Koenig, H. G. (2019). Illness perception and high readmission health outcomes. *Health Psychology Open, 6*(1), 1–11. https://doi.org/10.1177/2055102919844504

Schneiderman, J., Van Aswegen, H., & Becker, P. (2013). Health related quality of life of survivors of trauma six months after discharge. *South African Journal of Physiotherapy, 69*(1), 10–14. https://doi.org/10.4102/sajp.v69i1.366

Shepherd-Banigan, M. E., Shapiro, A., McDuffie, J. R., Brancu, M., Sperber, N. R., Van Houtven, C. H., Kosinski, A. S., Mehta, N. N., Nagi, A., & Williams, J. W. (2018). Interventions that support or involve caregivers or families of patients with traumatic injury: A systematic review. *Journal of General Internal Medicine, 33*(7), 1177–1186. https://doi.org/10.1007/s11606-018-4417-7

Siemonsma, P. C., Stuive, I., Roorda, L. D., Vollebregt, J. A., Walker, M. F., Lankhorst, G. J., & Lettinga, A. T. (2013). Cognitive treatment of illness perceptions in patients with chronic low back pain: A randomized controlled trial. *Physical Therapy, 93*(4), 435–448. https://doi.org/10.2522/ptj.20110150

Sluys, K. P., Shults, J., & Richmond, T. S. (2016). Health related quality of life and return to work after minor extremity injuries: A longitudinal study comparing upper versus lower extremity injuries. *Injury, 47*(4), 824–831. https://doi.org/10.1016/j.injury.2016.02.019

The Illness Perception Questionnaire. (2020). *The brief IPQ-acknowledgement*. https://ipq.h.uib.no/index.html (Original work published in Chinese)

Van Son, M. A. C., De Vries, J., Zijlstra, W., Roukema, J. A., Gosens, T., Verhofstad, M. H. J., & Den Oudsten, B. L. (2017). Trajectories in quality of life of patients with a fracture of the distal radius or ankle using latent class analysis. *Quality of Life Research, 26*(12), 3251–3265. https://doi.org/10.1007/s11136-017-1670-x

Vles, W. J., Steyerberg, E. W., Essink-Bot, M. L., Van Beeck, E. F., Meeuwis, J. D., & Leenen, L. P. (2005). Prevalence and determinants of disabilities and return to work after major trauma. *Journal of Trauma, 58*(1), 126–135. https://doi.org/10.1097/01.ta.0000112342.40296.1f

Vranceanu, A. M., Hageman, M., Strooker, J., Ter Meulen, D., Vrahas, M., & Ring, D. (2015). A preliminary RCT of a mind body skills based intervention addressing mood and coping strategies in patients with acute orthopaedic trauma. *Injury, 46*(4), 552–557. https://doi.org/10.1016/j.injury.2014.11.001

Willemse, H., van der Doef, M., & van Middendorp, H. (2019). Applying the common sense model to predicting quality of life in alopecia areata: The role of illness perceptions and coping strategies. *Journal of Health Psychology, 24*(11), 1461–1472. https://doi.org/10.1177/1359105317752826

Woodhouse, S., Hebbard, G., & Knowles, S. R. (2018). Exploring symptom severity, illness perceptions, coping styles, and well-being in gastroparesis patients using the common sense model. *Digestive Diseases and Sciences, 63*(4), 958–965. https://doi.org/10.1007/s10620-018-4975-x

Wu, L. Y., Lee, B. O, Hsu, C. T., Huang, K. H., & Bai, Y. L. (2014). Illness representations, stress, and quality of life in primary caregivers of individuals with injuries. *Journal of Nursing & Healthcare Research, 10*(3), 199–210. https://doi.org/10.6225/JNHR.10.3.199 (Original work published in Chinese)

Yao, K. P. G. (2000). Critiques on six generic health-related quality of life scales and suggestions on the further studies. *Psychological Testing, 42*(2), 111–138. (Original work published in Chinese)

Zatzick, D., Jurkovich, G., Rivara, F. P., Russo, J., Wagner, A., Wang, J., & Katon, W. (2013). A randomized stepped care intervention trial targeting posttraumatic stress disorder for surgically hospitalized injury survivors. *Annals of Surgery, 257*(3), 390–399. https://doi.org/10.1097/sla.0b013e31826bc313

4

Development and Psychometric Testing of the Registered Nurses' Perceptions of Rewarding Scale

Jaana SEITOVIRTA[1]* • Aku-Ville LEHTIMÄKI[2] • Katri VEHVILÄINEN-JULKUNEN[3] • Lasse MITRONEN[4] • Tarja KVIST[5]

ABSTRACT

Background: Rewarding is a powerful way to recognize, manage, and retain staff. However, the perceptions of registered nurses (RNs) toward rewarding have not yet been extensively examined in nursing studies. It is important to identify optimal and potentially innovative ways to reward RNs by taking their perceptions into consideration.

Purpose: The aim of this study was to develop and psychometrically test the Registered Nurses' Perceptions of Rewarding Scale (RNREWS).

Methods: A cross-sectional study design was used. The scale was developed in the three phases of item generation, content validity testing, and examination of psychometric properties. Tests of the scale included evaluation of content validity, exploratory factor analysis, parallel analysis, and internal consistency tests using Cronbach's alpha. Survey participants included 402 RNs working in Finnish healthcare in Autumn 2015.

Results: The RNREWS was found to have acceptable construct validity and good internal consistency. Exploratory factor analysis indicated that a 66-item scale with a 14-factor structure fits the data best. The final scale includes two subscales. The first is "reward type preferences" with 61 items covering 13 factors, and the second is "significance of rewarding" with five items covering one factor. The two sets of items accounted for 73.1% and 58.5% of the variance in responses and earned Cronbach's α values of .90 and .80, respectively.

Conclusions: The RNREWS is a valid and reliable instrument for acquiring knowledge regarding the perspective of RNs on rewarding in the nursing context. The results enhance the understanding of the range of rewards that may be implemented in the nursing profession and may assist human resources managers and administrators to formulate effective reward systems for their RNs to improve the rewarding and retention of nursing professionals. However, cultural equivalence and linguistic differences must be considered if this scale is to be applied in other countries or environments.

KEY WORDS:
registered nurse, reward, scale development, psychometric testing.

Introduction

Rewarding is a powerful way to recognize, manage, and retain staff. Various aspects of rewarding have been addressed by scholars in a diverse spectrum of disciplines, including management science (e.g., Armstrong & Murlis, 2007) and psychology (e.g., De Gieter, De Cooman, Pepermans, & Jegers, 2010). Hence, "rewards" are called many things, depending on the disciplinary context. For example, economists may refer to the "utility" (subjective value for a decision-maker) of a good or commodity, whereas psychologists may refer to "positive reinforcers" of behaviors or goals (Schultz, 2015).

In healthcare, the McCloskey/Mueller Satisfaction Scale developed by Mueller and McCloskey (1990) has been used to measure the dimensions of rewards (safety, social, and psychological) associated with nurse job satisfaction. Moreover, the Effort–Reward Imbalance Questionnaire by Siegrist (1996) has been used to explore links between job stress and both high job demands and low professional compensation in the form of money, social status, safety, and career opportunities. The Psychological Reward Satisfaction Scale by De Gieter et al. (2010) has been applied to address the impact of satisfaction with the pay and psychological rewards received from the head nurse and physicians. However, rewarding has not yet been extensively examined in nursing studies, and there is limited knowledge regarding the rewarding perceptions of the registered nurses (RNs) in particular. Moreover, no previously published instrument has been developed for assessing their "reward type preferences" or "significance of rewarding," which must be known to formulate optimal reward

[1]*PhD, RN, Department of Nursing Science, University of Eastern Finland, Finland* • [2]*MSc, Doctoral Student, School of Business, Department of Information and Service Economy, Aalto University, Finland* • [3]*PhD, RN, Professor, Department of Nursing Science, University of Eastern Finland, Finland* • [4]*DSc, Professor, Department of Marketing, School of Business, Aalto University, Finland* • [5]*PhD, RN, Associate Professor, Department of Nursing Science, University of Eastern Finland, Finland.*

strategies and systems for RNs. This study develops and tests the Registered Nurses' Perceptions of Rewarding Scale (RNREWS), a novel instrument that addresses these important but neglected aspects of reward management, especially in the nursing context. The RNREWS has been specifically developed to gauge the subjective perceptions of RNs regarding rewarding rather than measuring nurses' job satisfaction, associations between rewards and a positive or healthy work environment, or the psychological factors underlying rewards.

According to several studies, rewarding should be developed in a working-life-oriented manner and should take into account the viewpoints of staffs (Hulkko-Nyman, Sarti, Hakonen, & Sweins, 2012; Kurtzman et al., 2011; von Bonsdorff, 2011). RNREWS is intended to facilitate the abovementioned efforts. In the context of this study, reward was operationally defined in the noun form as something given in return for or received because of completed work, a good behavior, or a particular achievement and in the verb form as giving someone a reward. It was assumed that both financial and nonfinancial rewards should be recognized and included in a total reward package (National Health Service Employers, 2017). This study is a part of a research project on RNs' rewarding in public specialized medical care, public primary, and private healthcare settings in Finland.

Literature Review

Reward management

Reward management refers to the way an organization attracts competent personnel from the labor market and then motivates, leads, and commits to its staff (Armstrong & Murlis, 2007). It is crucial for healthcare organizations to design reward strategies that promote the job satisfaction and engagement of their nurses, attract recruits to nursing, and retain valuable staff members. Thus, an effective reward strategy is an important part of an efficient human resources strategy. A key component is a structured approach for setting rewards for an organization's staff. Reward systems may be used to define organizational values and norms and encompass all of the elements (e.g., policies, practices, and processes) of rewards. Many employees may not be aware of all of the rewards and benefits offered by their employer. Thus, clear formulation of a "total reward approach" may enhance employee perceptions of their rewards (National Health Service Employers, 2017). A total reward approach emphasizes the multidimensional nature of rewarding, combining various types of financial and nonfinancial reward elements. Typical financial rewards and benefits include, for example, basic pay and bonuses, performance-related pay, skill- and competency-based pay, additional pensions and holidays, and healthcare services. Nonfinancial rewards include, for example, training, ability to influence decision making, participation in workplace activities, work–life balance, work environment, responsibility, career opportunities, leadership, achievement and status, feedback, and recognition. Various reward models have been developed by scholars, but they usually include similar sets of financial and nonfinancial rewards. Generally, both financial and nonfinancial rewards, which combine all of the appreciated aspects of work, are considered valuable (Armstrong & Murlis, 2007).

Rewards in healthcare

Internationally, diverse reward types have been used in the healthcare field. Some of these include various forms of financial compensation such as salary, personal bonuses, pension benefits, access to fitness facilities (Kurtzman et al., 2011; Tourangeau, Cummings, Cranley, Ferron, & Harvey, 2010), and performance-based supplements, which have been reported to increase the quality and safety of work (Kurtzman et al., 2011). Other rewards are nonfinancial, including expressions of appreciation, written or verbal feedback (Dave, Dotson, Cazier, Chawla, & Badget, 2011; De Gieter et al., 2010), the provision of opportunities to develop professionally at work (Hulkko-Nyman et al., 2012), education (Seitovirta, Partanen, Vehviläinen-Julkunen, & Kvist, 2015; Seitovirta, Vehviläinen-Julkunen, Mitronen, De Gieter, & Kvist, 2017), and opportunities to influence and participate, for example, using one's skills in diverse ways (von Bonsdorff, 2011). Worktime arrangements such as flexible working hours (Dave et al., 2011) and personal control over work, for example, permission to take vacations when it is personally convenient (Li et al., 2011), are important complements to RNs' monthly salaries and other forms of financial compensation. Furthermore, nurses may find some aspects of their work content rewarding, for example, working in certain specialist areas such as elderly care settings (Bradbury-Jones, Irvine, Jones, Kakehashi, & Ogi, 2011; Hulkko-Nyman et al., 2012). A positive work environment, including the hospital's good reputation, is another potentially important type of nonfinancial reward (Dave et al., 2011). In addition, the provision of support from managers and the administration is meaningful (Morrison & Korol, 2014; Pasarón, 2013; Seitovirta et al., 2017) and plays an important role in retaining newly graduated nurses (Spence Laschinger, Wong, & Grau, 2012). Hence, the use of both financial and nonfinancial rewards in healthcare, coupled with a fair reward system, has been promoted by De Gieter et al. (2010) and Tourangeau et al. (2010).

There is international evidence that rewards significantly affect nursing outcomes and organizational commitment (Kurtzman et al., 2011; Morrison & Korol, 2014; Pasarón, 2013). Rewarding is seen as a contributory factor to coping with work-related stress (C. K. Chen, Lin, Wang, & Hou, 2009). Many rewards, particularly nonfinancial forms such as acknowledgement, may also reduce staff turnover, especially when nurses are supported by their managers (Dave et al., 2011; Morrison & Korol, 2014). Furthermore, praise and recognition strongly influence job satisfaction, satisfaction with nursing, and nurses' intent to leave (Duffield, Roche, Blay, & Stasa, 2011). As shown by von Bonsdorff (2011), research-based knowledge regarding the age-related reward preferences of nurses may assist healthcare managers and policymakers to design appropriate reward systems and thus encourage their employees to work longer. Other factors such as a positive work environment that supports professional nursing practices may further promote efforts to attract and retain nurses (Spence Laschinger et al., 2012). Several studies indicate that managers may strengthen the intentions of RNs to remain employed through actions such as praise and recognition (De Gieter et al., 2010; Tourangeau et al., 2010). In addition, nurses have a more positive work attitude when they are satisfied with the level of pay and psychological rewards that they receive from head nurses (F. Chen, Yang, Gao, Liu, & De Gieter, 2015).

Methods

The scale was developed in three phases: (1) item generation, (2) content validity testing, and (3) examination of psychometric properties (Figure 1). Tests of the scale included evaluation of content validity, exploratory factor analysis (EFA), parallel analysis, and internal consistency tests using Cronbach's alpha. Following the tests and modifications that were made based on the results of the abovementioned tests, the scale was applied in a cross-sectional survey of 402 RNs working in Finnish healthcare.

Phase 1: Item Generation

An empirical approach was adopted to operationalize rewarding in this study and other studies included on the project on the rewarding of nurses mentioned previously. First, a qualitative method was applied to probe the experiences of RNs to refine our understanding of practices that nurses find rewarding in real situations. A convenience sample was recruited, including 10 RNs from public specialized medical care organizations in 2011 and 20 RNs from public primary and private healthcare organizations in 2014. RNs' views were explored by applying content analysis to the responses of participants given in tape-recorded, semistructured individual interviews. The interviewed RNs reported positive experiences of rewarding in the form of several financial and nonfinancial rewards. These two surveys are described in our previous published studies (Seitovirta et al., 2015, 2017).

Next, to broaden our understanding of RNs' rewarding, we examined the treatment of rewarding in previous nursing research that was published in English during the period of 2009–2014 and listed in the CINAHL (EBSCO), Business Source Complete (EBSCO), Google Scholar, MEDLINE, and PubMed databases. The search terms used were "reward*," "nurs*," "incentive*" (the truncation operator * was used to list documents containing variations on a search term), "Nursing Manpower+" (the plus operator [+] collected extensions of its subordinate concepts), "exp reward" and "exp nurses" (expanding), and "nursing reward systems." Issues of the most relevant journals were also searched manually. After reviewing the titles, abstracts, and full texts of the hits obtained, 13 original studies that either examined nurses' rewarding or mentioned the reward concept in a nursing context were chosen for this study, together with the two previously mentioned interview studies. Eleven "reward types" (financial compensation, benefits, appreciation, feedback, opportunity to develop professionally at work, education, opportunity to influence and participate, worktime arrangements, work content, work environment, and managerial support) and the "significance of rewarding" were first identified and synthesized (Table 1) and then oper-

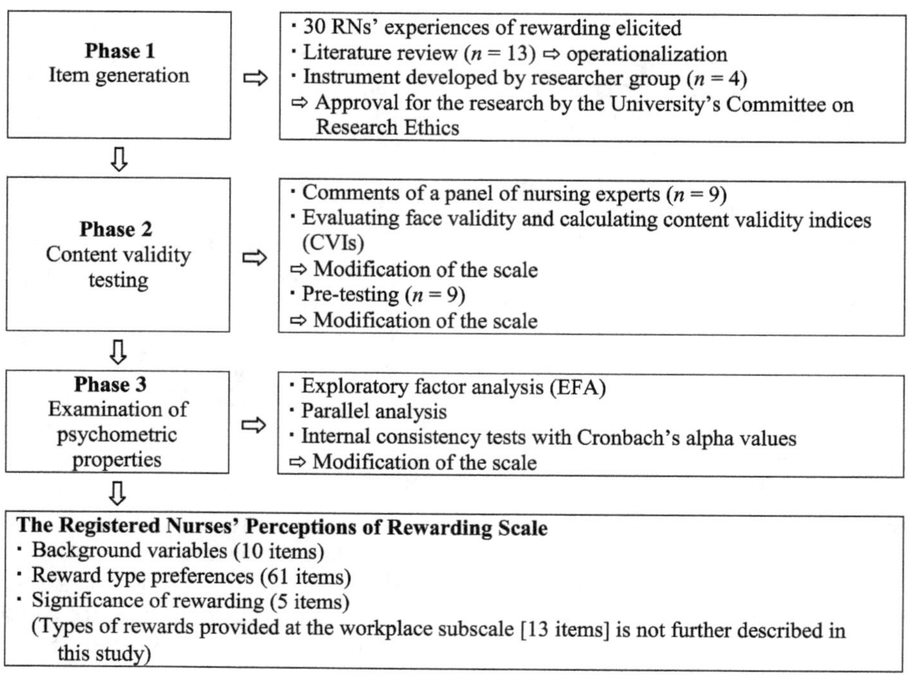

Figure 1. Developmental phases of the Registered Nurses' Perceptions of Rewarding Scale.

TABLE 1.
The Types of Rewards and Significance of Rewarding Derived From the Literature

Reward Types	Source Reference
Financial compensation	Tourangeau et al. (2010), Dave et al. (2011), von Bonsdorff (2011), Kurtzman et al. (2011), Hulkko-Nyman et al. (2012), Seitovirta et al. (2015, 2017)
Benefits	Tourangeau et al. (2010), Hulkko-Nyman et al. (2012), Seitovirta et al. (2015, 2017)
Appreciation	De Gieter et al. (2010), Tourangeau et al. (2010), Dave et al. (2011), von Bonsdorff (2011), Li et al. (2011), Hulkko-Nyman et al. (2012), Morrison & Korol (2014), Seitovirta et al. (2015, 2017)
Feedback	De Gieter et al. (2010), Tourangeau et al. (2010), von Bonsdorff (2011), Hulkko-Nyman et al. (2012), Seitovirta et al. (2015, 2017)
Opportunity to develop professionally at work	De Gieter et al. (2010), Li et al. (2011), Pasarón (2013), Seitovirta et al. (2015, 2017)
Education	Hulkko-Nyman et al. (2012), Seitovirta et al. (2015, 2017)
Opportunity to influence and participate	Tourangeau et al. (2010), von Bonsdorff (2011), Hulkko-Nyman et al. (2012), Seitovirta et al. (2015, 2017)
Worktime arrangements	Dave et al. (2011), Li et al. (2011), von Bonsdorff (2011), Hulkko-Nyman et al. (2012), Seitovirta et al. (2015, 2017)
Work content	C. K. Chen et al. (2009), Bradbury-Jones et al. (2011), Li et al. (2011), von Bonsdorff (2011), Hulkko-Nyman et al. (2012), Seitovirta et al. (2015, 2017)
Work environment	Dave et al. (2011), von Bonsdorff (2011), Spence Laschinger et al. (2012), Morrison & Korol (2014), Seitovirta et al. (2015, 2017)
Managerial support	De Gieter et al. (2010), Tourangeau et al. (2010), Spence Laschinger et al. (2012), Pasarón (2013), Morrison & Korol (2014), Seitovirta et al. (2015, 2017)
Significance of rewarding	C. K. Chen et al. (2009), De Gieter et al. (2010), Tourangeau et al. (2010), Dave et al. (2011), Duffield et al. (2011), Kurtzman et al. (2011), von Bonsdorff (2011), Hulkko-Nyman et al. (2012), Spence Laschinger et al. (2012), Pasarón (2013), Morrison & Korol (2014)

ationalized as items in the first version of the RNREWS. This first version, developed by our group of four researchers, included three subscales in total, entitled "reward type preferences" (57 items), "significance of rewarding" (six items), and "types of rewards provided at the workplace" (11 items). It also included eight items covering background variables. The last subscale was modified from a Finnish instrument (Nurmela, Hakonen, Hulkko, Kuula, & Vartiainen, 1999). Although this subscale was not judged to be entirely suitable for our study, we received permission from one of the cited authors to apply its content and associated information in the item design stage.

Phase 2: Content Validity Testing

The content validity of the first version of the scale was assessed in January 2015 by calculating content validity indices (CVIs; Polit & Beck, 2012) for the individual items (I-CVI) and the entire scale (S-CVI) using evaluations of face validity conducted by a panel of nine nursing experts. The panelists were RNs working in various healthcare organizations in Finland covering a wide range of nursing areas, who were selected to match those of participants in the main survey, as far as possible, in a small sample. The voluntary panelists were asked to rate the relevance (1 = *not relevant*, 2 = *somewhat relevant*, 3 = *quite relevant*, and 4 = *highly relevant*) of the 82 items. Following Polit and Beck (2012), I-CVIs were computed for items by summing the total number of 3 and 4 scores (quite relevant and highly relevant, respectively) and dividing by the total number of nursing experts (9). All of the nine panelists considered 81 of the 82 items to be highly relevant, so the I-CVI for each of these 81 items was 1.00, which is regarded as "excellent" (Polit & Beck, 2012). Three felt that the other item was only somewhat relevant, so the I-CVI for this item was .67, which is regarded as "fair." The experts were also asked to rate the clarity of each of the 82 individual items in advance (1 = *not at all clear*, 2 = *not very clear*, 3 = *quite clear*, and 4 = *very clear*). None of the 82 items was given a score of 1 by any of the experts, but 16 of the items were given a score of 2 by at least one of the experts. Thus, I-CVIs were 1.00 for 66 of the 82 items, .89 for 14 items, and .78 for two items. Earning an I-CVI of .78 or higher is deemed evidence of good content validity (Polit & Beck, 2012). In addition, we calculated the average I-CVIs for the relevance and clarity of all the items as indicators (S-CVI) of the content validity of the entire scale (Polit & Beck, 2012). Both of these S-CVIs were acceptable (.99 and .97, respectively).

In addition, the panelists gave oral and written comments. The scale was modified after the panel evaluation as follows: The order of the subscales was changed, two items were added (task-related supplement and well-functioning work environment), and three items were removed (nurse manager's oral support for my self-chosen education, access to paid-leave benefits, and rewards increase the good reputation of my employer). Thus, the modified second version of the scale included 81 items in total.

In the next phase, this 81-item version of the scale was pretested in paper-and-pencil format on a voluntary group of nine RNs working in the focal sectors of the planned survey (Rattray & Jones, 2007). The participants were recruited with the help of university researchers. The pretest was held at a Finnish university in April 2015. The participants were first asked to complete the questionnaire and record how long they took to answer. They were then asked to assess the questionnaire in terms of the intelligibility of the items, background variables, answer options, and instructions. In total, 38 written comments were received, most of which indicated that the scale was highly intelligible and that the instructions were clear. Frequencies and percentages of the scores for each question were calculated, and the variation in participant responses was examined to identify sources of measurement error. The written comments were carefully analyzed, and the scale was modified by adding five items under "reward type preferences," two items under "types of rewards provided at the workplace," and two items under "background variables." Thus, the third version included 90 items.

The final version of the RNREWS, reported here, included 67 positively worded items in total, covering "reward type preferences" (62 items) and "significance of rewarding" (five items). A 5-point Likert scale was used to score each item (1 = *strongly disagree*, 2 = *partly disagree*, 3 = *neither agree nor disagree*, 4 = *partly agree*, and 5 = *strongly agree*). In addition, an "I do not know" alternative (0) was included to avoid inappropriate use of the neutral point. The subscale "types of rewards provided at the workplace" (covered by 13 items, e.g., task-related supplements, employment stability, opportunity to develop professionally at work, and feedback, and scored using a trichotomous scale: *yes*, *no*, and *I don't know*) is not further described here because it will be used in a further planned study.

The final background variables (10 items) were gender, age (years), healthcare sector (public specialized medical care/public primary/private), working experience in the current organization (years or months), working experience as an RN (rounded to the nearest half-year), service type (permanent/fixed term), employment type (full/part time), working hours (day/shift work), assessment of current job satisfaction (Levels 1–10), and assessment of current quality of care (Levels 1–10).

Phase 3: Examination of Psychometric Properties

All data analyses were performed using SPSS Version 21.0 (IBM, Armonk, NY, USA). Assessments based on histograms and stem-and-leaf plots indicated that the model residuals were distributed sufficiently closely to normality for the applied statistical tests. EFA (principal axis factoring with varimax rotation) was applied rather than confirmatory factor analysis because we wanted to search for explanatory factors rather than confirm a presumed structure for the observed variables (Ramirez, Ford, Stewart, & Teresi, 2005). More specifically, principal axis factoring with varimax rotation was applied to decrease the number of variables, followed by Kaiser–Meyer–Olkin (KMO) and Bartlett's sphericity tests, with a cutoff point of .30 for the correlations and loadings (Green, Levy, Thompson, Lu, & Lo, 2012). The "reward type preferences" subscale was also subjected to parallel analysis using the 95th percentile rule (O'Connor, 2000). Cronbach's alpha values of all the resulting factors were calculated to evaluate internal consistency. "I don't know" responses were recorded together with missing responses as missing values.

Sample Description and Data Collection

A convenience sample totaling 596 voluntary RNs working in several clinical areas in one public specialized medical care organization (university hospital; n = 300), one public primary healthcare organization (n = 150), and two private healthcare organizations (n = 146) were invited to participate in a cross-sectional survey using the scale. The participants were anonymous and covered a wide range of clinical areas. Our choice of organizations was influenced by existing contacts and the possibility of collecting data from nurses in diverse clinical areas at the organizations' sites during Autumn 2015. The criteria for including participants were that they were working as an RN at one of the organizations during the time of the research, understood the Finnish language, and were not in a leadership position. Nurse leaders from the participating organizations informed their nurse managers about the study, who disseminated research invitation flyers and a paper-and-pencil format questionnaire with a postage-paid return envelope to nurses in their units during September 2015. There were 402 responses in total (188, 107, and 107 from RNs working in the public specialized medical care, public primary, and private healthcare organizations, respectively), with a response rate of 67.5%. In the current study, the RNREWS was developed and tested as a Finnish version. However, RNREWS was translated into English for dissemination purposes through a translation/back-translation comparison procedure by a Finnish–English bilingual expert.

Ethical Considerations

The research was approved by the Finnish University Committee on Research Ethics (Statement 2/2015). As ethical considerations based on human rights influenced all decision making throughout the research process, research permission was requested from all participating organizations in May 2015. All of the participating organizations were asked to designate contact persons to maintain participant anonymity. The cover letter of the study stated that participation was voluntary, that respondents' personal data would not be gathered, and that it would not be possible to identify any individual respondent at any point. Data security precautions and methods for scoring and reporting results were applied consistently.

Results

The number of participants ($N = 402$) met the recommended criteria, including a satisfactory subject-to-item ratio (6:1), for applying EFA to reduce item dimensionality and identify underlying latent structures. Characteristics of the RNs are presented in Table 2.

Construct Validity of the Registered Nurses' Perceptions of Rewarding Scale

The RNREWS was found to have acceptable construct validity and good internal consistency (Table 3). In the EFA of the structure of the scale, solutions with 10–14 factors were examined for the "reward type preferences" subscale (62 items), with 13 factors providing the best solution. Hence, 13 factors were computed in accordance with the groups formed using Kaiser's rule that factors with eigenvalues greater than 1 should be retained. However, principal axis factoring with the 95th percentile rule has been shown to generate results with a relatively high level of accuracy. Thus, a parallel analysis using the 95th percentile rule was performed (O'Connor, 2000). Eigenvalues obtained from both analyses (around the intersection point) are compared in Figure 2, showing that the 11th factor was the last factor for which the eigenvalue obtained using the 95th percentile rule was lower than the value obtained using Kaiser's rule. This indicates that the 11-factor solution is the most suitable. However, the primary aim of this study was to develop a psychometric scale, so every item should ideally be associated unequivocally with only one factor. Therefore, we adopted the 13-factor solution.

Following these analyses, the "reward type preferences" subscale was reduced from 62 to 61 items, covering the 13 factors of appreciation and feedback from work community; opportunity to develop, influence, and participate; patient/customer work; benefits; work content; performance-based pay; basic salary and supplements; education; managerial support; support for professional development; worktime arrangements; work environment and working atmosphere; and employers' values and reputation (Table 3). All of the 13 factors extracted had eigenvalues greater than 1, and the solution explained 73.13% of the total variation in responses. The KMO and Bartlett's sphericity tests yielded

TABLE 2.

Characteristics of the Participants (N = 402)

Characteristic	*n*	%
Gender		
Female	354	88.1
Male	43	10.7
Missing	5	1.2
Age (years)		
< 30	45	11.2
30–39	106	26.4
40–49	112	27.9
50–59	107	26.6
≥ 60	21	5.2
Missing	11	2.7
Place of work		
Public specialized medical care	188	46.8
Public primary healthcare	107	26.6
Private healthcare	107	26.6
Work experience in the current organization (years)		
< 1	39	9.7
1–3	93	23.1
4–9	119	29.6
10–19	117	29.1
≥ 20	32	8.0
Missing	2	0.5
Experience as an RN (years)		
< 1	11	2.7
1–3	52	12.9
4–9	59	14.7
10–19	157	39.1
≥ 20	121	30.1
Missing	2	0.5
Service type		
Permanent	338	84.1
Fixed term	63	15.7
Missing	1	0.2
Employment		
Full time	362	90.1
Part time	39	9.7
Missing	1	0.2
Working hours		
Daywork	103	25.6
Shift work	294	73.1
Missing	5	1.3
Assessment of current job satisfaction		
Total	397	98.8
Missing	5	1.2
Assessment of current quality of care		
Total	397	98.8
Missing	5	1.2

Note. RN = registered nurse.

TABLE 3.

Results of the 14-Factor Exploratory Factor Analysis Solution for the "Reward Type Preferences" and "Significance of Rewarding" (N = 402)

Subscale (Factor)/Item (66 Items)	*n*	Loading	*α*	Eigenvalue
Reward type preferences (Factors 1–13)				
1. Appreciation and feedback from work community	375		.91	1.06
• Appreciation from the work community		.57		
• Appreciation from the nurse manager		.73		
• Appreciation from senior management		.71		
• Nurses' appreciation in the society		.48		
• Feedback from the work community		.53		
• Feedback from the doctors		.66		
• Feedback from the nurse manager		.74		
• Feedback from the senior management		.73		
2. Opportunity to develop, influence, and participate	372		.88	1.17
• Adequate human resources		.38		
• Opportunity to develop professionally at work		.44		
• Employer's support (with worktime arrangements) for spontaneous training		.50		
• Opportunity to influence one's own work		.60		
• Opportunity to influence the functioning of the work community		.77		
• Opportunity to participate in making decision related to work		.85		
• Opportunity to participate in developing work		.80		
3. Patient/customer work	389		.88	1.09
• Work with patient/customer		.50		
• Appreciation from patients/customers		.81		
• Appreciation from relatives of the patients/customers		.81		
• Feedback from the patients/customers		.87		
• Feedback from relatives of the patients/customers		.85		
4. Benefits	323		.90	3.01
• Extensive occupational health services offered by the employer (healthcare)		.33		
• Exercise benefits offered by the employer		.52		
• Cultural benefits offered by the employer		.50		
• Commuting cost benefits offered by the employer		.74		
• Housing benefits offered by the employer		.70		
• Dining benefits offered by the employer		.73		
• Recreational/well-being days during working hours		.51		
• Christmas/birthday/years of service or other gifts given by the employer		.60		
5. Work content	384		.83	1.44
• Employment stability		.29		
• Present job description		.57		
• Responsibility at work		.75		
• Independence of work		.72		
• Variety of work		.67		
• Quality of work		.49		
• Teamwork		.49		
6. Performance-based pay	321		.89	4.46
• Initiative or other similar lump-sum payment		.72		
• Personal payment for student tutoring		.74		
• Personal performance-based pay		.74		
• Common performance-based pay of a work unit		.56		
7. Basic salary and supplements	360		.77	21.19
• Basic salary		.42		
• Personal supplement		.64		
• Experience-related supplement		.63		
• Task-related supplement		.61		

(continues)

TABLE 3.

Results of the 14-Factor Exploratory Factor Analysis Solution for the "Reward Type Preferences" and "Significance of Rewarding" (N = 402), Continued

Subscale (Factor)/Item (66 Items)	*n*	Loading	α	Eigenvalue
8. Education	389		.86	1.27
• Training organized by the employer		.63		
• External training paid for by the employer		.66		
• Access to desired training		.67		
9. Managerial support	368		.83	1.93
• Senior management's leadership style		.49		
• Nurse manager's leadership style		.75		
• Nurse manager's presence/visibility in daily work		.61		
• Nurse manager's nursing background		.37		
10. Support for professional development	352		.74	1.40
• Opportunity to advance in one's career		.34		
• Regular development discussions with one's nurse manager		.47		
• Professional literature and magazines at work		.70		
• Receiving work supervision		.61		
11. Worktime arrangements	377		.77	1.74
• Opportunity to participate in work shift planning		.44		
• Flexibility of working hours		.64		
• Opportunity to get unpaid leave		.58		
12. Work environment and working atmosphere	397		.88	2.58
• Well-functioning work environment		.72		
• Working atmosphere in the workplace		.73		
13. Employer values and reputation	378		.77	2.27
• Values represented by the employer		.37		
• Good reputation of the employer		.46		
Significance of rewarding (Factor 14)	393		.80	2.93
• To work enjoyment		.69		
• To work motivation		.77		
• To coping at work		.78		
• To commitment to employer		.63		
• To staying in the RN profession		.59		

Note. N = 402: number of missing values, including both missing data and "I don't know" responses.

values of .9 and $p < .001$, respectively. The final number of items was 61 because one item, "nurse manager's background in a field other than nursing," earned an overly low communality value of .169 and was thus dropped. In the 13-factor solution, 60 of the 61 items had loadings exceeding .30 on multiple factors (and every item correlated with at least one other item with a correlation coefficient exceeding .30), with the exception of "employment stability," which had a loading of .29. However, this item was retained because it matched the corresponding factor ideally. The "significance of rewarding" subscale (five items) yielded only one factor with an eigenvalue greater than 1. The rotated factor loadings varied from .59 to .78 (Table 3). The solution explained 58.5% of the variation in responses and yielded KMO and Bartlett's sphericity test values of .8 and $p < .001$, respectively.

Internal Consistency of the Registered Nurses' Perceptions of Rewarding Scale

The RNREWS was found in the evaluation of reliability to have good internal consistency, with Cronbach's α values ranging from .74 to .91 for the 61 items of the "reward type preferences" subscale and .80 for the five items of the "significance of rewarding" subscale (Table 3).

As shown in Table 3, fewer than 10% of the values were missing for each of the variables except for three: initiative or other similar lump-sum payment (13.7%), personal performance-based pay (11.7%), and housing benefits offered by the employer (11.4%). Data are assumed to be missing completely at random within the variables, following Hair, Black, Babin, and Anderson (2014).

Discussion

This study respected the strict procedures advocated by Streiner and Kottner (2014) for scale development. A review of multidisciplinary scientific articles and a wide-ranging approach to the phenomenon of RNs' rewarding deepened the understanding of researchers of this subject during the

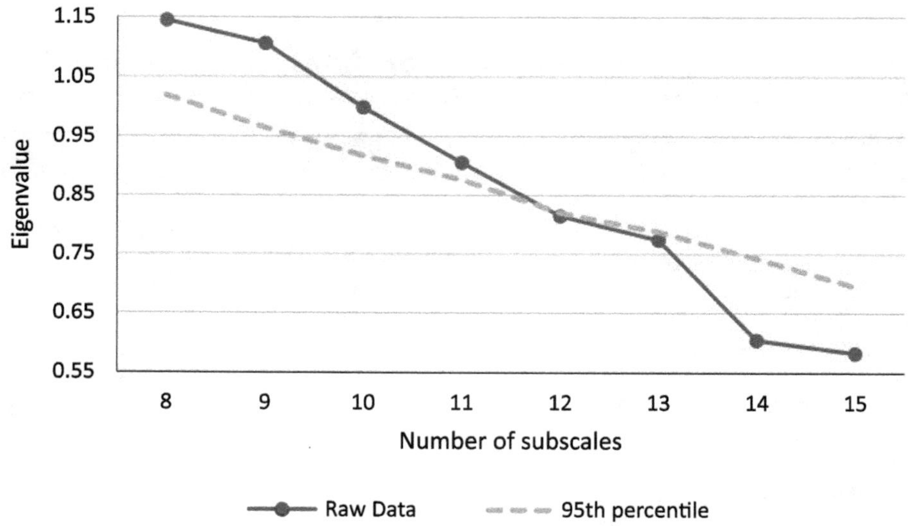

Figure 2. Comparison of eigenvalues obtained from principal axis factoring using Kaiser's rule (raw data) and parallel analysis (95th percentile) for the "reward type preference" subscale.

instrument development process. The success of the operationalization was assessed using reliability and validity tests (Rattray & Jones, 2007), the results of which indicate that the developed scale measures the issue that it is intended to measure. Face validity assessments are subjective and thus the weakest measure of validity (DeVon et al., 2007). However, in this study, these assessments provided insights into how potential participants may interpret and answer the items and evidence that the scale truly measures the types of reward that RNs prefer and the significance of rewarding RNs in their work settings. A panel of nursing experts (n = 9; DeVon et al., 2007) and CVIs (Polit & Beck, 2012) were used to further evaluate the validity of the scale and its individual items. Furthermore, the questionnaire was subjected to a pretest (n = 9) to assess it in terms of the intelligibility of the items, background variables, answer options, and instructions (Rattray & Jones, 2007).

The number of participants in our survey (N = 402, response rate = 67.5%) met the recommended criteria, including a satisfactory subject-to-item ratio (6:1), for applying the EFA to evaluate a scale's psychometric properties (Rattray & Jones, 2007). Moreover, the KMO and Bartlett's sphericity tests indicated that the data set was suitable for factor analysis. In addition, satisfactory internal consistency (Cronbach's α) values were obtained, indicating that all of the items measure the same thing and are strongly intercorrelated (DeVon et al., 2007). In addition, we cooperated with an expert statistician during the analytical process to identify and evaluate sources of measurement error, thereby increasing the reliability of the study. The literature suggests that parallel analysis provides an approach to determining the optimal number of factors that is superior to Kaiser's simple rule of retaining factors with an eigenvalue exceeding 1 (e.g., Green et al., 2012). However, no available method specifies precisely how many factors should be formed, and the final decision is influenced by the research problem. Therefore, if the initial scale and chosen EFA method conflict, a compromise between the best factor solution and usability is needed. Following the recommendations by Rattray and Jones (2007), we attempted to minimize the missing data problem through careful planning and pretesting as well as by offering a neutral point option and the alternative option "I don't know" to avoid respondent irritation and nonresponse bias. Nevertheless, any scale that addresses abstract concepts will always include a certain degree of bias, as they are unable to measure the focal concept perfectly. Our newly developed scale appears to fit its intended purpose because it showed acceptable construct validity and good internal consistency. In addition, the use of a panel of nursing experts, pretesting, and a sufficiently large sample allowed us to assess its research utility rigorously and to show that it provided sufficient validity and reliability.

Limitations and Future Studies

This research is affected by several limitations. First, RNREWS was developed and tested in a Finnish healthcare context. Thus, cultural equivalence and linguistic differences must be considered if the scale is to be applied in another country or environment (Ramirez et al., 2005). Notably, we were not able to use a subsample to explore the test–retest relationship because of participant anonymity, and we found no suitable validated and standardized scale in the literature. Nevertheless, the criterion-related validity should be tested in the future (Polit & Beck, 2012). Moreover, the presented RNREWS reliability and validity statistics inevitably apply solely to the particular set of study participants and circumstances under which the scale was administered (Streiner & Kottner, 2014). Finally, RNREWS was used for the first time in this study, and although it appeared to have good reliability, it should be further validated using confirmatory factor analysis to confirm the factor structure of the modified scale.

Conclusions

The findings provide preliminary evidence that the 66-item RNREWS is a valid and reliable scale for acquiring knowledge on the rewarding of RNs in the nursing context in Finland. The results highlight the potential to harmonize RN rewarding policies using a rigorously evaluated scale rooted in interviewed RNs' experiences of rewarding, a relevant literature review, an evaluation by an expert panel, pretests, and a survey with a sufficiently large sample. The use of these phases allowed the rigorous assessment of research utility and showed that the developed scale provides sufficient validity and reliability. In addition, the wide-ranging approach to the phenomenon of rewarding used in this study deepened the scholarly understanding of this issue during the scale development process. Finally, RNREWS has the potential to enhance understanding of the range of rewards that may be implemented in the nursing profession and to assist human resources managers and administrators to formulate effective reward strategies and systems for their RNs. This may represent an important initial step toward effective rewarding in the nursing profession.

Acknowledgments

We thank those who participated in this study in the public specialized, public primary, and private healthcare organizations as well as the nursing staff, nurse managers, nurse leaders, head nurses, and senior management who made this study possible.

References

Armstrong, M., & Murlis, H. (2007). *Reward management. A handbook of remuneration strategy and practice* (Rev. 5th ed.). London, England: Kogan Page Limited.

Bradbury-Jones, C., Irvine, F., Jones, C., Kakehashi, C., & Ogi, A. (2011). A comparison of elderly care nursing in the UK and Japan. *Nursing Older People, 23*(9), 31–35. https://doi.org/10.7748/nop2011.11.23.9.31.c8781

Chen, C. K., Lin, C., Wang, S. H., & Hou, T. H. (2009). A study of job stress, stress coping strategies, and job satisfaction for nurses working in middle-level hospital operating rooms. *The Journal of Nursing Research, 17*(3), 199–211. https://doi.org/10.1097/JNR.0b013e3181b2557b

Chen, F., Yang, M., Gao, W., Liu, Y., & De Gieter, S. (2015). Impact of satisfactions with psychological reward and pay on Chinese nurses' work attitudes. *Applied Nursing Research, 28*(4), e29–e34. https://doi.org/10.1016/j.apnr.2015.03.002

Dave, D. S., Dotson, M. J., Cazier, J. A., Chawla, S. K., & Badget, T. F. (2011). The impact of intrinsic motivation on satisfaction with extrinsic rewards in a nursing environment. *Journal of Management and Marketing in Healthcare, 4*(2), 101–107. https://doi.org/10.1179/175330311X12943314049493

De Gieter, S., De Cooman, R., Pepermans, R., & Jegers, M. (2010). The Psychological Reward Satisfaction Scale: Developing and psychometric testing two refined subscales for nurses. *Journal of Advanced Nursing, 66*(4), 911–922. https://doi.org/10.1111/j.1365-2648.2009.05199.x

DeVon, H. A., Block, M. E., Moyle-Wright, P., Ernst, D. M., Hayden, S. J., Lazzara, D. J., ... Kostas-Polston, E. (2007). A psychometric toolbox for testing validity and reliability. *Journal of Nursing Scholarship, 39*(2), 155–164. https://doi.org/10.1111/j.1547-5069.2007.00161.x

Duffield, C. M., Roche, M. A., Blay, N., & Stasa, H. (2011). Nursing unit managers, staff retention and the work environment. *Journal of Clinical Nursing, 20*(1–2), 23–33. https://doi.org/10.1111/j.1365-2702.2010.03478.x

Green, S. B., Levy, R., Thompson, M. S., Lu, M., & Lo, W. J. (2012). A proposed solution to the problem with using completely random data to assess the number of factors with parallel analysis. *Educational and Psychological Measurement, 72*(3), 357–374. https://doi.org/10.1177/0013164411422252

Hair, J. F., Black, W. C., Babin, B. J., & Anderson, R. E. (2014). *Multivariate data analysis* (7th ed.). Harlow, England: Pearson Education Limited.

Hulkko-Nyman, K., Sarti, D., Hakonen, A., & Sweins, C. (2012). Total rewards perceptions and work engagement in elder-care organizations: Findings from Finland and Italy. *International Studies of Management and Organization, 42*(1), 24–49. https://doi.org/10.2753/IMO0020-8825420102

Kurtzman, E. T., O'Leary, D., Sheingold, B. H., Devers, K. J., Dawson, E. M., & Johnson, J. E. (2011). Performance-based payment incentives increase burden and blame for hospital nurses. *Health Affair, 30*(2), 211–218. https://doi.org/10.1377/hlthaff.2010.0573

Li, J., Galatsch, M., Siegrist, J., Müller, B. H., & Hasselhorn, H. M.; European NEXT Study Group. (2011). Reward frustration at work and intention to leave the nursing profession—Prospective results from the European longitudinal NEXT study. *International Journal of Nursing Studies, 48*(5), 628–635. https://doi.org/10.1016/j.ijnurstu.2010.09.011

Morrison, K. B., & Korol, S. A. (2014). Nurses' perceived and actual caregiving roles: Identifying factors that can contribute to job satisfaction. *Journal of Clinical Nursing, 23*(23–24), 3468–3477. https://doi.org/10.1111/jocn.12597

Mueller, C. W., & McCloskey, J. C. (1990). Nurses' job satisfaction: A proposed measure. *Nursing Research, 39*(2), 113–116.

National Health Service Employers. (2017). *Total reward in the NHS.* Retrieved from http://www.nhsemployers.org/your-workforce/pay-and-reward/reward/the-business-case-for-reward

Nurmela, K., Hakonen, N., Hulkko, K., Kuula, T., & Vartiainen, M. (1999). *How does results oriented pay function in Finland?* Espoo, Finland: Laboratory of Work Psychology and Leadership, Helsinki University of Technology. (Original work published in Finnish)

O'Connor, B. P. (2000). SPSS and SAS programs for determining the number of components using parallel analysis and Velicer's MAP test. *Behavior Research Methods, Instruments, and Computers, 32*(3), 396–402. https://doi.org/10.3758/BF03200807

Pasarón, R. (2013). Nurse practitioner job satisfaction: Looking for successful outcomes. *Journal of Clinical Nursing, 22*(17–18), 2593–2604. https://doi.org/10.1111/j.1365-2702.2012.04331.x

Polit, D. F., & Beck, C. T. (2012). *Nursing research: Generating and assessing evidence for nursing practice* (9th ed.). Philadelphia, PA: Lippincott Williams & Wilkins.

Ramirez, M., Ford, M. E., Stewart, A. L., & Teresi, J. A. (2005). Measurement issues in health disparities research. *Health Services Research, 40*(5, Pt. 2), 1640–1657. https://doi.org/10.1111/j.1475-6773.2005.00450.x

Rattray, J., & Jones, M. C. (2007). Essential elements of questionnaire design and development. *Journal of Clinical Nursing, 16*(2), 234–243. https://doi.org/10.1111/j.1365-2702.2006.01573.x

Schultz, W. (2015). Neuronal reward and decision signals: From theories to data. *Physiological Reviews, 95*(3), 853–951. https://doi.org/10.1152/physrev.00023.2014

Seitovirta, J., Partanen, P., Vehviläinen-Julkunen, K., & Kvist, T. (2015). Registered nurses' experiences of rewarding in a Finnish University Hospital—An interview study. *Journal of Nursing Management, 23*(7), 868–878. https://doi.org/10.1111/jonm.12228

Seitovirta, J., Vehviläinen-Julkunen, K., Mitronen, L., De Gieter, S., & Kvist, T. (2017). Attention to nurses' rewarding—An interview study of registered nurses working in primary and private healthcare in Finland. *Journal of Clinical Nursing, 26*(7–8), 1042–1052. https://doi.org/10.1111/jocn.13459

Siegrist, J. (1996). Adverse health effects of high-effort/low reward conditions. *Journal of Occupational Health Psychology, 1*(1), 27–41.

Spence Laschinger, H. K., Wong, C. A., & Grau, A. L. (2012). The influence of authentic leadership on newly graduated nurses' experiences of workplace bullying, burnout and retention outcomes: A cross-sectional study. *International Journal of Nursing Studies, 49*(10), 1266–1276. https://doi.org/10.1016/j.ijnurstu.2012.05.012

Streiner, D. L., & Kottner, J. (2014). Recommendations for reporting the results of studies of instrument and scale development and testing. *Journal of Advanced Nursing, 70*(9), 1970–1979. https://doi.org/10.1111/jan.12402

Tourangeau, A. E., Cummings, G., Cranley, L. A., Ferron, E. M., & Harvey, S. (2010). Determinants of hospital nurse intention to remain employed: Broadening our understanding. *Journal of Advanced Nursing, 66*(1), 22–32. https://doi.org/10.1111/j.1365-2648.2009.05190.x

von Bonsdorff, M. E. (2011). Age-related differences in reward preferences. *The International Journal of Human Resource Management, 22*(6), 1262–1276. https://doi.org/10.1080/09585192.2011.559098

5

Effects of Auricular Acupressure on Sleep Quality, Anxiety and Depressed Mood in RN-BSN Students with Sleep Disturbance

Ke-Hsin Chueh[1] • Chia-Chuan Chang[2] • Mei-Ling Yeh[3]*

ABSTRACT

Background: Students in 2-year registered nurse to Bachelor of Science in nursing (RN-BSN) programs usually work full-time and study part-time. Sleep disturbance, anxiety, and depression are known to be common health problems among these students. Prior research has described the effectiveness of auricular acupressure (AA) in reducing sleep disturbance and improving mood.

Purpose: The aim of this study was to evaluate the effect of using a 4-week AA program that adheres to a magnetic pellet on the shenmen acupoint on sleep quality, anxiousness, and depressed moods in nursing students with sleep disturbance.

Methods: This study used a one-group, quasi-experimental design with repeated measures. Eligible students were recruited from an RN-BSN program offered by a university in northern Taiwan, and all were currently experiencing sleep disturbance. A 4-week AA intervention that applied a magnetic pellet on the shenmen acupoint was used. The Pittsburgh Sleep Quality Index, Beck Anxiety Inventory, and Beck Depression Inventory-II were used to measure sleep quality and mood outcomes each week during the 4-week intervention. Improvements in sleep quality, anxiety, and depressed moods were analyzed using the generalized estimating equation.

Results: Thirty-six participants with a mean age of 32 years were enrolled as participants. After adjusting for confounding factors, continuous and significant improvements in sleep quality, anxiety, and depressed mood ($p < .05$) were observed throughout the intervention, with 4-week improvements in sleep quality, anxiety, and depressed mood averaging 26.7%, 43.5%, and 25%, respectively.

Conclusions/Implications for Practice: This study showed the efficacy of using a 4-week AA that applies a magnetic pellet on the shenmen acupoint in terms of improving sleep quality, anxiousness, and depressed mood in RN-BSN students experiencing sleep disturbances. Especially, the emotional mood of participants improved significantly as early as the first week. The 4-week AA for reducing sleep disturbance, and improving students' anxiety, and depressed moods may be applied on primary healthcare.

Key Words:
RN-BSN students, sleep quality, anxiety, depression, auricular acupressure.

Introduction

Around 54.5% of college students in Taiwan (Wu, Li, & Chang, 2015), 17% in Canada (Lee, Shin, Suen, Park, & Ernst, 2008; Tavernier & Willoughby, 2014), and 39% in New Zealand (Samaranayake, Arroll, & Fernando, 2014) have been reported as experiencing sleep disturbance. Moreover, approximately 70% of registered nurses in Taiwan experience sleep disturbance (Lee, Chen, Meg Tseng, Lee, & Huang, 2015). In addition, 94% of nurses in 2-year registered nurse to Bachelor of Science in nursing (RN-BSN) programs reportedly experience sleep disturbance (Chueh & Chang, 2014). Working full-time while studying part-time may be the main causal factor of sleep disturbance. Sleep disturbance is associated with psychological distress in RN-BSN students (Chueh & Chang, 2014). Particularly, sleep disturbance is known to be concomitant with psychological distresses (American Psychiatric Association, 2013) such as anxiety and depression (Cho et al., 2013; Samaranayake et al., 2014). About 17.3% and 19.7% of college students in New Zealand have been identified with anxiety and depression, respectively (Samaranayake et al., 2014).

According to a systematic review, auricular acupressure (AA) is one of the most effective interventions for managing sleep problems (Lee et al., 2008). Previous studies support the positive effects on sleep quality of applying AA on single or multiple acupoints (Lee et al., 2008; Suen, Wong, & Leung, 2002; Wang et al., 2005; Wang, Yeh, Chung, & Yang, 2008). Shenmen is the most commonly proposed acupoint for improving sleep quality (Lee et al., 2008). This acupoint could be used alone to reduce sleep problems (Cheung, Chan, & Yip, 2015), calm the mind (Arai et al., 2013), and relieve anxiety (Kuo, Tsai, Chen, & Tzeng, 2016). However, studies that use the shenmen acupoint as a standalone intervention to treat sleep disturbance and that measure its effect repeatedly remain limited in Taiwan. This study investigated the effects on ameliorating sleep disturbance and improving

[1]PhD, RN, Associate Professor, Department of Nursing, Fu Jen Catholic University • [2]PhD, RN, Assistant Professor, Department of Nursing, Fu Jen Catholic University; and Deputy Director, Fu Jen Catholic University Hospital • [3]PhD, DMS, RN, Professor, Graduate Institute of Integration of Traditional Chinese Medicine with Western Nursing, National Taipei University of Nursing and Health Sciences.

psychological status of a 4-week AA intervention that applied a magnetic pellet on the shenmen acupoint.

Literature Review

Long-term sleep disturbance may lead to insomnia, which may impose a high societal expense and cause negative impacts on work productivity, economic welfare, accident rates, and health-related quality of life (Léger & Bayon, 2010). Furthermore, sleep disturbance has been associated in college students with gender, psychosocial function, and intrapersonal stress (Tavernier & Willoughby, 2014). In addition, circadian rhythm disorders and lack of activity exacerbate sleep disturbance (Samaranayake et al., 2014). A longitudinal study revealed that sleep disturbance predicted increases in the prevalence of subsequent anxiety and depression (Shanahan, Copeland, Angold, Bondy, & Costello, 2014). Sleep disturbance may be one of the core symptoms used to diagnose anxiety and depressed mood (American Psychiatric Association, 2013). In addition, anxiety and depressed mood may be the most prevalent causes of sleep disturbance (Samaranayake et al., 2014).

In Taiwan, students who are enrolled in 2-year RN-BSN programs also work full-time in the hospital. Hence, they are often under great pressure from both their studies and shift work (Lin, Chueh, & Lin, 2015) and sometimes take medicine for their sleep problems (Chueh & Chang, 2014). One study reported that 94% of 2-year RN-BSN students in Taiwan experience sleep disturbance (Chueh & Chang, 2014), which is a significantly higher ratio than the ratios among the general population of women (Cheng, 2002) and among nurses in clinics or hospitals (Chien et al., 2013). Other factors that are related to sleep disturbance in student nurses include age, body mass index (BMI), physical health, life stresses, regular exercise, workload, and the use of substances such as cigarettes, alcohol, coffee, and sleeping pills (Chueh & Chang, 2014; Lin et al., 2015).

Within traditional Chinese medicine, AA is held to modulate and alleviate poor health conditions by stimulating specific acupoints on the auricle and meridians that are distributed to other parts of the body to treat various conditions (Lee et al., 2008; Wang, Chen, Yeh, & Lin, 2010). Both physical and psychological problems are due to imbalances in internal energy or the blockage of energy flows (Cheung et al., 2015). AA is a noninvasive, simple, hygienic, and low-cost therapeutic method (Wang et al., 2010).

A systematic review study found that AA may be effective on sleep disturbance when applied on the shenmen (HT7, MA-TF1) acupoint either alone or in combination with AA applications to the heart (CO15), subcortex (AT4), kidney (MA-SC), liver (CO12), spleen (CO13), or occiput (AT3; Lee et al., 2008) acupoints. In addition, AA has been recommended as an intervention for sleep disturbance among the adult population (Lian & Yan, 1990; Suen et al., 2002; Wang et al., 2005, 2008). Using AA to stimulate only the shenmen acupoint may balance or unblock internal energy flows (Cheung et al., 2015) and tranquilize the mind (Arai et al., 2013). Significant change has been found in brain activity after 10-minute stimulation at the shenmen acupoint, which was associated with reduced sleep arousal, enhanced mood, and relieved anxiety (Cheung et al., 2015; Kuo et al., 2016). Although the reported efficacy of using AA to treating sleep disturbance has varied, the shenmen acupoint may be the most effective of all the previously studied acupoints.

Magnetic pellets or semen vaccariae are common materials that are used in noninvasive AA interventions (Lee et al., 2008; Suen et al., 2002). Magnetic pellets that are used in AA therapy courses must be "renewed" about every 3 days (Suen et al., 2002). AA that employs semen vaccariae must also replace the plaster about every 3–7 days (Wang et al., 2005, 2008). However, pressure must be applied regularly on the semen vaccariae on the acupoint (Wang et al., 2005, 2008) or even reinforced 1 hour before nighttime sleep (Lian & Yan, 1990). AA with magnetic pearls may promote the circulation of qi and blood in the meridians, regulate organ functions, and improve the general physiological functions of the body. Using magnetic pearls may be less traumatic and requires no pressing if the effect of magnetotherapy is present (Suen et al., 2002). Compared with magnetic pellets, semen vaccariae are less effective in reducing sleep disturbance (Suen et al., 2002). AA with one magnetic pellet may be administered feasibly and conveniently.

This study aimed to evaluate the effects of applying AA using a magnetic pellet on the shenmen acupoint only for 4 weeks in improving the sleep quality and psychological status of 2-year RN-BSN students. Significant differences over time in terms of sleep quality, anxiety, and depression, after adjusting the baseline data, were hypothesized.

Methods

Study Design and Sample

The present research was designed as a one-group, quasi-experimental study with repeated measures. A 4-week AA with a magnetic pellet on the shenmen acupoint was provided to the study participants. The baseline was monitored immediately before the intervention, and the outcome measures were assessed weekly.

Participants were recruited from the RN-BSN program of a university in northern Taiwan. All participants were screened according to the following criteria: (a) enrolled in the same nursing department of the university for at least 1 month and (b) score of > 5 on the Pittsburgh Sleep Quality Index (PSQI) taken within the past week. Students who regularly used hypnotic medication such as sleeping pills or tranquilizers or who had performed regular rotational shift work during the previous 6 months were excluded. Using repeated measurements of data to estimate sample size (Rosner, 2006), the minimum sample size was determined to be at least 32 for one group for an effect size of 0.2, α of

.05, and β of .2. With a 10% attrition rate taken into consideration, a target of 35 participants was set.

Figure 1 shows the flowchart of the research design and the allocation of participants. Fifty sleep-disordered students received explanations of the study purpose, procedure, and intervention and were scheduled to receive the 4-week AA intervention. Of these, 37 (74%) returned the signed informed consent form and the completed demographic data sheet, PSQI, Beck Anxiety Inventory (BAI), and Beck Depression Inventory-II (BDI-II) questionnaire. Demographics and PSQI, BAI, and BDI-II were collected before the intervention and used as baseline data. Moreover, PSQI, BAI, and BDI-II were collected weekly to track the intervention effect (Posttests I–IV). One participant was excluded from the study because of her absence at Posttest II, leaving 36 participants who completed the 4-week AA.

All participants received the first-week AA intervention with a magnetic pellet in a classroom setting. The shenmen acupoint is located near the top of the auricle and at the center of the tip of the triangular fossa, as shown in Figure 2. A seed-embedding method with a magnetic pellet (Hong Kong, China) was adopted to prolong the duration of stimulation. A magnetic pellet was taped on the shenmen acupoint of one ear (initially, the right ear), where it remained for 1 week. After 1 week, the pellet was removed, and a new pellet was taped on the other ear. The AA intervention procedure lasted for 4 weeks. Two researchers who were well trained by a traditional Chinese medicine physician embedded all of the magnetic pellets. Furthermore, these two researchers checked the participants' compliance to the intervention protocol and the accuracy of their AA performance. In the event that a magnetic pellet fell off or was removed prematurely, one of the

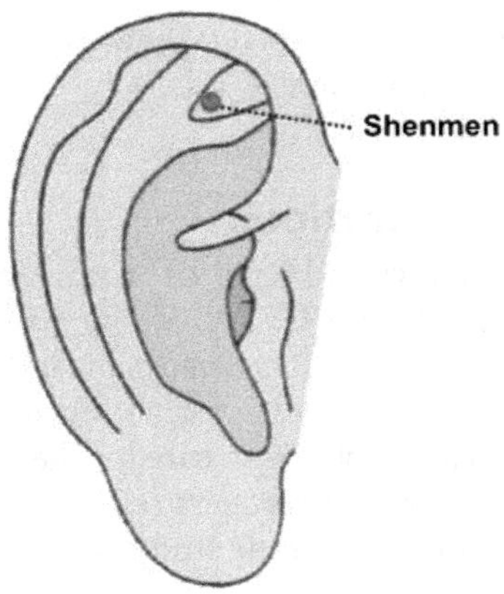

Figure 2. Location of the shenmen acupoint.

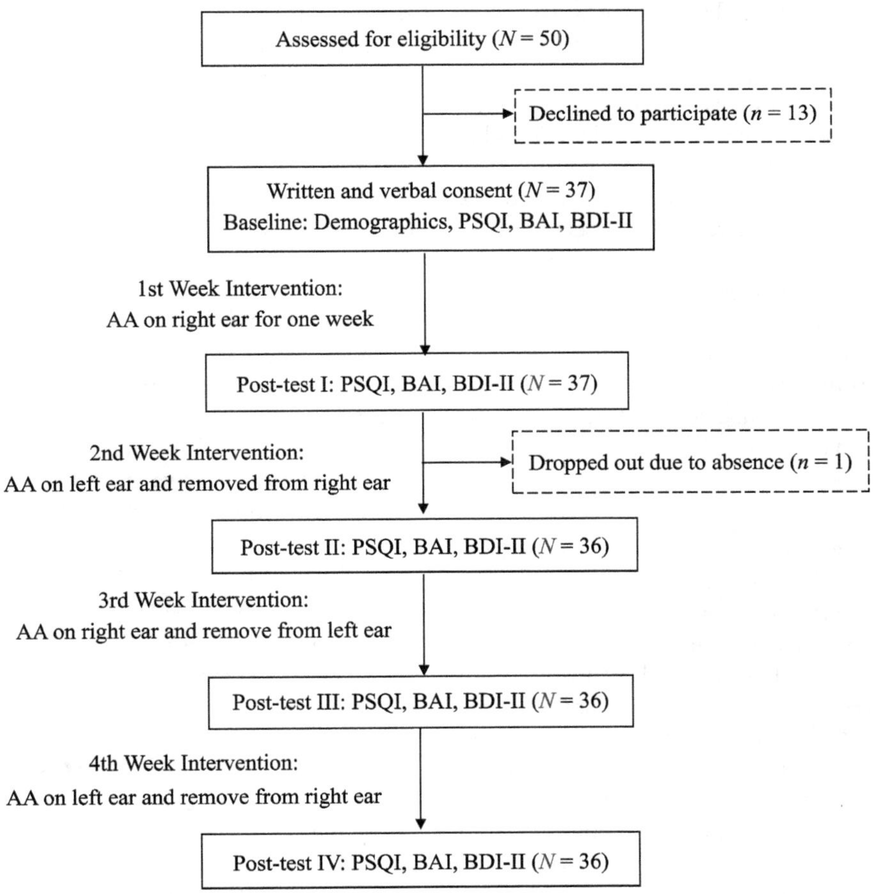

Figure 1. Flowchart of research design and allocation of participants. *Note.* PSQI = Pittsburgh Sleep Quality Index; BAI = Chinese version of the Beck Anxiety Inventory; BDI-II = Chinese version of the Beck Depression Inventory-II.

two researchers would embed a new pellet on the same acupoint as soon as possible.

Ethical Considerations

The institutional review board of a university approved this study (No. C10004R). All of the participants were volunteers and provided written consent. Participants received written and verbal information about the study as well as instructions on how to care for the magnetic pellet. They could contact the researchers regarding questions and were free to withdraw from the study at any time.

Outcome Measures

The questionnaire contained four parts, which gathered data respectively on the sleep quality, anxiety mood, depressed mood, and demographics of the participants.

Sleep quality

Sleep quality was measured using the PSQI developed by Buysse, Reynolds, Monk, Berman, and Kupfer (1989). The PSQI contains 19 items and generates seven components, including subjective sleep quality, sleep latency, sleep duration, habitual sleep efficiency, sleep disturbance, use of sleeping medication, and daytime dysfunction during the past month. The scores for each component range from 0 to 3, and the sum of the global score ranges from 0 to 21. A higher global score is associated with lower sleep quality. A global score of less than 6 indicates a good sleeper, with a good diagnostic sensitivity of 89.6% and a specificity of 86.5% (Buysse et al., 1989). The overall reliability coefficient (α) of the PSQI is .85 (Yao, Yu, Cheng, & Chen, 2008), and a test–retest reliability (r) of .74 over a 1-month period was also found (Chung & Tang, 2006). To measure the sleep quality of participants more precisely, this study modified the PSQI to assess sleep quality over the most recent week rather than the most recent month. The Cronbach's α of the PSQI in this study was .81.

Anxiety

The Chinese version of the BAI was adapted to measure level of anxiety. The BAI is a 21-item self-report inventory that is used to measure the severity of anxiety in psychiatric populations. The responses are rated on a scale from "not at all" (0) to "severely—I could barely stand it" (3) for each symptom of anxiety over the past week, with total possible scores ranging from 0 to 63 and higher scores associated with more severe levels of anxiety. BAI scores between 0 and 7, 8 and 15, 16 and 25, and 26 and 63 were interpreted in this study to represent "minimal," "mild," "moderate," and "severe" levels of anxiety, respectively. The original BAI showed high internal consistency (α = .92) and high test–retest reliability (r = .75; Beck, Epstein, Brown, & Steer, 1988). The Cronbach's α of the BAI in this study was .95.

Depressed mood

The Chinese version of the BDI-II was employed to measure level of depression. The BDI-II has 21 items, each of which is composed of four self-evaluative statements that are scored from 0 to 3, with higher scores associated with higher levels of depression. Responses are summed to yield a range of total possible scores between 0 and 63. BDI-II scores between 0 and 13, 14 and 19, 20 and 28, and 29 and 63 were interpreted in this study to represent "normal," "mild," "moderate," and "severe" levels of depression, respectively. The original BDI-II showed high internal consistency (α = .91) and high test–retest reliability (r = .93; Beck, Steer, Ball, & Ranieri, 1996). The Cronbach's α of the BDI-II in this study was .97.

Demographics

Demographics including age, length of service, and BMI as well as information on sleep disturbance and psychological distress factors, including self-aware workload, physical health, regular exercise, life stress, daily smoking, and alcohol and coffee consumption, were self-reported before the start of invention. The abovementioned factors were scored using visual analog scales (VAS; 100-mm horizontal line; Wewers & Lowe, 1990), with higher VAS scores associated with poorer situations or conditions for the related sleep disturbance or psychological distress factor. Factors were scored as follows: workload, 0 (no) to 10 (heavy); physical health, 0 (not healthy) to 10 (totally healthy); daily exercise, 0 (not regular) to 10 (totally regular); stress in daily life, 0 (no) to 10 (heavy); daily smoking, 0 (no) to 10 (heavy); daily alcohol consumption, 0 (no) to 10 (high); and daily coffee consumption, 0 (no) to 10 (high). The participants marked their scores on linear VASs.

Data Analysis

Data analysis was carried out using IBM SPSS 20.0 software for Windows. Demographics were all metric data. Descriptive statistical analysis was conducted on the PSQI, BAI, and BDI-II scores as well as on demographics and on the rates of improvement. Afterward, inferential statistical analysis, including the Spearman rho correlation, verified the respective relationships between the PSQI, BAI, and BDI-II scores with demographics at baseline. Finally, the differences in weekly intervention effect for PSQI, BAI, or BDI-II scores were analyzed using generalized estimating equation after controlling for the confounding factors of demographics.

Results

Table 1 shows the distribution and relationship of the 36 participants at baseline. All of the participants were women, with an average age of 32.0 (± 5.5) years, ranging from 23 to 48 years. Their average BMI was 23.4 (± 6.5) kg/m^2, and their mean length of service was 10.0 (± 5.0) years. The average PSQI score was 10.1 (± 3.1). The mean BAI score

TABLE 1.
Distributions and Relationships at Baseline (N = 36)

Parameter	*M*	*SD*	PSQI	BAI	BDI
PSQI (score)	10.1	3.1	–		
BAI (score)	9.2	8.9	.70***	–	
BDI-II (score)	14.0	9.0	.76***	.91***	–
Age (years)	32.0	5.5	.10	−.15	−.15
Body mass index (kg/m^2)	23.4	6.5	.24	.07	.21
Length of service (years)	10.0	5.0	.04	−.04	−.10
Workload (score)	6.2	2.3	.11	.31	.25
Physical health (score)	4.6	2.0	−.25	−.42*	−.51**
Regular exercise (score)	2.8	2.3	−.09	.23	.16
Life stress (score)	7.1	1.8	−.01	.28	.22
Smoking (score)	0.3	1.0	−.19	−.06	−.06
Alcohol consumption (score)	0.6	1.1	−.16	−.04	−.00
Coffee consumption (score)	4.5	3.3	.34*	.20	.22

Note. Higher scores for sleep disturbance and psychological distress factors were associated with worse situations/conditions. *p* Value was tested using the Spearman's rho correlation. PSQI = Pittsburgh Sleep Quality Index; BAI = Chinese version of the Beck Anxiety Inventory; BDI-II = Chinese version of the Beck Depression Inventory-II.
*$p < .05$. **$p < .01$. ***$p < .001$.

was 9.2 (± 8.9), with 22 (61.1%), 6 (16.7%), 7 (19.4%), and 1 (2.8%) participants having a "minimal," "mild," "moderate," and "severe" levels of anxiety mood, respectively. The average BDI-II score was 14.0 (± 9.0), with 22 (61.1%), 4 (11.1%), 6 (16.7%), and 4 (11.1%) participants having "normal," "mild," "moderate," and "severe" levels of depressed mood, respectively. In addition, the PSQI score was associated positively with the BAI score ($p < .001$), the BDI-II score ($p < .001$), and the amount of coffee consumed ($p < .05$). The BAI score was associated positively with the BDI-II score ($p < .001$) and negatively with physical health status ($p < .05$). Furthermore, the BDI-II score was associated negatively with physical health status ($p < .01$). Age, BMI, length of service, workload, regular exercise, life

TABLE 2.
Results of the Generalized Estimating Equation for Outcome Measures (N = 36)

Variable	Estimate	*SE*	*z*	*p*
Pittsburgh Sleep Quality Index (PSQI)				
Intercept	10.11	0.55	336.13	<.001
Posttest I	−0.89	0.47	3.66	.060
Posttest II	−1.67	0.47	12.85	<.001
Posttest III	−2.03	0.47	19.02	<.001
Posttest IV	−2.70	0.47	35.58	<.001
Beck Anxiety Inventory (BAI)				
Intercept	9.17	1.43	41.04	<.001
Posttest I	−1.94	0.83	5.55	.020
Posttest II	−2.17	0.83	6.89	.009
Posttest III	−3.58	0.83	18.85	<.001
Posttest IV	−4.00	0.83	23.49	<.001
Beck Depression Inventory-II (BDI-II)				
Intercept	14.03	1.60	76.58	<.001
Posttest I	−2.03	0.90	5.06	.030
Posttest II	−2.72	0.90	9.12	.003
Posttest III	−4.08	0.90	20.51	<.001
Posttest IV	−3.56	0.90	15.55	<.001

Note. Adjusted according to significantly related factors at baseline, including PSQI, BAI, BDI-II, coffee consumption, and physical health. Reference group: baseline.

stress, smoking, and alcohol consumption showed no significant association with the PSQI, BAI, or BDI-II score.

As shown in Table 2, the average score of PSQI was 9.2 (± 3.2), 8.4 (± 3.9), 8.1 (± 3.3), and 7.4 (± 3.0) at Posttests I–IV, respectively. The relationship between the mean PSQI score and time interaction was analyzed after controlling for BAI, BDI-II, and coffee consumption at baseline. The results showed a significant decrease in the PSQI score at Posttest II versus baseline (1.67 points lower, $p < .001$), Posttest III versus baseline (2.03 points lower, $p < .001$), and Posttest IV versus baseline (2.70 points lower, $p < .001$). The total PSQI score increased 26.7% between baseline and Posttest IV.

As also shown in Table 2, the average score of BAI was 7.2 (± 8.9), 7.0 (± 7.9), 5.6 (± 8.1), and 5.2 (± 8.4) at Posttests I–IV, respectively. The relationship between the mean BAI score and time interaction was analyzed after controlling for PSQI, BDI-II, and physical health status at baseline. The results show a significant decrease in the BAI score at Posttest I versus baseline (1.94 points lower, $p = .020$), Posttest II versus baseline (2.17 points lower, $p = .009$), Posttest III versus baseline (3.58 points lower, $p < .001$), and Posttest IV versus baseline (4.00 points lower, $p < .001$). Furthermore, the BAI score increased by 43.5% between baseline and Posttest IV.

Moreover, as shown in Table 2, the average score of BDI-II was 12.0 (± 10.2), 11.3 (± 9.7), 9.9 (± 9.0), and 10.5 (± 10.2) at Posttests I–IV, respectively. Next, the relationship between the mean BDI-II score and time interaction was analyzed after controlling for PSQI, BAI, and physical health status at baseline. The results showed significant decreases in the BDI-II score at Posttest I versus baseline (2.03 points lower, $p = .030$), Posttest II versus baseline (2.72 points lower, $p = .003$), Posttest III versus baseline (4.08 points lower, $p < .001$), and Posttest IV versus baseline (3.56 points lower, $p < .001$). Furthermore, the BDI-II score increased by 25.0% between baseline and Posttest IV.

Discussion

The 2-year RN-BSN students with sleep disturbance who participated in this study averaged 32 years old. The average score of sleep quality at baseline was 10.1 (± 3.1), which is similar with a score of 9.8 (± 3.2) for a similar population that was obtained by Chueh and Chang (2014). The 38.9% that were identified in this study as experiencing at least a mild level of anxiety mood is lower than the percentage of female nurses diagnosed with sleep disturbances in Taiwan (56.9%; Lin et al., 2015) and of female medical students in Pakistan (43.7%; Rab, Mamdou, & Nasir, 2008). However, the anxiety rate in this study is higher than that among female medical students in Saudi Arabia (34.9%; Ibrahim, Al-Kharboush, El-Khatib, Al-Habib, & Asali, 2013). Moreover, 38.9% of the participants in this study had a level of depression greater than "mild." This prevalence is higher than that among general female workers (20%; Cho et al., 2013). Furthermore, participants with higher coffee consumption had worse sleep quality, and those with poor physical health exhibited more severe anxiety and depressed moods. These results are similar to findings in other studies (Lin et al., 2015; Sawah et al., 2015). As reported, sleep disturbance coexists with psychotic symptoms (Freeman et al., 2015), which may account for the high correlation between sleep disturbance and anxiety and depressed moods.

This study provides evidence that the 4-week AA with a magnetic pellet on the shenmen acupoint is an effective alternative intervention for improving sleep quality. During the 4-week AA intervention, the sleep quality, anxiety, and depression of participants were generally ameliorated, with overall improvement rates of 26.7%, 43.5%, and 25%, respectively. This supports the finding of a previous systematic review that AA improves the clinical effective rate, including increased total sleep time, increased sleep efficiency, lower PSQI scores, shortened sleep-onset latency, and reduced number of awakenings in comparison with placebo or sham interventions (Lan et al., 2015). However, as the participants in this study had experienced sleep disturbance for an extended period, sudden and drastic improvement in their sleep quality would be difficult to achieve under any circumstances. Therefore, future research may measure not only sleep quality but also other sleep status variables such as total sleep time, time in bed, and sleep efficiency. This study further suggests that school nurses should encourage students with sleep disturbance to complete the entire 4-week AA to achieve a significant improvement in sleep.

At the end of the first-week intervention, both anxiety and depressed moods had improved significantly over baseline. The shenmen acupoint is generally effective in reducing arousal (Cheung et al., 2015) and in calming the mind (Arai et al., 2013). Furthermore, the literature indicates that applying AA on the shenmen acupoint (HT7, MA-TF1) effectively relieved anxiety in healthy female students before an anatomy examination (Klausenitz, Hesse, Hacker, Hahnenkamp, & Usichenko, 2016). AA on the shenmen acupoint (HT7, MA-TF1) is used mainly to treat diseases of the nervous system, including insomnia, depression, anxiety, and dementia (Feng, Zeng, Ren, & Liang, 2014). This study revealed a similar finding. Moreover, AA applied on the shenmen point (HT7, MA-TF1) for 1 week only reduced negative emotional states, especially anxiety. These findings thus support that AA is a faster and more effective intervention for alleviating anxiety and depressed moods than for enhancing sleep quality.

This study has several limitations. First, students who were absent were not included, whereas highly motivated students were not excluded. This selection bias may undermine the generalizability of the findings. Therefore, future studies that use probability approaches for sampling should be designed to ensure external validity. Second, the lack of a control group reduces the rigor of the obtained evidence. Factors that affect sleep quality in nursing students are complicated. Therefore, a control group design should be used in future evidence-based studies of this topic. Third, although sleep quality, anxiety, and depressed moods improved under the AA intervention, whether effects persisted beyond the 4-week intervention is unknown. Thus, we recommend conducting a longitudinal study to determine whether the improvement is short-term or sustained over the long term.

Conclusions

AA offers an efficient and noninvasive intervention for relieving sleep disturbance. The findings of this study support the effectiveness of a 4-week AA that applies a magnetic pellet on the MA-TF1 in terms of improving sleep quality and alleviating anxiety and depressed moods in 2-year RN-BSN students with sleep disturbance. The improvement rates between the first and fourth weeks of the AA intervention were 26.7% for sleep quality, 43.5% for anxiety, and 25% for depression.

Relevance to Clinical Practice

Two-year RN-BSN students with sleep disturbance often experience both anxiety and depressed moods. Therefore, school nurses and other health professionals should encourage students with sleep disturbance to undertake this 4-week AA because of the potential benefit of this intervention on sleep quality, anxiety, and depression. To obtain a high rate of improvement, an AA intervention of at least 4 weeks is recommended.

Acknowledgment

We are grateful for research funding from the Ministry of Science and Technology (NSC-100-2314-B-030-003).

References

American Psychiatric Association. (2013). *Diagnostic and statistical manual of mental disorders* (5th ed.). Washington, DC: Author.

Arai, Y. C., Sakakima, Y., Kawanishi, J., Nishihara, M., Ito, A., Tawada, Y., & Maruyama, Y. (2013). Auricular acupuncture at the "shenmen" and "point zero" points induced parasympathetic activation. *Evidence-Based Complementary and Alternative Medicine, 2013,* 945063. doi:10.1155/2013/945063

Beck, A. T., Epstein, N., Brown, G., & Steer, R. A. (1988). An inventory for measuring clinical anxiety: Psychometric properties. *Journal of Consulting and Clinical Psychology, 56*(6), 893–897. doi:10.1037/0022-006X.56.6.893

Beck, A. T., Steer, R. A., Ball, R., & Ranieri, W. (1996). Comparison of Beck Depression Inventories -IA and -II in psychiatric outpatients. *Journal of Personality Assessment, 67*(3), 588–597. doi:10.1207/s15327752jpa6703_13

Buysse, D. J., Reynolds, C. F. III, Monk, T. H., Berman, S. R., & Kupfer, D. J. (1989). The Pittsburgh Sleep Quality Index: A new instrument for psychiatric practice and research. *Psychiatry Research, 28*(2), 193–213. doi:10.1016/0165-1781(89)90047-4

Cheng, Y. Y. (2002). *A study on quality of sleep of Taiwanese from the survey of social development trends.* Retrieved from http://www.stat.gov.tw/public/Data/4122719141571.pdf

Cheung, M. C., Chan, A. S., & Yip, J. (2015). Microcurrent stimulation at shenmen acupoint facilitates EEG associated with sleepiness and positive mood: A randomized controlled electrophysiological study. *Evidence-Based Complementary and Alternative Medicine, 2015,* 182837. doi:10.1155/2015/182837

Chien, P. L., Su, H. F., Hsieh, P. C., Siao, R. Y., Ling, P. Y., & Jou, H. J. (2013). Sleep quality among female hospital staff nurses. *Sleep Disorders, 2013,* 283490. doi:10.1155/2013/283490

Cho, H. S., Kim, Y. W., Park, H. W., Lee, K. H., Jeong, B. G., Kang, Y. S., & Park, K. S. (2013). The relationship between depressive symptoms among female workers and job stress and sleep quality. *Annals of Occupational and Environmental Medicine, 25*(1), 12. doi:10.1186/2052-4374-25-12

Chueh, K. H., & Chang, C. C. (2014). Relationship between presleep arousal status and sleep quality among the female RN-BSN nursing students. *Fu-Jen Journal of Medicine, 12*(4), 253–262. doi:10.3966/181020932014121204005 (Original work published in Chinese)

Chung, K. F., & Tang, M. K. (2006). Subjective sleep disturbance and its correlates in middle-aged Hong Kong Chinese women. *Maturitas, 53*(4), 396–404. doi:10.1016/j.maturitas.2005.07.001

Feng, S. W., Zeng, F., Ren, Y. L., & Liang, F. R. (2014). Discussion on disease spectrum treated with acupuncture at shenmen (HT 7) and its compatibility based on bibliometrics. *Chinese Acupuncture & Moxibustion, 34*(6), 561–564. (Original work published in Chinese)

Freeman, D., Sheaves, B., Goodwin, G. M., Yu, L. M., Harrison, P. J., Emsley, R., ... Espie, C. A. (2015). Effects of cognitive behavioural therapy for insomnia on the mental health of university students: Study protocol for a randomized controlled trial. *Trials, 16,* 236. doi:10.1186/s13063-015-0756-4

Ibrahim, N., Al-Kharboush, D., El-Khatib, L., Al-Habib, A., & Asali, D. (2013). Prevalence and predictors of anxiety and depression among female medical students in King Abdulaziz University, Jeddah, Saudi Arabia. *Iranian Journal of Public Health, 42*(7), 726–736.

Klausenitz, C., Hesse, T., Hacker, H., Hahnenkamp, K., & Usichenko, T. (2016). Auricular acupuncture for pre-exam anxiety in medical students: A prospective observational pilot investigation. *Acupuncture in Medicine, 34*(2), 90–94. doi:10.1136/acupmed-2015-010887

Kuo, S. Y., Tsai, S. H., Chen, S. L., & Tzeng, Y. L. (2016). Auricular acupressure relieves anxiety and fatigue, and reduces cortisol levels in post-caesarean section women: A single-blind, randomised controlled study. *International Journal of Nursing Studies, 53,* 17–26. doi:10.1016/j.ijnurstu.2015.10.006

Lan, Y., Wu, X., Tan, H. J, Wu, N., Xing, J. J., Wu, F. S., ... Liang, F. R. (2015). Auricular acupuncture with seed or pellet attachments for primary insomnia: A systematic review and meta-analysis. *BMC Complementary and Alternative Medicine, 15,* 103. doi:10.1186/s12906-015-0606-7

Lee, C. Y., Chen, H. C., Meg Tseng, M. C., Lee, H. C., & Huang, L. H. (2015). The relationships among sleep quality and chronotype, emotional disturbance, and insomnia vulnerability in shift nurses. *The Journal of Nursing Research, 23*(3), 225–235. doi:10.1097/jnr.0000000000000095

Lee, M. S., Shin, B. C., Suen, L. K., Park, T. Y., & Ernst, E. (2008). Auricular acupuncture for insomnia: A systematic review. *International Journal of Clinical Practice, 62*(11), 1744–1752. doi:10.1111/j.1742-1241.2008.01876.x

Léger, D., & Bayon, V. (2010). Societal costs of insomnia. *Sleep Medicine Reviews, 14*(6), 379–389. doi:10.1016/j.smrv.2010.01.003

Lian, N., & Yan, Q. (1990). Insomnia treated by auricular pressing therapy. *Journal of Traditional Chinese Medicine, 10*(3), 174–175.

Lin, Y. H., Chueh, K. H., & Lin, Y. N. (2015). Work stress and anxiety among clinical female nurses with sleep disturbance. *VGH Nursing, 32*(5), 154–165. doi:10.6142/VGHN.32.2.154 (Original work published in Chinese)

Rab, F., Mamdou, R., & Nasir, S. (2008). Rates of depression and anxiety among female medical students in Pakistan. *Eastern Mediterranean Health Journal, 14*(1), 126–133.

Rosner, B. (2006). *Fundamentals of biostatistics* (6th ed.). Belmont, CA: Thomson Brooks.

Samaranayake, C. B., Arroll, B., & Fernando, A. T. III. (2014). Sleep disorders, depression, anxiety and satisfaction with life among young adults: A survey of university students in Auckland, New Zealand. *The New Zealand Medical Journal, 127*(1399), 13–22.

Sawah, M. A., Ruffin, N., Rimawi, M., Concerto, C., Aguglia, E., Chusid, E., ... Battaglia, F. (2015). Perceived stress and coffee and energy drink consumption predict poor sleep quality in podiatric medical students: A cross-sectional study. *Journal of the American Podiatric Medical Association, 105*(5), 429–434. doi:10.7547/14-082

Shanahan, L., Copeland, W. E., Angold, A., Bondy, C. L., & Costello, E. J. (2014). Sleep problems predict and are predicted by generalized anxiety/depression and oppositional defiant disorder. *Journal of the American Academy of Child & Adolescent Psychiatry, 53*(5), 550–558. doi:10.1016/j.jaac.2013.12.029

Suen, L. K., Wong, T. K., & Leung, A. W. (2002). Effectiveness of auricular therapy on sleep promotion in the elderly. *The American Journal of Chinese Medicine, 30*(4), 429–449. doi:10.1142/S0192415X0200051X

Tavernier, R., & Willoughby, T. (2014). Bidirectional associations between sleep (quality and duration) and psychosocial functioning across the university years. *Developmental Psychology, 50*(3), 674–682. doi:10.1037/a0034258

Wang, H. H., Kuo, Y. L., Lee, H. T., Chung, U. L., Wu, S. M., & Sun, J. L. (2005). The effectiveness of auricular-acupuncture in the treatment of insomnia in nurses at a regional hospital. *Journal of Evidence-Based Nursing, 1*(4), 283–291. doi:10.6225/JEBN.1.4.283 (Original work published in Chinese)

Wang, H. H., Yeh, M. L., Chung, U. L., & Yang, C. H. (2008). Improving sleep quality: The efficacy of auricular acupressure. *Journal of Evidence-Based Nursing, 4*(3), 243–250. doi:10.6225/JEBN.4.3.243 (Original work published in Chinese)

Wang, Y. Z., Chen, H. H., Yeh, M. L., & Lin, S. D. (2010). Auricular acupressure combined with multimedia instruction or alone for quitting smoking in young adults: A quasi-experimental study. *International Journal of Nursing Studies, 47*(9), 1089–1095. doi:10.1016/j.ijnurstu.2010.02.009

Wewers, M. E., & Lowe, N. K. (1990). A critical review of visual analogue scales in the measurement of clinical phenomena. *Research in Nursing & Health, 13*(4), 227–236. doi:10.1002/nur.4770130405

Wu, S. C., Li, M. H., & Chang, S. P. (2015). Investigation of the sleep quality in the Ling Tung University. *Journal of Sport, Leisure and Hospitality Research, 10*(2), 60–72. (Original work published in Chinese)

Yao, K. W., Yu, S., Cheng, S. P., & Chen, I. J. (2008). Relationships between personal, depression and social network factors and sleep quality in community-dwelling older adults. *The Journal of Nursing Research, 16*(2), 131–139. doi:10.1097/01.JNR.0000387298.37419.ff

6

Exploring a Nursing Home-Specific, Interdisciplinary, Function-Focused, Communicative Framework Based on Situation, Background, Assessment and Recommendation

Min Sun PARK[1] • Su Jung LEE[2] • Young Rim CHOI[2] • Sung Ok CHANG[3]*

ABSTRACT

Background: Improved methods of communication are needed among professionals in related fields to address the increasing complexity of clinical situations and various levels of functioning experienced by older adults who live in nursing homes.

Purpose: The purpose of this study was to explore function-focused clinical communication among nurses and providers based on the Situation, Background, Assessment, Recommendation (SBAR) approach toward interdisciplinary collaboration to maintain function among nursing home residents and to identify the characteristics of SBAR flows in nursing homes.

Methods: Detailed interviews with 28 interdisciplinary professionals working in four nursing homes were conducted. Directed qualitative content analysis was used to identify the internal attributes of SBAR-based communication. Case analysis was conducted to identify SBAR flows.

Results: Four themes emerged as key factors for function-focused interdisciplinary staff communication in nursing homes. Effective nursing care to maintain function among nursing home residents requires accurate awareness of abnormal circumstances. Knowledge of assessment and resident background are needed to address situations requiring intervention and identify the problems underlying a resident's current state. The optimal therapeutic environment is created by sharing roles and tasks among practitioners through referrals. Twelve generalized situations requiring function-focused communication (i.e., dislocation of body line because of joint contracture, change in walking, difficulty of moving because of pain, difficulty in eating, fever, change in sleep pattern, change in excretion pattern, change in weight, change in condition, change in problematic behavior, decrease in cognitive function, and change in relationships) and the related nurse-centered SBAR pathways were identified.

Conclusions/Implications for Practice: These results represent a first prototype for developing practical communication guidelines for nursing-home-specific function-focused care and provide new insights into the interdisciplinary approach.

Key Words:
older adults, communication, interdisciplinary studies, nursing homes, SBAR.

Introduction

As geriatric syndromes have multiple causes and underlying diseases, assessment and intervention require input from multiple experts in related fields (Colón-Emeric et al., 2017). Increased clinical complexity is difficult to manage with the application of only a single domain of expertise and instead requires responses based on interdisciplinary team consensus and cooperation (Colón-Emeric et al., 2017; Renz & Carrington, 2016). Nursing homes are residential long-term care facilities in the community that rely on the constant coordination of multiple disciplines. Residents comprise older individuals who experience dementia and whose function is impaired by two or more complications (Lee et al., 2019; Williams et al., 2018). Previous research on interdisciplinary collaboration in the nursing home setting revealed that providing care to residents who might have experienced fractures requires the synthesis of judgments of interdisciplinary teams based on nurses' medical knowledge of osteoporosis, physical therapists' knowledge of range of motion (ROM), and social workers' knowledge of social isolation (Park, Kim, et al., 2019; Park, Lee, & Chang, 2019). Therefore, developing ways to improve communication among interdisciplinary health professionals is key to improved quality of nursing home care (Alexander, 2015).

Proper communication among related professionals when providing function management has a direct impact on care outcomes for patients with dementia (Shaw et al., 2018; Townsend-Gervis et al., 2014). In addition, effective information sharing

[1]PhD, RN, Assistant Professor, Department of Nursing, Cheongju University, Cheongju, Republic of Korea • [2]PhD, RN, Research Professor, College of Nursing, Korea University, Seoul, Republic of Korea • [3]PhD, RN, Professor, College of Nursing, and BK21 FOUR R&E Center for Learning Health Systems, Korea University, Seoul, Republic of Korea.

within the team avoids duplicate interventions, thereby reducing wasted practitioner time and effort during the care process (Xyrichis et al., 2018). In particular, the quality of connections among practitioners, the degree of information flow, and the various perspectives involved in planning care are the key factors that determine care outcomes (Colón-Emeric et al., 2017; Renz & Carrington, 2016). Thus, observations of subtle functional changes in older adults should be shared within interdisciplinary teams and cooperatively interpreted for the care plan (Colón-Emeric et al., 2017; Park, Lee, & Chang, 2019). However, previous research and nursing home practice have not emphasized care processes based on such cooperative intercommunication.

The Situation, Background, Assessment, Recommendation (SBAR) tool has been recommended by the World Health Organization to promote standardized, structured communication (Institute for Healthcare Improvement, 2019). The SBAR is a handoff tool that organizes information clearly and concisely to facilitate collaborative communication (Panesar et al., 2016). The SBAR is regarded as a clear and safe communication method for problem solving among different disciplines in the medical environment and a simple way of sharing patient information with other medical professionals (Ashcraft & Owen, 2017; Cornell et al., 2013). The SBAR was developed for use in urgent and time-sensitive medical situations (Thomas et al., 2009; Townsend-Gervis et al., 2014). Thus, research to date has focused mainly on nurse–physician and nurse–nurse interactions, with little literature related to prolonged communication across various fields based on interdisciplinary approaches (Griffiths et al., 2014; Renz & Carrington, 2016; Townsend-Gervis et al., 2014). Thus, the SBAR should be extended to the nursing home environment. In contrast to the urgent clinical situations in general hospitals, nursing homes require sustained sharing of clinical information among professionals to provide appropriate care.

In fact, nursing home care differs slightly from physician-centered, general hospital level care, which focuses on comprehensive professional medical services. To maximize and preserve function in older adult residents, nurses should play a key practitioner role (H. J. Kim et al., 2016; S. J. Kim et al., 2014). In this context, beyond the dichotomous communication between nurses and physicians, communication occurs among nurses and practitioners to find the best solutions to address functional problems of residents. Furthermore, to develop an appropriate SBAR, it is essential to understand how interdisciplinary practitioners make decisions, what assessments and interventions they use, and what they typically refer to other disciplines. The purpose of this study was to explore nurses' and related practitioners' communications about the clinical care necessary to maintain function in nursing home residents and to explore the characteristics of SBAR flows in nursing home settings.

Methods

The first step was a directed qualitative content analysis to extract the internal attributes of the core concept based on the SBAR framework. The second step was an SBAR-based case analysis to further understand these information flows and identify how information is shared within an interdisciplinary nursing home team.

Data Collection

Data were collected from August to November 2017. Because the practical knowledge and accumulated know-how gained from the actual experience of practitioners may be used to determine the quality of data obtained through the interviews, the researchers used a purposive sampling method to acquire sufficient data until theoretical saturation was reached. Using semistructured questionnaires, each interview was conducted 1–2 times and was audio recorded. Data were collected using one-on-one interviews with 28 staff members working in four nursing homes of different size categories. The interviewees consisted of seven nurses, six social workers, five physical therapists, one occupational therapist, four nutritionists, and five care helpers. Average participant age was 46 years, ranging from 27 to 63 years, and the average length of experience providing care in nursing homes was 6 years.

The in-depth interviews began with general, open-ended questions about the interdisciplinary approach to care that focused on function in nursing home residents (e.g., "Please explain to me the collaborative approach among related occupations in your nursing home when providing care to improve the quality of life of resident by managing their functions."). After a general question, the researcher asked questions focusing on the four stages of SBAR, a predetermined category, which probed the practitioners' experience and knowledge of background, assessment, and recommendation in situations where function management requires interdisciplinary collaborative approaches. Furthermore, the researchers asked the staff about referring function-related situations to the relevant practitioners to initiate communication.

Data Analysis

Step 1: A directed qualitative content analysis

A directed content analysis approach, a more structured process than conventional content analysis, was undertaken to verify the developed theoretical framework and expand knowledge and understanding of phenomena that have not been actively studied (Hsieh & Shannon, 2005). The researcher became familiar with the interview data by reading the transcript several times. The researcher reviewed the interview data to identify repeated thoughts, ideas, and phrases, and codes were generated to represent these meaningful concepts. Using the existing framework, the researcher began to analyze the key concepts and variables as the initial coding categories. In this study, four categories of SBAR were used as an initial framework to explore the stages of interdisciplinary communication in nursing homes. The researchers repeatedly reviewed and revised the coded data through discussions within the research team, with the results used as the themes and subthemes (Hsieh & Shannon, 2005).

Step 2: Case analysis for identifying Situation, Background, Assessment, Recommendation flows in nursing homes

The SBAR-based case analysis was conducted to explore how information is transmitted among interdisciplinary practitioners in nursing homes and to clarify the relationships between the various disciplines. In the interviews, 39 cases of SBAR were collected and analyzed, and each was categorized into the four stages of SBAR. The professional in the referring role, the professional in the receiving role, and the information shared between them were analyzed.

Data Credibility

Padgett's (1998) strategy was used to assess the reliability and rigor of the data and the processes of the qualitative research. The researchers were experienced in qualitative research on older adults, were familiar with nursing home facilities, and had long-term contacts with practitioners in nursing homes. All research data were collected via audio recordings, and the transcripts were double-checked with other researchers to ensure reliability. The researchers conducted constant communication and verification with their peers to avoid analysis bias and compared the themes and subthemes they had respectively extracted. The analysis procedures and methods for all of the qualitative studies were undertaken under the supervision of another qualitative researcher, and the final results were verified and evaluated by a qualitative expert with extensive research experience.

Ethical Considerations

The research began after approval by the institutional review board of the affiliated university (1040548-KU-IRB-17-122-A-1). The researchers also received permission from the participating facilities and obtained written informed consent from participants, who were informed of their autonomy in participation and their right to withdraw from the study at any time.

Results

Step 1: A Directed Qualitative Content Analysis

The directed qualitative content analysis of the interview revealed four themes related to the nature and content of SBAR regarding the function-focused care approach among interdisciplinary practitioners in nursing homes and suggested practical communicative care strategies based on the interdisciplinary assessments and interventions in actual nursing home circumstances (Table 1).

Theme 1. Situation: Recognizing abnormal resident situations/circumstances

Recurring situations relevant to SBAR were extracted from the interviews in the form of situational phenomena requiring interdisciplinary intervention in the practice dimension. In these situations, unusual interventions by interdisciplinary staff who provide direct care to residents were inevitable, and the participants mentioned that the ability of the practitioner to recognize the associated problematic situations was an important factor. The complex subthemes for which functional intervention is recommended included situations of both gradual deterioration and subtle changes in functioning.

1. **Gradual deterioration in function.** In particular, the gradual progression of joint contracture could cause problems for both patients and providers: "*After entering nursing homes, there was an elderly resident whose legs became progressively more rigid. Now it is difficult for them to bend or move joints by loosening legs bent in an X-shape. The nurse recognized that there was a possibility*

Table 1

Emerged Themes and Subthemes

No.	Theme	Subtheme
Theme 1	Situation: Recognizing abnormal resident situations/circumstances	1. Gradual deterioration in function 2. Subtle changes in function
Theme 2	Background: Tracking information related to situations requiring intervention	1. Usual functional status and life patterns 2. Related past medical history
Theme 3	Assessment: Identifying practical issues that practitioners should check in relation to the current situation	1. Functional degradation compared with the past 2. Newly detected unusual symptoms or abnormal behaviors 3. Changed input or intervention 4. Recent unusual events
Theme 4	Recommendation: Sharing the roles and tasks of each practitioner	1. Requesting other occupations for assessments and interventions based on their distinct knowledge 2. Suggesting a better way to improve the quality of life of residents to other practitioners

of a fracture occurring when the resident's joints had to be moved, such as when providing positional change or diaper change" (a nurse with 11 years of experience).

2. **Subtle changes in function.** In particular, a care helper who provided 24-hour close assistance to the resident would often perceive subtle functional changes when the resident was walking or eating: "*There was a resident who liked walking as an exercise. When I observed him from behind a few days ago, his walking posture seemed a little different from normal and I felt something strange. He limped and did not want to walk. Also, he seemed to walk with his hips pulled back*" (a care helper with 10 years of experience).

Theme 2. Background: Tracking information related to situations requiring intervention

Based on SBAR, the participants reported that the background for interventions was compiled from past and present information about residents; this information helped practitioners identify problems requiring functional intervention. In other words, the background corresponded to the knowledge dimension. In addition, practitioners commonly stated that there might be differences in the degree to which appropriate information could be collected, depending on the level of awareness of the problem. Subthemes derived from actual experience in nursing homes consisted of the usual functional status and life patterns of residents related to their past medical history.

1. **Usual functional status and life patterns.** Practitioners stated that it was necessary to focus on symptoms of aging including functional discomfort, which helped them better understand residents' normal functional conditions and lifestyle patterns. Factors to be specifically identified included physical and cognitive functional status, habits (sleep, excretion, and dietary patterns), preferences, responses to care (the degree of cooperation with practitioners), and recent condition: "*There was a resident who enjoyed walking around the unit three times every morning. I used to check his physical function carefully if he tried to rest instead of undertaking his normal walking exercise*" (a care helper with 10 years of experience).
2. **Related past medical history.** Most practitioners noted that underlying diseases (dementia, Parkinson's disease, osteoporosis) and past surgical history (hip replacement) could be key background information, as these may have a continuing impact on cognitive and physical function: "*Operations such as hip arthroplasty can damage the overall functions of the resident. Rehabilitation such as walking exercise to recover physical functions is necessary for them, and changes in cognitive functions should also be checked*" (a nurse with 10 years of experience).

Theme 3. Assessment: Identifying practical issues that practitioners should check in relation to the current situation

In the interviews, it was found that, based on SBAR, assessments are evaluations of elements related to problematic situations that require verification by practitioners. In nursing-home-based function-focused care, the assessed elements represented the extent to which changes in life patterns or symptoms occurred in activities of daily living. The practitioners reported that level of assessment may change according to information gathered about a problematic situation. Thus, it could be said that, in the SBAR framework, the theme of assessment also belongs in the knowledge dimension. The subthemes that emerged relevant to identifying functional changes among residents at the assessment stage were as follows:

1. **Functional degradation compared with the past.** Practitioners who observe the daily life of residents are able to evaluate the degree of change in ROM, walking, and the amount of food eaten, although they may have difficulty applying accurate numerical indicators to these variables: "*When I evaluated the range of motion (ROM) of both knees, the elderly resident shouted that he was sick and that his bent knee joints could not be moved at all*" (a nurse with 11 years of experience) and "*During the assisted meal, when the resident ate food, much saliva flowed out of his mouth, and more than half of his food came out of his mouth*" (a social worker with 11 years of experience).
2. **Newly detected unusual symptoms or abnormal behaviors.** Participants reported the necessity of observation not only of physical function, such as patterns of excretion and sleep, but also of cognitive function, such as changes in memory and problematic behavior: "*The resident had walked out of the bed about 3–4 times in the last 3 days, wanting to go to the restroom all night*" (a care helper with 10 years of experience) and "*The resident was angry and showed problematic behavior such as violent language and threatening behavior in the ward*" (a social worker with 4 years of experience).
3. **Changed input or intervention.** Practitioners must assess changes in medication type and dosage, diet and snacks, and the types and timing of provided programs: "*Recently, the resident has not eaten much more than half of the provided meals even though I changed his diet from rice to porridge*" (a nutritionist with 2 years of experience).
4. **Recent unusual events.** Practitioners noted that changes in physical and cognitive function as well as changes in social functions such as relationships with family and practitioners or worrying events should not be overlooked: "*A few days ago, there was a conflict between two residents because of where they were seated in the program. They sat next to each other and continued their fighting. The social worker separated them to stop their fight*" (a social worker with 3 years of experience).

Theme 4. Recommendation: Sharing the roles and tasks of each practitioner

The recommendation based on the SBAR was to divide tasks among the related professions and share appropriate care when referring to other practitioners in the interdisciplinary

Table 2
Extracted Practice Strategies Expected in Function-Focused Referral Situations in SBAR

Function-Focused Situation	Sending Position	Accepting Position	Practice Strategies Expected When Referring to Another Discipline
Dislocation of body line because of joint contracture	NS	PT	Checking safe range of motion
Change in walking	NS	PT	Checking safe range of walking exercises
	CH	NS	Assessing physical functions based on medical knowledge (fracture, swelling, etc.)
	PT	NS	Assessing pain and requesting hospital care
	PT	CH	Educating residents on how to walk safely in daily activities
Difficulty of moving because of pain	NS	PT	Relieving pain
Difficulty of eating	NS	NT	Providing an alternative or preferred diet
	CH	NS	Checking changes in the mouth Assessing swallowing and chewing problems
	CH	SW	Asking the family to make the resident's favorite food
	CH	NT	Providing proper snacks and implementing a proper diet
	OT	NS	Checking current medications
	OT	NT	Providing an alternative diet
	OT	CH	Providing proper assistance during meals
	OT	SW	Considering the resident's preferred colors when providing programs
	SW	NS	Assessing oral wounds as well as teeth and chewing problems
	SW	OT	Assessing oral wounds as well as teeth and chewing problems
	SW	NT	Requesting a proper diet
	CH	NS	Assessing chewing problems
	CH	NS	Assessing digestive problems
	NT	NS	Assessing chewing problems
	NT	CH	Continuous observing and reporting during meal assistance
Fever	CH	NS	Assessing physical functions based on medical knowledge
Change in sleep pattern	CH	NS	Intervening with medication and requesting hospital care
Change in excretion pattern	NS	CH	Observing and reporting urinary symptoms and urine patterns
	CH	NS	Intervening with medication
	NS	NT	Changing diet
Change in weight	NT	NS	Identifying increases and decreases in body weight
	NT	SW	Managing nutritional status and requesting nutritional support
Change in condition	PT	NS	Checking vital signs at the time of problem
	SW	NS	Checking vital signs at the time of problem
	SW	CH	Continuous observing and reporting of the resident's condition
Change in problematic behavior	SW	NS	Checking changes in behavior patterns Encouraging the resident to go the hospital and take medication
	CH	NS	Intervening with medication
	SW	NS	Considering hospitalization Writing up behavioral patterns

(continues)

Table 2

Extracted Practice Strategies Expected in Function-Focused Referral Situations in SBAR, Continued

Function-Focused Situation	Sending Position	Accepting Position	Practice Strategies Expected When Referring to Another Discipline
Decrease in cognitive function	NS	PT	Assessing fall risk Providing physical therapy in a place suitable for physical function
	SW	CH	Continuous observing and reporting on changes in activities of daily living and changes in cognitive functions
	SW	NS	Checking changes in cognitive functions Requesting a focus case conference
Change in relationships	SW	CH	Observing and reporting relationships with the surrounding older adults
	SW	NS	Requesting coordination so that problems do not occur

Note. SBAR = Situation, Background, Assessment, Recommendation; NS = nurse; PT = physical therapist; OT = occupational therapist; SW = social worker; NT = nutritionist; CH = care helper.

team to develop the most appropriate care plan. The ultimate goal of practitioners' interactions was the best care outcomes and management of function for nursing home residents; this was achieved by synthesizing the professional interventions of each discipline through the exchange of requests and suggestions (Table 2). These elements, which belonged to the share and distribution dimension of interdisciplinary communication, included requesting other occupations for assessments and interventions based on their distinct knowledge and suggesting to other practitioners better ways to improve the quality of life of residents.

1. **Requesting other occupations for assessments and interventions based on their distinct knowledge.** Practitioners generally requested more in-depth assessments and interventions based on the expertise of other disciplines or requested constant monitoring and reporting of a problematic situation: "*The occupational therapist requested the nurse to check for any recently changed medications or doses*" (an occupational therapist with 2 years of experience) and "*In the program, I noticed that the condition of the resident had deteriorated. Thus, I requested the care helper to continuously observe the resident in the ward and to promptly report any problems to the nurse*" (a social worker with 1 year of experience).
2. **Suggesting a better way to improve the quality of life of residents to other practitioners.** Practitioners suggested interventions to improve the quality of daily life for nursing home residents that did not occur to other occupational groups: "*If the resident has a large number of medications to take, the occupational therapist will suggest the nurse to divide the appropriate number of medications by type of drug before and after meals*" (an occupational therapist with 2 years of experience) and "*The nurse suggested that the physical therapist identify ways of minimizing damage to the joints and the extent of the safe range of motion, even when residents cannot move their joints within the normal range*" (a nurse with 11 years of experience).

Step 2: Case Analysis for Identifying Situation, Background, Assessment, Recommendation Flows in Nursing Homes

From the case analysis for identifying SBAR flows in nursing homes, the researchers extracted 39 SBAR cases related to interdisciplinary function-focused communications from the 28 practitioner interviews. In addition, the researchers classified the general function-focused communications of the 39 SBAR cases into 12 categories. The left vertical row in Table 2 presents 12 general categories of function-focused situation requiring interdisciplinary communication. In SBAR, the communication situation addressing "difficulty of eating" was found to be the most common, corresponding to 15 of the 39 SBAR cases. The next most common general function-focused communicative situation, "change in walking," corresponded to four of the 39 SBAR cases (Table 2).

The results of the case analysis of the positions of senders and acceptors based on SBAR are shown in Table 2. Senders were generally practitioners who determined that situations required functional intervention and requested input from relevant occupations. Of the 39 SBAR cases, the sender was a social worker in 11 cases, a care helper in 10 cases, and a nurse in seven cases. Social workers and care helpers asked nurses for assessments based on professional medical knowledge. Nurses asked physical therapists mainly about walking, ROM, and pain. Acceptors were generally practitioners who were able to advise with expertise beyond the sender's level of care, provide more in-depth assessments and interventions, and observe subtle changes to solve the problem. Of the 39 SBAR cases, the accepting practitioner was a nurse in 17 cases and a care helper in seven cases.

The results of the SBAR case analysis of the interdisciplinary practice strategies expected on referral to other disciplines are shown in Table 2. Nurses were expected to evaluate functional status primarily based on medical knowledge. Example observations that reflected SBAR communication included weight gain and loss, wounds in the mouth, fractures, swelling, pain, digestion, excretion, medications, and hospital care. Care helpers were expected to observe and report on residents' actual condition and activities of daily living. The physical therapist was expected to employ knowledge about physical movement such as ROM, strength, pain, and fall risk. The occupational therapist was expected to employ practical strategies that made the daily activities of residents more comfortable through stimulation of physical and cognitive sensations. Social workers were expected to employ knowledge about a resident's internal and external resources such as personality and preference, key related people, family relationships, and economic support. Nutritionists were expected to employ their knowledge of eating such as appropriate and preferred diets and eating problems. Representative examples of nursing-home-specific interdisciplinary function-focused communications based on SBAR are presented in Table 3.

Flows of nursing-home-specific interdisciplinary function-focused communication in terms of the number of SBAR cases based on Table 2 are presented in Figure 1. Of the 39 SBAR cases, the highest number (eight) involved care helpers asking the nurses to communicate. The next highest number of cases were social workers asking nurses (six), followed by nurses asking physical therapists (four).

Discussion

To the best of the authors' knowledge, this study is the first attempt to explore interactive communication in the context of interdisciplinary function-focused approaches in nursing homes conducted by identifying the nurse and related practitioners' clinical communications and interpreting the characteristics of the SBAR flows. Thus, this study provides new perspectives on nursing home interdisciplinary communications in areas including exchanges of specialized and common knowledge and the transfer of information on welfare in daily

Table 3
Representative Examples of Nursing-Home-Specific Interdisciplinary Function-Focused Communications Based on SBAR

Function-Focused Situation/SBAR	Sample
Changes in walking	
Situation	*When I (physical therapist) looked at the back of the resident walking, one foot was everted. Compared to usual, today she seemed to walk uncomfortably and bent over her waist a lot.*
Background	*Cognitively, the elderly had enough cognitive ability to communicate and was good at expressing pain. Physically, the resident walked independently using a walker. She had the habit of sitting down sufficiently hard in a wheelchair making a noise.*
Assessment	*I stopped her walking to check if she was able to stand, and she could stand alone for five minutes. I took the resident to her bed and asked where the pain was, and she complained of back pain.*
Recommendation	1. The physical therapist informs the nurse that the resident's physical condition is worse than before and requests hospital treatment if the resident continues to experience back pain. 2. The physical therapist also requests the care helper to assist the resident to sit down slowly when sitting in a wheelchair.
Difficulty of eating	
Situation	*When I (care helper) recently helped feeding the elderly person, I found that he was worse than usual and left much more food than before. I was worried that nutritional problems would arise if he was continuously unable to eat.*
Background	*Since, usually the elderly had a big appetite and could eat a general diet, the elderly had been judged as having no particular problems with their digestive function.*
Assessment	*The weight of the elderly decreased by 3 kg compared to the previous month. When I looked inside his mouth, I saw a scar, which seemed to be a little torn and tingling.*
Recommendation	1. The care helper asked the nurse to provide an appropriate ointment that can be applied in the mouth. 2. The care helper asked the social worker to ask the family member to bring food that the resident likes. 3. The care helper asked the nutritionist to provide the resident with adequate snacks to increase their weight. If necessary, the care helper will request the nurse and nutritionist for a dietary change from general meals to a liquid diet.

Note. SBAR = Situation, Background, Assessment, Recommendation.

Figure 1

Situation, Background, Assessment, Recommendation (SBAR) flows of nursing-home-specific interdisciplinary function-focused communication

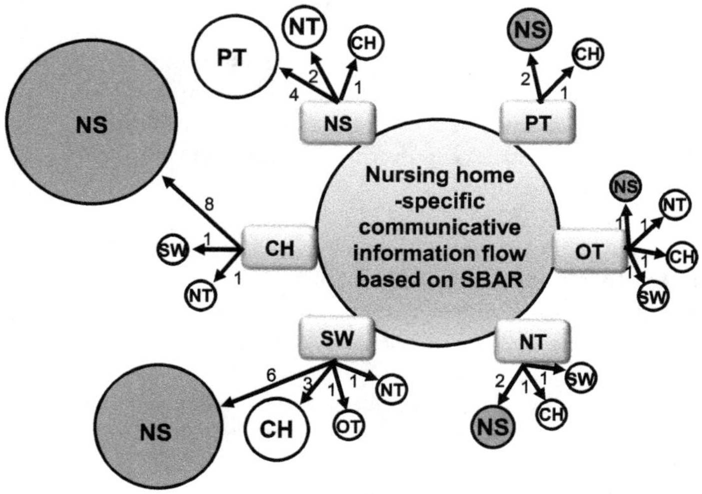

Note. Thirty-nine cases of SBAR in total. NS = nurse; PT = physical therapist; OT = occupational therapist ; SW = social worker; Nutritionist; CH = care helper. Square represents sending postion, circle represent accepting position. The size of the circle reflects the number of cases of SBAR extracted from the results of this study. The number of SBAR cases is indicated by the number next to the arrow.

life, proper diet, and rehabilitation, which spans different yet related fields, as well as perspectives on nursing in nursing home settings, as opposed to hospital settings, which focus more on disease treatment.

Overall, the four themes developed here proposed communicative strategies that are practical and available in current clinical practice and based on the characteristics of the interdisciplinary approach specific to the nursing home context, which differs from that of general hospitals. Moreover, the results highlight the necessity of continuous connectivity among the practice, knowledge, and share and distribution dimensions based on continuous relationships among interdisciplinary practitioners. In particular, 12 general situations requiring function-focused intervention were extracted, with the recommendation that practitioners should be able to communicate with each other interactively if such problems develop (Resnick et al., 2013). From this perspective, there was a similar discussion in the previous study on the importance of practitioners' abundant real-world experience in the "practice domain" for the development of effective practical care strategies (H. S. Kim, 2010; Park et al., 2018).

In addition, the results of the analysis of the SBAR flows covered all SBAR cases extracted from the interviews, enabling the clarification of entire work roles of related practitioners at a glance, and provided practice strategies for coordinating residents' care plans at each step with other disciplines (Park, Kim, et al., 2019). As shown in Table 2, the number of nurses (19) in the accepting position was the highest by far, followed by care helpers (7), nutritionists (5), physical therapists (4), and social workers (3). On the other hand, the sending position featured similar numbers of social workers (11), care helpers (10), and nurses (7). This finding implies that interdisciplinary practitioners in nursing homes may determine and prioritize problems and set care plans using assessments based on professional nurse-centered medical knowledge. In particular, as the target residents of nursing homes are those older than 80 years old with various symptoms associated with multicomplex underlying diseases, including impaired physical and cognitive function, obtaining the baseline assessment of nurses is indispensable (Asadi et al., 2019; Park, Kim, et al., 2019; Park, Lee, & Chang, 2019; Shin, 2019). As shown in Figure 1, a pathway of communication involving the nurse may be derived when interdisciplinary practitioners communicate in nursing home settings. This result is consistent with the role of nurses as key practitioners and core information providers in nursing homes, as supported in previous studies (Park, Kim, et al., 2019; Park, Lee, & Chang, 2019; Park et al., 2018).

As nursing homes are complex adaptive systems in which interdisciplinary practitioners maintain continuous two-way communications, research on related intercommunication activities has been difficult until recently (Anderson et al., 2003; Griffiths et al., 2014). For this reason, there has been a need to explore the information exchange and information transfers that occur among a variety of related interdisciplinary areas beyond those between nurses and physicians or between nurses and the nursing team. Thus, the new framework of communication derived in this study suggested a prototype platform for the development of standardized SBAR in community nursing home settings by identifying effective communicative examples and patterns among interdisciplinary practitioners, including professional care, rehabilitation, and nursing.

This study was affected by several limitations. First, although the numbers of facilities (4) and interdisciplinary practitioners (28) participating in this study were relatively small, this study, which targeted practitioners providing care to approximately 500 older adult residents, is significant considering its wide-ranging diversity in terms of the sizes and characteristics of the facilities included. In addition, researchers tried to generalize the final 39 cases by eliminating redundant function-focused communicative cases derived from more than 30 in-depth interviews with interdisciplinary practitioners. Finally, the researchers suggest that further research into interdisciplinary practical communicative knowledge may be refined by studying more facilities, particularly in areas with differing cultural backgrounds.

Conclusions

The results of this research support the idea that, in nursing home practice, the quality of interactive communications between interdisciplinary professionals is based on an external communicative framework and internal information flows. In addition, the extracted SBAR framework and pathways of information flow may be applied when teaching communication methods to nurses and related practitioners in long-term care facilities to improve the quality of interdisciplinary collaborative care focused on managing function among residents. This method of communication regarding residents who complain of multiple discomforts in nursing homes should avoid dichotomies of communication between different occupations; transform them to provide optimal interventions, especially for top-priority problems; and be based on collaborative consensus among all related practitioners. The original framework of nursing-home-specific interdisciplinary communication developed here may be used as a guide containing representative communicative examples for new practitioners in various fields, including beginner nurses, and may serve as a first prototype for developing interdisciplinary communicative guidelines focused on the various needs and discomforts of older adults living in nursing homes.

Acknowledgments

The research was supported by the Basic Science Research Program through the National Research Foundation of Korea (NRF) funded by the Ministry of Education, Science and Technology (NRF-2017R1A2B4007896). This research was supported by the Research Institute of Korea University College of Nursing, Seoul, Republic of Korea.

Author Contributions

Study conception and design: SOC, MSP
Data collection: MSP, SJL, YRC
Data analysis and interpretation: All authors
Drafting of the article: MSP, SOC
Critical revision of the article: SOC, MSP

References

Alexander, G. L. (2015). Nurse assistant communication strategies about pressure ulcers in nursing homes. *Western Journal of Nursing Research, 37*, 984–1004. https://doi.org/10.1177/0193945914555201

Anderson, R. A., Issel, L. M., & McDaniel, R. R. Jr. (2003). Nursing homes as complex adaptive systems: Relationship between management practice and resident outcomes. *Nursing Research, 52*, 12–21.

Asadi, N., Memarian, R., & Vanaki, Z. (2019). Motivation to care: A qualitative study on Iranian nurses. *The Journal of Nursing Research, 27*(4), e34. https://doi.org/10.1097/jnr.0000000000000294

Ashcraft, A. S., & Owen, D. C. (2017). Comparison of standardized and customized SBAR communication tools to prevent nursing home resident transfer. *Applied Nursing Research, 38*, 64–69. https://doi.org/10.1016/j.apnr.2017.09.015

Colón-Emeric, C. S., Corazzini, K., McConnell, E. S., Pan, W., Toles, M., Hall, R., Cary, M. P. Jr., Batchelor-Murphy, M., Yap, T., Anderson, A. L., Burd, A., Amarasekara, S., & Anderson, R. A. (2017). Effect of promoting high-quality staff interactions on fall prevention in nursing homes: A cluster-randomized trial. *JAMA Internal Medicine, 177*, 1634–1641. https://doi.org/10.1001/jamainternmed.2017.5073

Cornell, P., Gervis, M. T., Yates, L., & Vardaman, J. M. (2013). Improving shift report focus and consistency with the situation, background, assessment, recommendation protocol. *Journal of Nursing Administration, 43*, 422–428. https://doi.org/10.1097/NNA.0b013e31829d6303

Griffiths, D., Morphet, J., Innes, K., Crawford, K., & Williams, A. (2014). Communication between residential aged care facilities and the emergency department: A review of the literature. *International Journal of Nursing Studies, 51*, 1517–1523. https://doi.org/10.1016/j.ijnurstu.2014.06.002

Hsieh, H. F., & Shannon, S. E. (2005). Three approaches to qualitative content analysis. *Qualitative Health Research, 15*(9), 1277–1288. https://doi.org/10.1177/1049732305276687

Institute for Healthcare Improvement. (2019). *SBAR communication technique*. http://www.ihi.org/Topics/SBARCommunicationTechnique/Pages/default.aspx

Kim, H. J., Choi, J. E., Kim, M. S., Kim, S. J., & Chang, S. O. (2016). Nurses' clinical decision-making for preserving nursing home residents' remaining abilities. *Journal of Clinical Nursing, 25*, 1326–1335. https://doi.org/10.1111/jocn.13206

Kim, H. S. (2010). *The nature of theoretical thinking in nursing* (3rd ed.). Springer.

Kim, S. J., Kim, M. S., Kim, H. J., Choi, J. E., & Chang, S. O. (2014). Nursing home nurses' ways of knowing about peaceful deaths in end-of-life care of residents: Personal knowledge and strategies. *Journal of Hospice and Palliative Nursing, 16*, 438–445. https://doi.org/10.1097/NJH.0000000000000093

Lee, S. J., Kim, M. S., Jung, Y. J., & Chang, S. O. (2019). The effectiveness of function-focused care interventions in nursing homes: A systematic review. *The Journal of Nursing Research, 27*(1), 1–13. https://doi.org/10.1097/jnr.0000000000000268

Padgett, D. K. (1998). Does the glove really fit? Qualitative research and clinical social work practice. *Social Work, 43*, 373–381. https://doi.org/10.1093/sw/43.4.373

Panesar, R. S., Albert, B., Messina, C., & Parker, M. (2016). The effect of an electronic SBAR communication tool on documentation of acute events in the pediatric intensive care unit. *American Journal of Medical Quality, 31*, 64–68. https://doi.org/10.1177/1062860614553263

Park, M. S., Kim, G.-T., Lee, S. J., Kim, M. S., Jeong, E.-H., & Chang, S. O. (2019). Sequential two-stage network and thematic analysis for exploring an interdisciplinary care approach in nursing homes. *Computers, Informatics, Nursing: CIN, 37* (9), 473–481. https://doi.org/10.1097/CIN.0000000000000530

Park, M. S., Lee, S. J., & Chang, S. O. (2019). Exploring a nursing home-specific interdisciplinary approach: Toward palliative care for the demented and complex-disabled elderly. *Journal of Hospice and Palliative Nursing, 21*(6), E9–E15. https://doi.org/10.1097/NJH.0000000000000579

Park, M. S., Lim, S. Y., Kim, E. Y., Lee, S. J., & Chang, S. O. (2018). Examining practical nursing experiences to discover ways in which to retain and invigorate the remaining functions of the elderly with a demented and complex disability in nursing homes. *Japan Journal of Nursing Science: JJNS, 15*, 77–90. https://doi.org/10.1111/jjns.12174

Renz, S. M., & Carrington, J. M. (2016). Nurse-physician communication in long-term care: Literature review. *Journal of Gerontological Nursing, 42*, 30–37. https://doi.org/10.3928/00989134-20160615-04

Resnick, B., Galik, E., & Boltz, M. (2013). Function focused care approaches: Literature review of progress and future possibilities. *Journal of the American Medical Directors Association, 14*, 313–318. https://doi.org/10.1016/j.jamda.2012.10.019

Shaw, C., Williams, K. N., & Perkhounkova, Y. (2018). Educating nursing home staff in dementia sensitive communication: Impact on antipsychotic medication use. *Journal of the American Medical Directors Association, 19*, 1129–1132. https://doi.org/10.1016/j.jamda.2018.09.030

Shin, J. H. (2019). Nursing staff characteristics on resident outcomes in nursing homes. *The Journal of Nursing Research, 27*(1), 1–9. https://doi.org/10.1097/jnr.0000000000000269

Thomas, C. M., Bertram, E., & Johnson, D. (2009). The SBAR communication technique: Teaching nursing students professional communication skills. *Nurse Educator, 34*, 176–180. https://doi.org/10.1097/NNE.0b013e3181aaba54

Townsend-Gervis, M., Cornell, P., & Vardaman, J. M. (2014). Interdisciplinary rounds and structured communication reduce re-admissions and improve some patient outcomes. *Western Journal of Nursing Research, 36*, 917–928. https://doi.org/10.1177/0193945914527521

Williams, K. N., Perkhounkova, Y., Jao, Y.-L., Bossen, A., Hein, M., Chung, S., Starykowicz, A., & Turk, M. (2018). Person-centered communication for nursing home residents with dementia: Four communication analysis methods. *Western Journal of Nursing Research, 40*(7), 1012–1031. https://doi.org/10.1177/0193945917697226

Xyrichis, A., Reeves, S., & Zwarenstein, M. (2018). Examining the nature of interprofessional practice: An initial framework validation and creation of the InterProfessional Activity Classification Tool (InterPACT). *Journal of Interprofessional Care, 32*(4), 416–425. https://doi.org/10.1080/13561820.2017.1408576

7

Effects of Smoking and Physical Activity on the Pulmonary Function of Young University Nursing Students in Cáceres (Spain)

Sergio RICO-MARTÍN[1]* • Jorge M. DE NICOLÁS-JIMÉNEZ[2] • Mariana MARTÍNEZ-ÁLVAREZ[3] • Sergio CORDOVILLA-GUARDIA[4] • Esperanza SANTANO-MOGENA[5] • Julián F. CALDERÓN-GARCÍA[6]

ABSTRACT

Background: The simultaneous effect of physical activity (PA) and smoking on pulmonary function in young people remains unclear.

Propose: The aim of this study was to determine the influence of smoking and PA on pulmonary function in young university students in Cáceres, Spain.

Methods: A sample of 120 young nursing students was studied (60 smokers and 60 nonsmokers). All subjects underwent spirometry with a COPD-6 portable device, and their level of PA was quantified using the International Physical Activity Questionnaire. The influence of PA and smoking on pulmonary function was determined by comparing hypotheses.

Results: Significant differences were observed between smokers and nonsmokers in terms of percent forced expiratory volume in 1 second, percent forced expiratory volume in 6 seconds, lung age, and the difference between lung age and chronological age (LA–CA) in those who practiced mild PA. In the subjects who performed moderate and vigorous PA, these differences were not noted. In the intragroup analysis, significant differences were observed in smokers in terms of percent forced expiratory volume in 1 second, percent forced expiratory volume in 6 seconds, lung age, and LA–CA; however, in the control group, differences were only observed in terms of lung age and LA–CA. These findings were confirmed in the multivariate analysis.

Conclusions/Implications for Practice: Our findings confirmed a deterioration in pulmonary function in smokers who did not perform moderate or vigorous PA. The level of PA performed was positively related to pulmonary function in smokers, whereas in nonsmokers, improvements were only significant in LA–CA.

KEY WORDS:
pulmonary function, smokers, physical activity, young, nursing students.

Introduction

Although the incidence of smoking has decreased during the past few years (Ng et al., 2014), smoking remains one of the main risk factors for preventable morbidity and mortality in the world (Lim et al., 2012). According to the National Institute of Statistics of Spain, it is estimated that 22.98% of the population smokes daily, with a somewhat lower incidence (18.51%) in young people under 24 years old. Most smokers begin at the age of 14 years, and a large number of these individuals already consume cigarettes on a regular basis when they reach the age of majority. This age range represents a vital stage in which there is a consolidation of personality that leads to the maintenance of healthy habits and lifestyles throughout life.

Tobacco smoke affects the airways and lungs of young people who smoke actively or are passively exposed on a regular basis and is associated with adverse health problems in the upper and lower respiratory tract, including higher rates of asthma and reduced pulmonary function (Gibbs, Collaco, & McGrath-Morrow, 2016). In healthy adults, tobacco smoke has been shown to be the main cause of chronic obstructive pulmonary disease (COPD) and chronic respiratory symptoms such as chronic cough, increased production of phlegm, wheezing, and shortness of breath (Forey, Thornton, & Lee, 2011). In addition, tobacco smoke causes a decrease in pulmonary function (Simmons et al., 2005).

The medical literature clearly shows the beneficial effects of physical activity (PA) on health, reducing the risk of morbidity and mortality of many diseases and helping maintain and/or improve individuals' independence and functional capacities (Fogelholm, 2010). Cohort studies have indicated that the regular practice of PA may be effective in both the prevention and treatment of chronic respiratory diseases, including asthma and COPD (Lahti, Holstila, Lahelma, & Rahkonen, 2014). Furthermore, a positive relationship has been confirmed between

[1]*PhD, RN, Associate Professor, Department of Nursing, Nursing and Occupational Therapy College, University of Extremadura, Cáceres, Spain* • [2]*PhD, MD, Primary Attention Doctor, Zona Centro Health Center, Extremadura Health Service, Cáceres, Spain* • [3]*PhD, RN, Associate Professor, Department of Nursing, Faculty of Medicine, University of Extremadura, Badajoz, Spain* • [4]*PhD, RN, Associate Professor, Department of Nursing, Nursing and Occupational Therapy College, University of Extremadura, Cáceres, Spain* • [5]*RN, Teaching Assistant, Department of Nursing, Nursing and Occupational Therapy College, University of Extremadura, Cáceres, Spain* • [6]*PhD, RN, Professor, Department of Nursing, Nursing and Occupational Therapy College, University of Extremadura, Cáceres, Spain.*

physical exercise and spirometric parameters (Gimeno-Santos et al., 2014; Paulo, Petrica, & Martins, 2013), although some studies have not confirmed this relationship (Smith et al., 2016).

Because smoking and PA are largely incongruent behaviors (Kaczynski, Manske, Mannell, & Grewal, 2008) and the simultaneous effect on pulmonary function in young people remains unclear (Campbell Jenkins et al., 2014; Holmen, Barrett-Connor, Clausen, Holmen, & Bjermer, 2002; Michalak, Gatkiewicz, Pawlicka-Lisowska, & Poziomska-Piatkowska, 2012), the objective of this study was to determine the influence of smoking and PA on pulmonary function in young university students (aged 18–24 years) in Cáceres, Spain. The hypothesis is that PA may have a beneficial effect on lung capacity in young people who smoke.

Methods

Design and Population

This cross-sectional, descriptive, association study was conducted on a sample of 120 healthy young people (94 women and 26 men) between 18 and 24 years old. The recruitment was performed during the months of March and April 2017. The subjects were first-, second-, and third-year nursing students from the Cáceres university campus. Figure 1 illustrates the sample selection process. Before the inclusion of participants, a questionnaire was conducted to determine the number of students who smoked on a regular basis (n = 66). The sample was categorized into two groups of 60 subjects according to whether they were current smokers or had never smoked. The group of current smokers (n = 60) accounted for 91% of the total active smokers. Nonsmoking subjects were randomly selected from the total of nonsmoking students. All of the participants were informed of the nature of the investigation and gave their written consent to participate. The study was designed in accordance with the Declaration of Helsinki, and the protocol was approved by the local ethics committee (No. 18000574).

The exclusion criteria in this study were as follows: (a) presence of asthma, (b) presence of catarrh or constipation at the time of the study, (c) presence of diseases that affect lung capacity, (d) presence of thoracic deformity, and (e) being a former smoker.

Data were collected from all of the participants on age, gender, and disease history. A physical examination was conducted to determine weight, height, body mass index, heart rate, and arterial oxygen saturation. For smokers, the following variables were recorded: age when they started smoking (years), how long they had smoked (years), number of cigarettes consumed daily, pack-years, amount of time between getting up in the morning and the first cigarette (minutes), and type of cigarette usually consumed (rolled or manufactured).

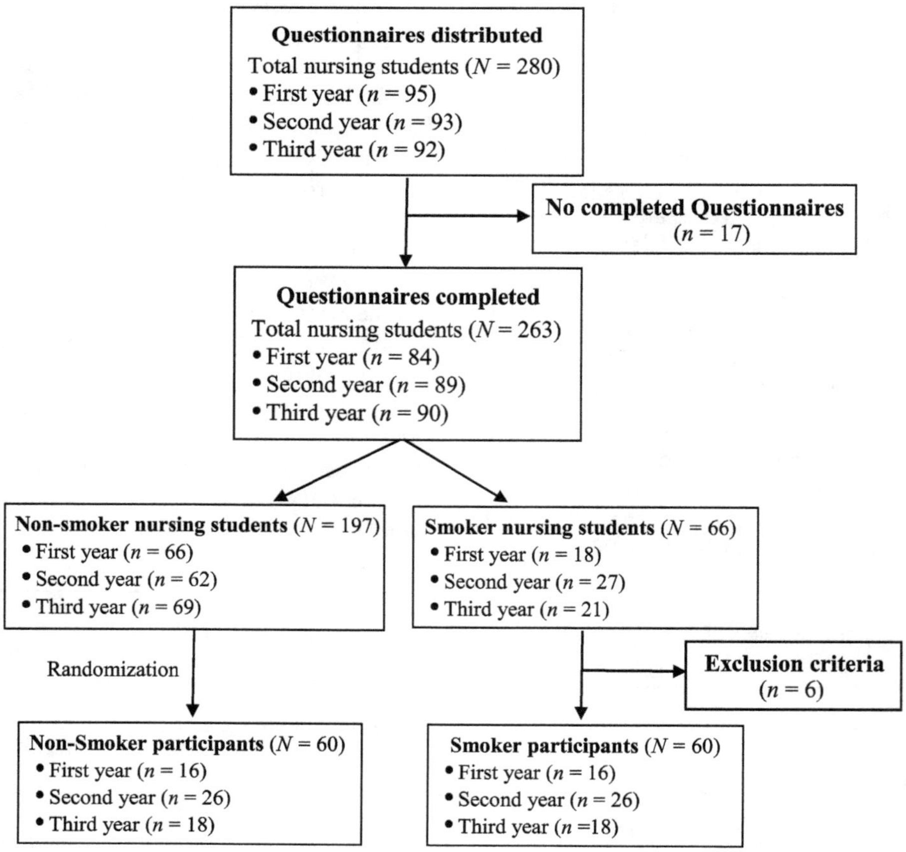

Figure 1. Sample selection process.

The Fagerström test, which is used worldwide to assess the degree of physical dependence on tobacco smoking, was used to assess level of nicotine addiction (Fagerstrom & Schneider, 1989). This test has six items, with a total score ranging from 0 to 10. Scores were categorized into low dependence (≤ 4), medium dependence (5–6), and high dependence (≥ 7). The Spanish version was previously validated, and the reliability coefficient was .66 (Becoña & Vázquez, 1998). The Richmond test was used to determine the degree of motivation to stop smoking (Richmond, Kehoe, & Webster, 1993). This test has four items, with a total possible score ranging from 0 to 10. Motivation is considered low when the score is between 0 and 5, moderate when the score is between 6 and 8, and high when the score is 9 or 10.

Pulmonary Function Assessment

Each participant underwent forced spirometry with a COPD-6 portable spirometer (Vitalograph). The diagnostic utility of this device was previously validated (Represas Represas et al., 2010) and has been recently used in several studies to determine pulmonary function (Figueira Gonçalves et al., 2017; Kjeldgaard, Lykkegaard, Spillemose, & Ulrik, 2017). The recommendations of the Spanish Society of Pneumology and Thoracic Surgery were followed for the spirometry tests conducted in this study (García-Río et al., 2013). Three maneuvers were performed for each patient, which met the criteria of acceptability and reproducibility, and the best device was selected for each parameter. Nasal clamps were not used, and no bronchodilator test was performed. The values of percent forced expiratory volume in 1 second (FEV_1%), percent forced expiratory volume in 6 seconds (FEV_6%), and FEV_1/FEV_6 (%) adjusted for age, gender, height, and lung age were measured using the device. The difference between lung age and chronological age (LA–CA) was calculated for each of the participants. The tests were performed by the same operator, who had been trained in the same laboratory (the Nursing and Occupational Therapy College of Cáceres).

Assessment of Physical Activity

The level of PA was quantified using the International Physical Activity Questionnaire-Short Form (Craig et al., 2003). This questionnaire consists of seven questions and is used to measure the intensity of PA performed over a 1-week period in different aspects of people's lives (work, household tasks, transportation, and leisure). This questionnaire classifies PA into three categories: mild, moderate, and vigorous. The International Physical Activity Questionnaire-Short Form questionnaire has shown adequate validity for use with Spanish university students (Rodriguez-Muñoz, Corella, Abarca-Sos, & Zaragoza, 2017).

Statistical Analysis

All values were expressed in terms of mean and standard deviation, medians (interquartile ranges), frequency, and percentage. Before applying the standard tests, the Kolmogorov–Smirnov test of goodness of fit was performed to verify whether the data had a normal distribution, and the Levene test was used to determine if the distribution of the samples assumed equal variances. The comparative study of smokers and nonsmokers was performed with the *t* test for independent samples when the data were parametric, and the Mann–Whitney *U* test was used when the data were not parametric. The groups were stratified according to the level of PA performed, and the Kruskal–Wallis test was used for intragroup comparisons.

TABLE 1.
Baseline Characteristics of the Groups

	Nonsmoker (n = 60)		Smoker (n = 60)		
Characteristic	Median	Interquartile Range	Median	Interquartile Range	p
Age[a] (years)	20	20–22	20.5	19–22	.931
Gender: male[a] (n and %)	14	23	13	22	.827
Weight[a] (kg)	62.5	55–69	60	56–67	.777
Height[a] (cm)	165	157–171	164	160–170	.542
BMI[a] (kg/m^2)	22.6	20.8–24.8	22.5	20.7–24.8	.867
Heart rate[b] (beats per minute; M and SD)	77	12	77	10	.936
SaO_2[a] (%)	99	99–99	99	99–99	.151
	n	%	n	%	p
Physical activity[c]					
Mild	12	20	15	25	.430
Moderate	28	46	34	56	.273
Vigorous	20	33	11	18	.060

Note. BMI = body mass index; SaO_2 = arterial oxygen saturation.
[a]Comparison by Mann–Whitney *U* test. [b]Comparison by independent *t* test. [c]Comparison by Pearson χ^2 test.

The Pearson chi-square test was used to compare categorical variables.

A multivariate logistic regression analysis was performed to measure the association between independent variables and the dependent variable. The quartile with the worst spirometric values provided the cutoff points for FEV_1% (≤ 92%), FEV_6% (≤ 90%), FEV_1%/FEV_6% (≤ 100%), and lung year (≥ 33 years). The cutoff point for LA–CA was ≥ 1 year, that is, having a pulmonary age that is higher than chronological age. Two adjusted models were used to perform the multivariate analysis. Model 1 was adjusted by smoking, PA level, years, gender, body mass index, and packs consumed per year. Afterward, the participants were stratified into two groups (smokers and nonsmokers). A multivariate analysis adjusted by PA level, years, gender, body mass index, and packs consumed per year was performed. Data were expressed as odds ratio (*OR*) and 95% confidence interval (CI).

The significance threshold was $p < .05$ for all the statistical tests. Statistical analysis was performed using IBM SPSS Version 24 (IBM Corporation, Armonk, NY, USA).

Results

This study included 120 young nursing students (22% male) between 19 and 24 years old as participants. The main characteristics of the smoking and nonsmoking participants are shown in Table 1. Vigorous PA was more frequent in the nonsmoker group than the smoker group (33% vs. 18%, respectively). No significant differences were found in any of the variables analyzed.

Table 2 shows the data related to consumption of tobacco in the smoking group. The average time smoking was 5 ± 3 years, and the average proportion of packs consumed per year was 2 ± 2. Regarding nicotine dependence, most showed low dependence (78%), and most had a low motivation to quit (45%).

Table 3 shows the results of the comparative study between the groups regarding spirometry variables. Significant differences were observed between both groups ($p < .05$), with the group of nonsmokers obtaining better results in FEV_1%, lung age, and LA–CA. Table 3 also shows the relationship between pulmonary function in both groups, stratified according to PA level. Significant differences ($p < .05$) were observed in the spirometric values of FEV_1%, FEV_6%, lung age, and LA–CA in those who practiced mild PA. In the nonsmoking group, with the exception of FEV_6%, these differences were not detected in those participants who performed moderate or vigorous PA, even with better spirometric values. In the intragroup analysis, significant differences were observed in FEV_1%, FEV_6%, lung age, and LA–CA in smokers. However, in the control group, differences were only found in lung age and LA–CA. In the smoking group, these differences were mainly seen between the mild PA group and the moderate PA group and between the mild PA group and the vigorous PA group, whereas differences in the group of nonsmokers existed between the mild PA group and the vigorous PA group and between the vigorous PA group and the moderate PA group.

Table 4 shows the assessment results of the multivariate logistic regression models for the association between smoking and PA levels with spirometric variables. With regard to the unadjusted model, being a smoker was associated with worse FEV_1% (*OR* = 2.72, 95% CI [1.11, 6.69]). Nevertheless, FEV_1% (*OR* = 0.32, 95% CI [0.12, 0.87]) and FEV_6% (*OR* = 0.33, 95% CI [0.12, 0.88]) for moderate PA and FEV_1% (*OR* = 0.18, 95% CI [0.04, 0.67]), FEV_6% (*OR* = 0.29, 95% CI [0.08, 0.95]), lung age (*OR* = 0.17, 95% CI [0.04, 0.65]), and LA–CA (*OR* = 0.07, 95% CI [0.01, 0.30]) for vigorous PA were shown to be protective factors for pulmonary function. Finally, according to Model 1, smoking was not associated with any of the spirometry variables analyzed. In contrast, moderate and vigorous PA were shown to be a protective factor for pulmonary function outcomes, except for FEV_1%/FEV_6%.

TABLE 2.
Characteristics Related to the Consumption of Tobacco in the Smoking Group (N = 60)

Characteristic	*M*	*SD*
Age when started smoking (years)	16	2
Smoking time (years)	5	3
Cigarettes smoked per day	8	5
Packs per year	2	2
Amount of time[a] (minutes)	117	113
	n	%
Type of cigarette		
Rolled	36	60
Manufactured	24	40
Nicotine dependence		
Low	47	78
Medium	13	22
Psychological dependence		
Low	14	23
Medium	33	55
High	13	22
Social dependence		
Low	6	10
Medium	32	53
High	22	37
Gestural dependence		
Low	38	63
Medium	22	37
Degree of motivation to stop smoking		
Low	27	45
Moderate	19	32
High	14	23

[a]Between getting up in the morning and the first cigarette.

Table 5 shows the results for the stratified multivariate analysis that was carried out between smokers and nonsmokers. In the context of both models (unadjusted and adjusted), for the smoking group, moderate and vigorous levels of PA were identified as protective factors for the lung function outcomes FEV_1, FEV_6, lung age, and LA–CA. However, for the nonsmoking group, only vigorous PA was identified as a protective factor, for LA–CA ≥ 1 year.

Discussion

This study found a beneficial effect for moderate and vigorous PA on pulmonary function (FEV_1%, FEV_6%, lung age, and age difference) in a population of nursing students who smoked. There were no significant differences in lung function values between smoker and nonsmoker groups for those participants who practiced moderate or vigorous PA. However, for those participants who practiced mild PA, no beneficial effect was found on pulmonary function in the smoker group, which showed lower spirometric values for FEV_1% and FEV_6% and higher lung age and LA–CA.

Spirometry is a basic test for the study of pulmonary function and is necessary for evaluating and monitoring respiratory diseases (García-Río et al., 2013). The quality of this test may be affected by the difficulties faced in correctly obtaining the forced vital capacity (FVC). Therefore, the FEV_6 has been accepted as an alternative parameter (Jing, Huang, Cui, Xu, & Shen, 2009). This substitution simplifies the spirometry technique, improving accuracy in the diagnosis of airway obstruction in nonspecialized environments (López-Campos, Soriano, & Calle, 2014). In recent years, several portable spirometers have been designed and marketed to obtain FEV_1, FEV_6, and their quotient, which, because of their easy handling and cost-effectiveness, are increasingly being used in primary care (Derom et al., 2008). The COPD-6 device is a valid screening tool for COPD and may be used by personnel who have received a brief training session (Represas-Represas et al., 2016). The diagnostic utility of this device has been validated (Represas Represas et al.,

TABLE 3.

Comparative Study Between the Groups, Stratified According to PA Level Regarding Spirometry Variables

	Nonsmoker (n = 60)		Smoker (n = 60)		
Variable	Median	Interquartile Range	Median	Interquartile Range	p
FEV_1^a (%)	99.0	94.0–103.0	94.5	91.0–99.0	.010
Mild PA	98.0	90.5–104.2	90.0	83.0–94.0	.019
Moderate PA	99.0	93.2–102.0	95.0	91.2–101.5	.335
Vigorous PA	100.5	96.0–105.0	99.0	97.0–104.0	.741
p^b	.150		< .001[c,d]		
FEV_6^a (%)	96.0	91.0–102.0	95.0	86.0–102.0	.235
Mild PA	94.5	91.0–101.5	85.0	79.0–93.0	.012
Moderate PA	95.0	91.2–101.5	95.5	88.2–102.7	.848
Vigorous PA	99.0	90.0–110.0	105.0	96.0–111.0	.407
p^b	.472		< .001[c,d]		
FEV_1/FEV_6^a (%)	106.0	100.0–108.0	104.0	100.0–107.0	.073
Mild PA	106.5	98.0–108.7	105.0	98.0–107.0	.377
Moderate PA	106.0	98.0–108.7	104.0	100.0–107.0	.500
Vigorous PA	105.0	102.0–108.0	102.0	100.0–106.0	.068
p^b	.884		.696		
Lung age[a] (years)	24.0	21.0–31.0	30.0	25.0–35.0	.002
Mild PA	26.0	20.2–35.7	39.0	31.0–46.0	.009
Moderate PA	24.0	22.0–32.7	30.0	24.2–33.2	.439
Vigorous PA	21.5	20.0–24.0	27.0	21.0–28.0	.080
p^b	.045[d]		< .001[c,d]		
LA–CA[a] (years)	2.5	0.0–9.0	10.0	2.0–14.0	.001
Mild PA	7.0	1.0–15.7	18.0	10.0–27.0	.009
Moderate PA	4.0	0.5–10.0	8.0	1.7–13.0	.226
Vigorous PA	0.0	0.0–2.0	0.0	0.0–7.0	.433
p^b	.002[d,e]		< .001[c,d]		

Note. FEV_1 = forced expiratory volume in 1 second; FEV_6 = forced expiratory volume in 6 seconds; LA–CA = difference between lung age and chronological age; PA = physical activity.

[a]Comparison by Mann–Whitney *U* test. [b]Comparison by Kruskal–Wallis test. [c]Mild vs. moderate PA. [d]Mild vs. vigorous PA. [e]Moderate vs. vigorous PA.

TABLE 4.

Multivariate Logistic Regression Model of the Association Between Smoking and PA Levels With Spirometry Variables

	Unadjusted		Model 1	
Spirometry Variable	*OR*	95% CI	*OR*	95% CI
$FEV_1 \leq 92\%$				
Nonsmoker	1.00 (ref)		1.00 (ref)	
Smoker	2.72	[1.11, 6.69]*	1.51	[0.41, 5.52]
Mild PA	1.00 (ref)		1.00 (ref)	
Moderate PA	0.32	[0.12, 0.87]*	0.27	[0.08, 0.82]*
Vigorous PA	0.18	[0.04, 0.67]*	0.11	[0.02, 0.51]**
$FEV_6 \leq 90\%$				
Nonsmoker	1.00 (ref)		1.00 (ref)	
Smoker	2.23	[0.95, 5.25]	2.98	[0.79, 11.22]
Mild PA	1.00 (ref)		1.00 (ref)	
Moderate PA	0.33	[0.12, 0.88]*	0.25	[0.08, 0.78]*
Vigorous PA	0.29	[0.08, 0.95]*	0.15	[0.03, 0.64]*
$FEV_1/FEV_6 \leq 100$				
Nonsmoker	1.00 (ref)		1.00 (ref)	
Smoker	1.04	[0.46, 2.36]	0.48	[0.14, 1.58]
Mild PA	1.00 (ref)		1.00 (ref)	
Moderate PA	1.21	[0.45, 3.24]	1.23	[0.43, 3.49]
Vigorous PA	0.46	[0.12, 1.64]	0.46	[0.12, 1.75]
Lung age ≥ 33 years				
Nonsmoker	1.00 (ref)		1.00 (ref)	
Smoker	2.10	[0.89, 4.94]	1.01	[0.26, 3.85]
Mild PA	1.00 (ref)		1.00 (ref)	
Moderate PA	0.39	[0.15, 1.03]	0.28	[0.09, 0.88]*
Vigorous PA	0.17	[0.04, 0.65]*	0.07	[0.01, 0.38]**
LA–CA ≥ 1 year				
Nonsmoker	1.00 (ref)		1.00 (ref)	
Smoker	2.14	[0.91, 5.04]	2.93	[0.79, 10.88]
Mild PA	1.00 (ref)		1.00 (ref)	
Moderate PA	0.32	[0.08, 1.23]	0.20	[0.04, 0.89]*
Vigorous PA	0.07	[0.01, 0.30]***	0.03	[0.01, 0.18]***

Note. Model 1: adjusted by smoking, PA level, years, gender, body mass index, and packs consumed per year. FEV_1 = forced expiratory volume in 1 second; FEV_6 = forced expiratory volume in 6 seconds; LA–CA = difference between lung age and chronological age; PA = physical activity; ref = reference.
**p* < .05. ***p* < .01. ****p* < .001.

2010), and the device has been recently used in several studies to determine pulmonary function (Figueira Gonçalves et al., 2017; Kjeldgaard et al., 2017).

Respiratory health problems related to smoking do not usually manifest fully until later in life, and it is generally assumed that young smokers may not have respiratory problems because of the brief period in which they have been exposed to tobacco smoke. However, the results of this study found that, despite the relatively young age of the participants, the smokers exhibited decreased lung capacity and those that performed only mild PA exhibited significantly decreased lung capacity. Specifically, this was found in the variables $FEV_1\%$, $FEV_6\%$, lung age, and LA–CA. Exposure to tobacco smoke throughout life affects pulmonary function and health (Martinez, 2016), with effects varying based on type of smoke exposure and the stage at which individuals are exposed to smoke (Kuh & Ben-Shlomon, 2004). The first years of life represent a critical period of development (Shaheen, 1997) when exposure to smoke may significantly affect the development of pulmonary functions. Furthermore, whereas smoking during adulthood is classically associated with an accelerated decrease in FEV_1 (Allinson et al., 2016), smoking during adolescence may interfere with the final stages of lung development that influence both FEV_1 and FVC (Gold et al., 1996). Several studies conducted in young smokers have shown a decrease in lung capacity compared with nonsmokers. Merghany et al. studied 153 male adolescents aged 9–14 years in Khartoum, Sudan, and found that FEV_1 and FVC were significantly lower in the group that was exposed to tobacco smoke than in the control, nonsmoking group (Merghani & Saeed, 2013). Similar results (in FEV_1, FEV_1/FVC, and $FEV_{25\%-75\%}$) were observed by Bird and Staines-Orozco

TABLE 5.

Multivariate Logistic Regression Model of the Association Between Smoking and PA Levels With Spirometry Variables Stratified Into Smoker and Nonsmoker Groups

	Nonsmoker				Smoker			
	Unadjusted		Adjusted[a]		Unadjusted		Adjusted[a]	
Spirometry Variable	*OR*	[95% CI]	*OR*	[95% CI]	*OR*	[95% CI]	*OR*	[95% CI]
$FEV_1 \leq 92\%$								
Mild PA	1.00 (ref)		1.00 (ref)		1.00 (ref)		1.00 (ref)	
Moderate PA	0.65	[0.12, 3.31]	0.37	[0.02, 1.80]	0.20	[0.05, 0.76]*	0.18	[0.03, 0.93]*
Vigorous PA	0.33	[0.04, 2.36]	0.23	[0.02, 1.80]	0.11	[0.02, 0.72]*	0.02	[0.01, 0.93]*
$FEV_6 \leq 90\%$								
Mild PA	1.00 (ref)		1.00 (ref)		1.00 (ref)		1.00 (ref)	
Moderate PA	0.65	[0.12, 3.31]	0.26	[0.02, 2.69]	0.20	[0.05, 0.76]*	0.14	[0.03, 0.66]*
Vigorous PA	0.75	[0.13, 4.12]	0.15	[0.01, 2.10]	0.11	[0.02, 0.72]*	0.03	[0.01, 0.38]**
$FEV_1/FEV_6 \leq 100$								
Mild PA	1.00 (ref)		1.00 (ref)		1.00 (ref)		1.00 (ref)	
Moderate PA	1.11	[0.26, 4.63]	0.84	[0.18, 3.93]	1.31	[0.34, 6.08]	1.54	[0.35, 6.73]
Vigorous PA	0.22	[0.03, 1.47]	0.16	[0.02, 1.16]	1.03	[0.17, 5.94]	1.56	[0.22, 10.63]
Lung age ≥ 33 years								
Mild PA	1.00 (ref)		1.00 (ref)		1.00 (ref)		1.00 (ref)	
Moderate PA	1.00	[0.21, 4.76]	0.33	[0.04, 2.67]	0.20	[0.05, 0.76]*	0.18	[0.03, 0.93]*
Vigorous PA	0.33	[0.47, 2.36]	0.07	[0.01, 1.07]	0.11	[0.01, 0.72]*	0.02	[0.01, 0.51]*
LA–CA ≥ 1 year								
Mild PA	1.00 (ref)		1.00 (ref)		1.00 (ref)		1.00 (ref)	
Moderate PA	0.70	[0.15, 3.24]	0.24	[0.03, 1.67]	0.01	[0.00, 0.23]**	0.01	[0.00, 0.19]**
Vigorous PA	0.14	[0.02, 0.72]*	0.01	[0.01, 0.21]**	0.01	[0.00, 0.12]***	0.01	[0.00, 0.09]***

Note. FEV_1 = forced expiratory volume in 1 second; FEV_6 = forced expiratory volume in 6 seconds; LA–CA difference between lung age and chronological age; PA = physical activity; ref = reference.

[a]Adjusted by PA level, years, gender, body mass index, and packs consumed per year.

$^{*}p < .05$. $^{**}p < .01$. $^{***}p < .001$.

(2016) in a population of 300 students (137 boys) aged 13–15 years in Juárez, Mexico. Young nonsmokers exhibited significantly higher values than both passive and active smokers. Vianna et al. studied the effects of smoking on the pulmonary function of 2,063 young people with an average age of 24 years in Brazil and found a significant association between smoking and the FEV_1/FVC ratio (Vianna et al., 2008). In Spain, a similar study was conducted with 2,647 young people (1,275 men) with an average age of 32 years (Urrutia et al., 2005). The authors reported significantly lower values of FEV_1, FEV_1/FVC, and $FEF_{25\%-75\%}$ among young smokers. However, none of the studies mentioned considered PA as a factor of influence on pulmonary function in young people.

Previous studies have reported a positive relationship between the performance of physical exercise and spirometric parameters (Gimeno-Santos et al., 2014; Nystad, Samuelsen, Nafstad, & Langhammer, 2006; Paulo et al., 2013), although other studies have not found a significant relationship (Smith et al., 2016). In addition, the simultaneous effect of PA and smoking on pulmonary function in young people remains unclear. Holmen et al. studied this relationship in 6,811 students aged 13–18 years, observing a significant association between lung capacity (FVC and FEV_1) and level of physical exercise in those who have never smoked, but not in daily smokers (Holmen et al., 2002). Michalak et al. evaluated the influence of regular PA for 10 months in young smokers and nonsmokers aged 19–24 years, observing improvements in both the FVC and FEV_1 of both groups (Michalak et al., 2012). Campbell Jenkins et al. studied the relationship between physical inactivity and smoking in pulmonary function in a cohort of 5,301 African American adults aged 21–95 years, concluding that physically active smokers had higher pulmonary functions than the sedentary ones (Campbell Jenkins et al., 2014). This study observed that pulmonary capacity values ($FEV_1\%$, $FEV_6\%$, lung age, and LA–CA) improved in the smoker group when the intensity of the PA increased. However, in the nonsmoker group, improvements were only seen in the values for LA–CA. These findings suggest that moderate or vigorous PA may contribute to reducing smoking-related damage to pulmonary capacity.

This study is affected by several limitations. The design was cross-sectional and thus addresses associations only, not causality. In addition, this study used a convenience sample of first-, second-, and third-year nursing students from a university campus in Cáceres, Spain, who were included randomly depending on whether they smoked or not. This is the reason why the numbers of subjects classified into PA categories vary widely. Consequently, the participants may not be representative of university students in other degree programs or even in the same age range, suggesting that the findings may not be applicable to other populations. However, improving the health status of future health professionals was a primary motivation for this work. All of the participants were informed of their spirometric results, including lung age, as there is evidence that knowledge of lung age is a factor that motivates individuals to quit smoking (Ferguson, Enright, Buist, & Higgins, 2000). Furthermore, it has been shown that smoking among health professionals is an important factor affecting the attitudes of society toward this habit (Russell, Wilson, Taylor, & Baker, 1979). Improving the behavior of nursing professionals, as examples and models for the community, may be crucial to achieving behavioral changes in the general population (Aucoin, 1986; Kelly, Wills, & Sykes, 2017). A particular strength of this study was its use, as suggested by Campbell Jenkins et al. (2014), of different categories to assess PA to clarify its effects on lung function. In addition, the young age of the participants may reflect the initial changes in lung function because of tobacco use and the possible benefits of PA. All of these favor an early approach to discouraging smoking.

In conclusion, although the smokers who were assessed in this study were young in age and short-term smokers, the findings confirm that smokers have decreased pulmonary function, as compared with their nonsmoking peers, when they do not regularly perform moderate or vigorous PA. The findings of this study support that level of PA performed is positively related to pulmonary function in smokers, whereas in nonsmokers, the improvements were only significant in LA–CA.

Acknowledgment

We thank all of the students for their participation, which made this work possible.

References

Allinson, J. P., Hardy, R., Donaldson, G. C., Shaheen, S. O., Kuh, D., & Wedzicha, J. A. (2016). The presence of chronic mucus hypersecretion across adult life in relation to chronic obstructive pulmonary disease development. *American Journal of Respiratory and Critical Care Medicine, 193*(6), 662–672. https://doi.org/10.1164/rccm.201511-2210OC

Aucoin, R. A. (1986). Smoking behavior and the efficacy of nurses as role models. *Health Values, 10*(4), 25–29.

Becoña, E., & Vázquez, F. L. (1998). The Fagerström test for nicotine dependence in a Spanish sample. *Psychological Reports, 83*(3, Pt. 2), 1455–1458. https://doi.org/10.2466/pr0.1998.83.3f.1455

Bird, Y., & Staines-Orozco, H. (2016). Pulmonary effects of active smoking and secondhand smoke exposure among adolescent students in Juárez, Mexico. *International Journal of Chronic Obstructive Pulmonary Disease, 11*, 1459–1467. https://doi.org/10.2147/COPD.S102999

Campbell Jenkins, B. W., Sarpong, D. F., Addison, C., White, M. S., Hickson, D. A., White, W., & Burchfiel, C. (2014). Joint effects of smoking and sedentary lifestyle on lung function in African Americans: The Jackson heart study cohort. *International Journal of Environmental Research and Public Health, 11*(2), 1500–1519. https://doi.org/10.3390/ijerph110201500

Craig, C. L., Marshall, A. L., Sjöström, M., Bauman, A. E., Booth, M. L., Ainsworth, B. E., ... Oja, P. (2003). International physical activity questionnaire: 12-country reliability and validity. *Medicine & Science in Sports & Exercise, 35*(8), 1381–1395. https://doi.org/10.1249/01.MSS.0000078924.61453.FB

Derom, E., van Weel, C., Liistro, G., Buffels, J., Schermer, T., Lammers, E., ... Decramer, M. (2008). Primary care spirometry. *European Respiratory Journal, 31*(1), 197–203. https://doi.org/10.1183/09031936.00066607

Fagerstrom, K. O., & Schneider, N. G. (1989). Measuring nicotine dependence: A review of the Fagerstrom Tolerance Questionnaire. *Journal of Behavioral Medicine, 12*(2), 159–182. https://doi.org/10.1007/BF00846549

Ferguson, G. T., Enright, P. L., Buist, A. S., & Higgins, M. W. (2000). Office spirometry for lung health assessment in adults: A consensus statement from the National Lung Health Education Program. *Chest, 117*(4), 1146–1161.

Figueira Gonçalves, J. M., Pérez Méndez, L. I., Guzmán Sáenz, C., Diaz Pérez, D., Viña Manrique, P., & Pedrero Garcia, A. J. (2017). Impact of body mass index on the predictive capacity of the COPD-6 device in the detection of airflow obstruction. *Medicina Clinica, 149*(11), 483–487. https://doi.org/10.1016/j.medcle.2017.10.023

Fogelholm, M. (2010). Physical activity, fitness and fatness: Relations to mortality, morbidity and disease risk factors. A systematic review. *Obesity Reviews, 11*(3), 202–221. https://doi.org/10.1111/j.1467-789X.2009.00653.x

Forey, B. A., Thornton, A. J., & Lee, P. N. (2011). Systematic review with meta-analysis of the epidemiological evidence relating smoking to COPD, chronic bronchitis and emphysema. *BMC Pulmonary Medicine, 11*, 36. https://doi.org/10.1186/1471-2466-11-36

García-Río, F., Calle, M., Burgos, F., Casan, P., Del Campo, F., Galdiz, J. B., ... Puente-Maestu, L. (2013). Spirometry. Spanish Society of Pulmonology and Thoracic Surgery (SEPAR). *Archivos de Bronconeumologia, 49*(9), 388–401. https://doi.org/10.1016/j.arbres.2013.04.001

Gibbs, K., Collaco, J. M., & McGrath-Morrow, S. A. (2016). Impact of tobacco smoke and nicotine exposure on lung development. *Chest Journal, 149*(2), 552–561. https://doi.org/10.1378/chest.15-1858

Gimeno-Santos, E., Frei, A., Steurer-Stey, C., de Batlle, J., Rabinovich, R. A., Raste, Y., ... PROactive consortium. (2014). Determinants and outcomes of physical activity in patients with COPD: A systematic review. *Thorax, 69*(8), 731–739. https://doi.org/10.1136/thoraxjnl-2013-204763

Gold, D. R., Wang, X., Wypij, D., Speizer, F. E., Ware, J. H., & Dockery, D. W. (1996). Effects of cigarette smoking on lung function in adolescent boys and girls. *The New England Journal of Medicine, 335*(13), 931–937. https://doi.org/10.1056/NEJM199609263351304

Holmen, T. L., Barrett-Connor, E., Clausen, J., Holmen, J., & Bjermer, L. (2002). Physical exercise, sports, and lung function in smoking versus nonsmoking adolescents. *The European Respiratory Journal, 19*(1), 8–15. https://doi.org/10.1183/09031936.02.00203502

Jing, J.-Y., Huang, T.-C., Cui, W., Xu, F., & Shen, H.-H. (2009). Should FEV_1/FEV_6 replace FEV_1/FVC ratio to detect airway obstruction? A metaanalysis. *Chest Journal, 135*(4), 991–998. https://doi.org/10.1378/chest.08-0723

Kaczynski, A. T., Manske, S. R., Mannell, R. C., & Grewal, K. (2008). Smoking and physical activity: A systematic review. *American Journal of Health Behavior, 32*(1), 93–110. https://doi.org/10.5993/AJHB.32.1.9

Kelly, M., Wills, J., & Sykes, S. (2017). Do nurses' personal health behaviours impact on their health promotion practice? A systematic review. *International Journal of Nursing Studies, 76,* 62–77. https://doi.org/10.1016/j.ijnurstu.2017.08.008

Kjeldgaard, P., Lykkegaard, J., Spillemose, H., & Ulrik, C. S. (2017). Multicenter study of the COPD-6 screening device: Feasible for early detection of chronic obstructive pulmonary disease in primary care? *International Journal of Chronic Obstructive Pulmonary Disease, 12,* 2323–2331. https://doi.org/10.2147/COPD.S136244

Kuh, D., & Ben-Shlomon, Y. (2004). *A life course approach to chronic disease epidemiology* (2nd ed.). New York, NY: Oxford University Press.

Lahti, J., Holstila, A., Lahelma, E., & Rahkonen, O. (2014). Leisure-time physical activity and all-cause mortality. *PLoS One, 9*(7), e101548. https://doi.org/10.1371/journal.pone.0101548

Lim, S. S., Vos, T., Flaxman, A. D., Danaei, G., Shibuya, K., Adair-Rohani, H., ... Ezzati, M. (2012). A comparative risk assessment of burden of disease and injury attributable to 67 risk factors and risk factor clusters in 21 regions, 1990–2010: A systematic analysis for the Global Burden of Disease Study 2010. *The Lancet, 380*(9859), 2224–2260. https://doi.org/10.1016/S0140-6736(12)61766-8

López-Campos, J. L., Soriano, J. B., & Calle, M. (2014). Interregional changes in the performance and interpretation of spirometry in Spain: 3E study. *Archivos de Bronconeumologia, 50*(11), 475–483. https://doi.org/10.1016/j.arbr.2014.09.011

Martinez, F. D. (2016). Early-life origins of chronic obstructive pulmonary disease. *The New England Journal of Medicine, 375*(9), 871–878. https://doi.org/10.1056/NEJMra1603287

Merghani, T. H., & Saeed, A. M. (2013). The relationship between regular second-hand smoke exposure at home and indictors of lung function in healthy school boys in Khartoum. *Tobacco Control, 22*(5), 315–318. https://doi.org/10.1136/tobaccocontrol-2011-050169

Michalak, K., Gatkiewicz, M., Pawlicka-Lisowska, A., & Poziomska-Piatkowska, E. (2012). The influence of swimming activity on lung function parameters among smoking and non-smoking youth. *Polski Merkuriusz Lekarski: Organ Polskiego Towarzystwa Lekarskiego, 33*(193), 13–19.

Ng, M., Freeman, M. K., Fleming, T. D., Robinson, M., Dwyer-Lindgren, L., Thomson, B., ... Gakidou, E. (2014). Smoking prevalence and cigarette consumption in 187 countries, 1980–2012. *JAMA, 311*(2), 183–192. https://doi.org/10.1001/jama.2013.284692

Nystad, W., Samuelsen, S. O., Nafstad, P., & Langhammer, A. (2006). Association between level of physical activity and lung function among Norwegian men and women: The HUNT study. *The International Journal of Tuberculosis and Lung Disease, 10*(12), 1399–1405.

Paulo, R., Petrica, J., & Martins, J. (2013). Physical activity and respiratory function: Corporal composition and spirometric values analysis. *Acta Medica Portuguesa, 26*(3), 258–264.

Represas Represas, C., Botana Rial, M., Leiro Fernández, V., González Silva, A. I., del Campo Pérez, V., & Fernández-Villar, A. (2010). Assessment of the portable COPD-6 device for detecting obstructive airway diseases. *Archivos de Bronconeumologia, 46*(8), 426–432. https://doi.org/10.1016/j.arbres.2010.04.008 (Original work published in Spanish)

Represas-Represas, C., Fernández-Villar, A., Ruano-Raviña, A., Priegue-Carrera, A., Botana-Rial, M., & Study Group of "Validity of COPD-6 in non-specialized healthcare settings" (2016). Screening for chronic obstructive pulmonary disease: Validity and reliability of a portable device in non-specialized healthcare settings. *PLoS One, 11*(1), e0145571. https://doi.org/10.1371/journal.pone.0145571

Richmond, R. L., Kehoe, L. A., & Webster, I. W. (1993). Multivariate models for predicting abstention following intervention to stop smoking by general practitioners. *Addiction (Abingdon, England), 88*(8), 1127–1135. https://doi.org/10.1111/j.1360-0443.1993.tb02132.x

Rodriguez-Muñoz, S., Corella, C., Abarca-Sos, A., & Zaragoza, J. (2017). Validation of three short physical activity questionnaires with accelerometers among university students in Spain. *The Journal of Sports Medicine and Physical Fitness, 57*(12), 1660–1668. https://doi.org/10.23736/S0022-4707.17.06665-8

Russell, M. A., Wilson, C., Taylor, C., & Baker, C. D. (1979). Effect of general practitioners' advice against smoking. *British Medical Journal, 2*(6184), 231–235. https://doi.org/10.1136/bmj.2.6184.231

Shaheen, S. (1997). The beginnings of chronic airflow obstruction. *British Medical Bulletin, 53*(1), 58–70. https://doi.org/10.1093/oxfordjournals.bmb.a011606

Simmons, M. S., Connett, J. E., Nides, M. A., Lindgren, P. G., Kleerup, E. C., Murray, R. P., ... Tashkin, D. P. (2005). Smoking reduction and the rate of decline in FEV_1: Results from the lung health study. *European Respiratory Journal, 25*(6), 1011–1017. https://doi.org/10.1183/09031936.05.00086804

Smith, M. P., von Berg, A., Berdel, D., Bauer, C. P., Hoffmann, B., Koletzko, S., ... Schulz, H. (2016). Physical activity is not associated with spirometric indices in lung-healthy German youth. *European Respiratory Journal, 48*(2), 428–440. https://doi.org/10.1183/13993003.01408-2015

Urrutia, I., Capelastegui, A., Quintana, J. M., Muñiozguren, N., Basagana, X., Sunyer, J., & Spanish Group of the European Community Respiratory Health Survey (ECRHS-I). (2005). Smoking habit, respiratory symptoms and lung function in young adults. *European Journal of Public Health, 15*(2), 160–165. https://doi.org/10.1093/eurpub/cki113

Vianna, E. O., Gutierrez, M. R., Barbieri, M. A., Caldeira, R. D., Bettiol, H., & Da Silva, A. A. (2008). Respiratory effects of tobacco smoking among young adults. *The American Journal of the Medical Sciences, 336*(1), 44–49. https://doi.org/10.1097/MAJ.0b013e31815c3b47

8

The Relationship Between Work Environment Satisfaction and Retention Intention Among Nursing Administrators in Taiwan

Chiou-Fen LIN[1] • Chung-I HUANG[2] • Che-Ming YANG[3] • Meei-Shiow LU[4]*

ABSTRACT

Background: Nursing administrators are essential to ensuring the quality of healthcare provided in hospitals. The nursing manpower shortage that has affected hospitals in Taiwan over the past decade has weighed particularly heavily on nursing administrators, who are expected to maintain high levels of nursing care quality in frequently understaffed healthcare settings.

Purpose: The objective of this study was to explore the relationship between work environment satisfaction and nursing administrator retention in Taiwan.

Methods: This study used a cross-sectional, questionnaire-based survey to collect data from a sample population of nursing administrators. A set of indicators of quality nursing work environments was developed and included in the questionnaire. A total of 1,829 questionnaires were distributed, and the effective response rate was 95.57%.

Results: The average overall rate of satisfaction with the current work environment across all domains was 3.59 (SD = 0.61). The highest level of satisfaction was found in the domain of safe practice environment (M = 3.83, SD = 0.70), and the lowest was found in the domain of informatics (M = 3.38, SD = 0.91). Length of administrative position tenure was significantly correlated with retention. Each of the eight domains significantly influenced retention. The domain of support and caring was the most significant predictor of nursing administrator retention.

Conclusions/Implications for Practice: Length of administrator position tenure was significantly correlated with nursing administrator retention. Moreover, intention to stay among junior administrators was particularly affected by the support and caring domain. Therefore, it is recommended that nursing departments develop effective strategies to assist and encourage junior administrators to strengthen their career prospects and satisfaction.

KEY WORDS:
nursing administrator, work environment satisfaction, intention to stay.

Introduction

The International Council of Nurses has actively promoted the development of positive practice environments since its inception. Positive practice environments are characterized by innovative policy frameworks that focus on recruitment and retention, strategies for continuing education and promotion, adequate employee compensation, recognition programs, sufficient equipment and supplies, and a safe working environment (International Council of Nurses, 2007).

Because of their role in managing the nursing workforce, nursing administrators significantly affect the quality of healthcare provided by hospitals (Dehghani, Nasiriani, & Salimi, 2016). During the past decade, hospitals in Taiwan have been affected by significant nurse manpower shortages and a corresponding decline in the number of nursing administrators (Lin, Lu, & Huang, 2016).

The environment in which nurses practice is extremely hazardous. Nurses face biological, physical, chemical, psychosocial, and ergonomic hazards, among many others. To create a safe practice environment, all of these factors must be taken into account (Ma, Wang, & Chen, 2011; Yildirim & Yildirim, 2007). Kramer and Schmalenberg (2005) suggested that adequate nursing manpower is indicated when sufficient time and manpower are available to provide quality care.

Number of nurses is not a suitable single representative of nursing manpower adequacy. Factors such as workload, work environment, nursing manpower mix, nurse-to-patient ratio, working hours, nursing specialties and skill levels, and ratio of junior nurses must also be considered (Kaur, Kaur, Kalia, & Kumar, 2010). Moreover, nurse salary and welfare must be commensurate with salary and welfare.

In the professional specialization and team collaboration domain, Schmalenberg and Kramer (2008) pointed out that special attention must be paid to five factors that ensure excellent

[1]*PhD, RN, Professor, College of Nursing, School of Gerontology Health Management, Taipei Medical University, and Adjunct Nursing Consultant, Department of Nursing, Shuang Ho Hospital, Taipei Medical University* • [2] *PhD, Deputy Director, Center for Management and Development, and Adjunct Assistant Professor, School of Health Care Administration, Taipei Medical University* • [3]*PhD, Professor, College of Management and College of Humanities and Social Sciences, Taipei Medical University, and Director, Department of Nuclear Medicine, Taipei Medical University Shuang Ho Hospital* • [4]*MSN, RN, Endowed Professor, College of Nursing, Taipei Medical University, and Chairperson, Board of Controllers, Taiwan Union of Nurses Association.*

teamwork. These include the elevation of a nurse's professional ability, an organizational culture that cares for its employees and patients, robust professionalism, a framework to resolve conflicts, and the support and dedication of administrative superiors. In addition, the simplification of work and the use of informatics are essential to reduce workload. To this end, all aspects of nursing, including teaching, research, and clinical services, can and should be computerized (Chen, 2009). The literature indicates that providing resources for continuing education may be a significant contributing factor to the retention of senior staff, quality of patient care, and nurse satisfaction with their practice environment (Kramer & Schmalenberg, 2005). In the support and caring domain, collaborative, visible management and shared decision making have been shown to positively impact nurse retention (Force, 2005; Friese, 2005; Huang & Lu, 2015). Holden (2006) asserted that support, appreciation, and respect from superiors also play a critical role in nurse retention. Furthermore, work environment quality and job satisfaction have also been shown to significantly affect retention (Balouch & Hassan, 2014; Holston-Okae, 2017; Markey, Ravenswood, & Webber, 2012).

A research team at the Taiwan Union of Nurses Association (TUNA) developed a literature-based research framework in 2012 to assess the current quality of nursing work environments in hospitals. This framework measures environmental quality using the eight domains of practice environment safety; staff quality and quantity; workload, salary, and welfare; professional specialization and team collaboration; work simplification; informatics; personal growth and professional development; and support and caring. In 2013, further related research expanded the content of each domain to include indicators and scoring standards, which were subsequently published in *The Journal of Nursing Research* in 2016 (Lin et al., 2016).

The demand for nurses is increasing continuously because of Taiwan's rapidly aging population. Although it is known that young and inexperienced nurses rely on experienced nursing administrators to help implement clinical practices, few studies have targeted nursing administrators. Therefore, the objective of this study was to explore the relationship between work environment satisfaction and nursing administrator retention in Taiwan, with the intention of determining which factors predict nursing administrator retention.

Methods

Research Subjects

This study used a cross-sectional, questionnaire-based survey to collect data from a sample population consisting of nursing administrators working in Taiwan. The study sample was recruited from among participants in a series of nursing administrator training workshops organized by TUNA in 2016. The workshop participants, including nursing leaders, head nurses, supervisors, and directors, were given the survey at the beginning of each workshop. This study was approved by the joint institutional review board of Taipei Medical University (TMU-JIRB No. N201604013).

Research Instruments

The questionnaire used in this study included a set of indicators of nursing work environment quality that was developed by the research team based on findings published in the literature (Lin et al., 2016). The validity and reliability of this questionnaire were tested and confirmed. The set of indicators covered eight domains (see Table 1) and 65 items. The eight domains were safe practice environment (16 items); quality and quantity of staff (four items); workload, salary, and welfare (seven items); professional specialization and team collaboration (seven items); work simplification (five items); informatics (five items); personal growth and professional development (nine items); and support and caring (12 items). Level of satisfaction with each domain was measured using a Likert scale that ranged from 1 to 5, with 5 indicating the highest level of satisfaction.

In addition to work environment satisfaction, the questionnaire gathered information on participant characteristics and intention to stay. These characteristics, which were determined in prior studies using expert focus groups (Huang, Yu, & Yu, 2016; Lin et al., 2016), were treated as independent variables and included hospital location, hospital accreditation level, work unit, job position, educational level, duration in administrative positions, nursing seniority, gender, and marital status. Intention to stay was determined by the participant's self-stated willingness to remain employed in the nursing field during the subsequent 3-year period.

Data Collection and Analysis

The researchers distributed 1,829 questionnaires and retrieved 1,748 effective responses, with a respondent rate of 95.57%. IBM SPSS Statistics Version 19.0 (IBM, Inc., Armonk, NY, USA) was used for statistical analyses, and the significance level was set at $p < .05$. Inferential statistics included the chi-square test, independent t test, simple logistic regression, and multiple logistic regression.

Results

Participant Characteristics

Data were collected from 1,784 participants. Distributions of participant characteristics are shown in Table 2. The largest number of respondents was from northern Taiwan (n = 630, 36.0%). In terms of hospital accreditation level, most (n = 855, 48.9%) worked in regional hospitals. Nearly two thirds (31.5%) of participants worked in general wards. In terms of job position, most were head nurses (n = 779, 44.6%). Furthermore, most held bachelor's degrees (n = 1,091, 62.4%). In terms of duration as a nursing administrator, most had

TABLE 1.
Questions Used to Address Nursing Work Environment Quality

Domain	Question
1. Safe practice environment	How satisfied are you with the biological, physical, chemical, psychosocial, and ergonomic safety in your hospital's nursing practice environment?
2. Quality and quantity of staff	How satisfied are you with the percentage of nurses who are licensed as RNs, the percentage of nurses above the N2 level, the percentage of nurses who remain employed at your hospital for more than 2 years, and the percentage of nurses with graduate degrees and above in your hospital?
3. Workload, salary, and welfare	How satisfied are you with the statement that your hospital has sufficient nursing staff in proportion to service volume and provides reasonable salaries and benefits?
4. Professional specialization and teamwork collaboration	How satisfied are you with the statement that the multidisciplinary team members in your hospital respect each other and can work together?
5. Work simplification	How satisfied are you with the statement that your hospital continually simplifies nursing work procedures?
6. Informatics	How satisfied are you with the statement that your hospital uses informatics to increase efficacy, accuracy, and expediency?
7. Personal growth and professional development	How satisfied are you with the statement that your hospital cultivates excellence in nursing staff by allowing them to develop professional nursing roles and project a professional nursing image?
8. Support and caring	How satisfied are you with the statement that your hospital administrators' management style offers support and care for nursing staff to optimize their performance?

less than a year of experience (n = 370, 21.2%). With regard to nursing seniority, most had between 16 and 20 years of nursing practice experience (n = 481, 27.50%). Nearly all (98.2%) of the participants were female, and 71.8% were married. Finally, 89.1% indicated that they intended to stay in the nursing field, and only 6.8% (n = 118) indicated that they would not stay.

Duration of time spent in nursing administrative positions correlated significantly with intention to stay (chi-square test: $\chi^2 = 12.731$, $df = 5$, $p = .026$). Nursing administrators who had been in administrative positions for less than 1 year reported a lower willingness to remain in the nursing field over the coming 3-year period (n = 37, 31.4%).

Comparative Analyses Between Individual Characteristics and Work Environment Satisfaction

All of the participant characteristics were shown to significantly affect the domains of safe practice environment; workload, salary, and welfare; work simplification; and personal growth and professional development. Similar results were found for hospital accreditation level, job position, and nursing seniority for the professional specialization and team collaboration domain and the support and caring domain. In terms of the quality and quantity of staff domain, hospital accreditation level, educational level, and nursing seniority all showed significant effects. Finally, hospital accreditation level, duration in administrative positions, and nursing seniority all had significant effects on the informatics domain (Table 3).

Work Environment Satisfaction Scores in Terms of Quality Indicator Domains

The overall satisfaction across all of the eight domains averaged 3.59 (SD = 0.61). As detailed in Table 4, the domain of safe practice environment earned the highest average satisfaction score (M = 3.83, SD = 0.70), followed in descending order by support and caring (M = 3.75, SD = 0.75); personal growth and professional development (M = 3.67, SD = 0.76); quality and quantity of staff (M = 3.61, SD = 0.51); professional specialization and team collaboration (M = 3.62, SD = 0.77); workload, salary, and welfare (M = 3.45, SD = 0.87); work simplification (M = 3.43, SD = 0.81); and informatics (M = 3.38, SD = 0.91).

Correlation Between Intention to Stay and Work Environment Satisfaction

Analysis of data using a simple logistic regression model showed a significant effect of work environment satisfaction on intention to stay. Those participants who intended to stay had an average work environment satisfaction score of 3.63 (SD = 0.68), whereas the scores of those who intended to leave averaged 3.04 (SD = 0.70). Furthermore, these two groups significantly differed across all of the eight domains ($p < .001$), with the "stay" group scoring higher on each domain than the "leave" group. Significantly, the "leave" group had an average score below 3 on three domains: informatics (M = 2.78, SD = 0.95); work simplification (M = 2.82, SD = 0.96); and workload, salary, and welfare (M = 2.87, SD = 0.946). Univariate analyses showed that all of the domains were valid predictors of intention to stay and that quality and quantity of staff (OR = 0.51);

TABLE 2.

Participant Characteristics and Their Intention to Stay (N = 1,748)

			Stay (n = 1,630)		Not Stay (n = 118)			
Characteristic	n	%	n	%	n	%	χ^2	p
Hospital location (Taiwan)							5.294	.151
Northern	630	36.0	580	35.6	50	42.4		
Central	430	24.6	411	25.2	19	16.1		
Southern	508	29.1	472	29.0	36	30.5		
Eastern	178	10.2	165	10.1	13	11.0		
Missing	2	0.1	2	0.1	0	0.0		
Hospital accreditation level							4.894	.180
Medical center	368	21.1	350	21.5	18	15.3		
Regional hospital	855	48.9	795	48.8	60	50.8		
District hospital	447	25.5	409	25.1	38	32.2		
Specialty hospital	52	3.0	50	3.0	2	1.7		
Missing	26	1.5	26	1.6	0	0.0		
Work unit							8.430	.280
Department of nursing	321	18.4	303	18.6	18	15.3		
Outpatient department	86	4.9	82	5.0	4	3.4		
Emergency room	89	5.1	80	4.9	9	7.6		
Intensive care unit	240	13.7	217	13.3	23	19.5		
General ward	551	31.5	518	31.8	33	28.0		
Psychiatric ward	110	6.3	106	6.5	4	3.4		
Others	309	17.7	286	17.6	23	19.5		
Missing	42	2.4	38	2.3	4	3.4		
Job position							5.731	.220
Leader	430	24.6	402	24.7	28	23.7		
Deputy head nurse	341	19.5	319	19.6	22	18.6		
Head nurse	779	44.6	716	43.9	63	53.4		
Supervisor	103	5.9	100	6.1	3	2.5		
Director/deputy director	41	2.3	40	2.5	1	0.9		
Missing	54	3.1	53	3.2	1	0.9		
Educational level							1.598	.660
Vocational school diploma	6	0.4	6	0.4	0	0.0		
2-Year college degree	222	12.7	209	12.8	13	11.0		
Bachelor degree	1091	62.4	1013	62.1	78	66.1		
Graduate degree	399	22.8	376	23.1	23	19.5		
Missing	30	1.7	26	1.6	4	3.4		
Years in administrative positions							12.731	.026
< 1	370	21.2	333	20.4	37	31.4		
1–3	301	17.2	288	17.7	13	11.0		
4–6	283	16.2	262	16.1	21	17.8		
7–9	201	11.5	184	11.3	17	14.4		
10–14	237	13.5	223	13.7	14	11.9		
≥ 15	292	16.7	279	17.1	13	11.0		
Missing	64	3.7	61	3.7	3	2.5		
Nursing seniority (years)							7.733	.172
≤ 5	27	1.5	23	1.4	4	3.4		
6–10	178	10.2	162	9.9	16	13.6		
11–15	419	24.0	389	23.9	30	25.4		
16–20	481	27.5	448	27.5	33	28.0		
21–25	386	22.1	369	22.6	17	14.4		
> 25	241	13.8	224	13.8	17	14.4		
Missing	16	0.9	15	0.9	1	0.8		

(continues)

TABLE 2.
Participant Characteristics and Their Intention to Stay (N = 1,748), Continued

Characteristic	*n*	%	Stay (*n* = 1,630) *n*	%	Not Stay (*n* = 118) *n*	%	χ^2	*p*
Gender							1.770	.183
Male	24	1.4	24	1.5	0	0.0		
Female	1716	98.2	1598	98.0	118	100.0		
Missing	8	0.4	8	0.5	0	0.0		
Marital status							0.174	.917
Married	1255	71.8	1168	71.6	87	73.7		
Single	456	26.1	427	26.2	29	24.6		
Others	29	1.7	27	1.7	2	1.7		
Missing	8	0.4	8	0.5	0	0.0		
Intent to remain employed in nursing over the coming 3 years								
Yes	1630	93.2						
No	118	6.8						

informatics (*OR* = 0.48); and workload, salary, and welfare (*OR* = 0.46) were the most significant (Table 4).

Effects of Duration in Administrative Positions and Work Environment Satisfaction on Intention to Stay

As indicated previously, intention to stay had a significant correlation with the length of time that a nursing administrator had spent in administrative positions. The researchers conducted a multiple logistic regression on intention to stay against duration in administrative positions and each of the other domains of work environment satisfaction. The results indicate that only support and caring achieved statistical significance (Table 5).

Discussion

The results support the idea that work environment satisfaction is a valid predictor of intention to stay in the nursing field for nursing administrators, which is in line with Warshawsky, Wiggins, and Rayens (2016). In this study, the total overall score for work environment satisfaction averaged 3.59, which is slightly lower than the national average of 3.74, as found in a study conducted in 2013 (Lin et al., 2016). Although the safe practice environment domain reflected the highest level of satisfaction, the average for this domain only reached 3.83, which is significantly lower than the 4.1 obtained in 2013. The nursing administrators who indicated that they would leave the profession in the coming 3 years reported the greatest dissatisfaction in the domains of informatics; work simplification; and workload, salary, and welfare. This result differs from the findings of previous studies. In the previously mentioned 2013 national study, which surveyed all nurses in Taiwan, the three most cited reasons for dissatisfaction were as follows: Salary does not change to reflect work volume, there is a shortage of manpower, and salary is not commensurate with workload. This discrepancy between the current study and the 2013 study may be explained by the different effects of certain factors on retention in nursing administrators and general nurses, respectively. Therefore, the strategies implemented to retain these two tiers of nursing staff should be structured differently.

Nursing administrators expressed dissatisfaction with the informatics domain. There are several possible explanations for this result. First, nursing information systems lag behind other healthcare information systems in terms of development, and many development-related challenges remain unresolved (Hung, 2012). Second, advances in information and communication technologies have affected the process of computerization in ways that have adverse impacts on senior nurses and nursing administrators (Lin & Huang, 2014). Finally, introductions of nursing information systems frequently encounter heavy resistance from nursing staff (Chen, 2011; Gao, 2015; Wu & Hung, 2009).

The results of this study showed that work environment satisfaction differed significantly across hospital accreditation levels, with medical centers earning the highest average score. This result indicates that the work environment in tertiary care hospitals, on average, is superior to those in hospitals of other levels.

Leaders expressed the lowest satisfaction with their administrative jobs. Leaders are the lowest tier of nursing administrators and spend much of their time in direct patient care, which may make their situation psychologically similar to that of general nurses (Chang & Lin, 2016). In terms of educational level, nursing administrators with graduate degrees reported higher levels of satisfaction. The literature offers a possible explanation for this, in that administrators with higher levels of

TABLE 3.
Comparative Analyses of Individual Characteristics and Work Environment Satisfaction (N = 1,748)

			Domain 1			Domain 2			Domain 3			Domain 4		
Variable	*n*	%	Mean	*SD*	*p*	Mean	*SD*	*p*	Mean	*SD*	*p*	Mean	*SD*	*p*
Hospital accreditation level					.000			.000			.000			.000
① Medical center	368	21.1	4.05	0.64		3.97	0.72		3.42	0.85		3.84	0.73	
② Regional hospital	855	48.9	3.83	0.69		3.57	0.78		3.34	0.90		3.58	0.75	
③ District hospital	447	25.6	3.67	0.74		3.42	0.84		3.48	0.96		3.48	0.81	
④ Specialty hospital	52	3.0	3.75	0.68		3.48	0.85		3.45	0.87		3.62	0.75	
Post hoc			① > ②, ③, ④			① > ②, ③, ④; ② > ③			① > ②, ③			① > ②, ③		
Job position					.001			.406			.000			.024
① Leader	430	24.6	3.75	0.72		3.60	0.79		3.32	0.86		3.60	0.76	
② Deputy head nurse	341	19.5	3.86	0.70		3.60	0.80		3.39	0.89		3.66	0.79	
③ Head nurse	779	44.6	3.82	0.69		3.61	0.81		3.49	0.85		3.57	0.76	
④ Supervisor	103	5.9	4.04	0.69		3.75	0.86		3.65	0.90		3.63	0.79	
⑤ Director/deputy director	41	2.3	4.02	0.65		3.49	0.84		3.88	0.71		3.95	0.71	
Post hoc			① < ③						① < ③, ④, ⑤					
Educational level					.003			.000			.000			.066
① Vocational school diploma	6	0.3	3.5	0.84		2.83	0.98		3.33	1.03		3.50	0.55	
② 2-Year college degree	222	12.7	3.75	0.67		3.54	0.78		3.33	0.87		3.52	0.82	
③ Bachelor degree	1091	62.4	3.81	0.71		3.58	0.80		3.42	0.88		3.61	0.77	
④ Graduate degree	399	22.8	3.93	0.69		3.76	0.81		3.61	0.82		3.69	0.74	
Post hoc			④ > ③, ②			④ > ①, ②, ③			④ > ②, ③					
Years in administrative positions					.000			.053			.008			.100
① < 1	370	21.2	3.77	0.73		3.56	0.81		3.35	0.88		3.64	0.78	
② 1–3	301	17.2	3.79	0.69		3.55	0.78		3.44	0.88		3.55	0.80	
③ 4–6	283	16.2	3.73	0.71		3.57	0.82		3.40	0.85		3.54	0.71	
④ 7–9	201	11.5	3.84	0.71		3.64	0.81		3.47	0.87		3.66	0.75	
⑤ 10–14	237	13.6	3.87	0.69		3.63	0.83		3.48	0.86		3.58	0.81	
⑥ ≥ 15	292	16.7	4.00	0.64		3.74	0.80		3.60	0.85		3.69	0.78	
Post hoc			⑥ > ①, ②, ③						⑥ > ①					
Nursing seniority (years)					.000			.000			.000			.009
① ≤ 5	27	1.5	3.67	0.96		3.74	0.90		3.56	0.97		3.85	0.99	
② 6–10	178	10.2	3.78	0.72		3.54	0.87		3.31	0.93		3.65	0.76	
③ 11–15	419	24.0	3.78	0.73		3.53	0.82		3.35	0.86		3.56	0.74	
④ 16–20	481	27.5	3.77	0.70		3.56	0.80		3.41	0.88		3.57	0.77	
⑤ 21–25	386	22.1	3.88	0.65		3.68	0.76		3.52	0.84		3.61	0.78	
⑥ > 25	241	13.8	4.02	0.66		3.79	0.80		3.69	0.82		3.76	0.78	
Post hoc			⑥ > ②, ③, ④			⑥ > ③, ④			⑥ > ②, ③, ④					

education tend to possess greater problem-solving, leadership, and management abilities (Aiken et al., 2014).

In addition, the results indicate that duration in administrative positions significantly affects intention to stay in the nursing field. In this study, participants with less than a year of administrative experience were more likely to express an intention to leave than their more experienced peers. Nursing administrators face daunting challenges and must grapple with a burgeoning workload that is compounded by personnel shortages (Chang, Lu, & Lin, 2010; Lin, Huang, Kao, & Lu, 2013). Past studies indicate that nursing seniority affects the adoption of strategies. Senior administrators are more likely to adopt positive

Domain 5			Domain 6			Domain 7			Domain 8		
Mean	*SD*	*p*	Mean	*SD*	*p*	Mean	*SD*	*p*	Mean	*SD*	*p*
		.000			.000			.000			.000
3.66	0.80		3.75	0.83		3.96	0.69		3.92	0.69	
3.40	0.79		3.34	0.88		3.67	0.70		3.76	0.75	
3.30	0.82		3.18	0.94		3.45	0.83		3.60	0.77	
3.27	0.74		2.90	0.86		3.42	0.92		3.58	0.73	
① > ②, ③, ④			① > ②, ③, ④			① > ②, ③, ④			① > ②, ③, ④		
		.000			.316			.013			.000
3.29	0.82		3.33	0.89		3.6	0.72		3.70	0.73	
3.48	0.78		3.41	0.90		3.71	0.73		3.80	0.77	
3.42	0.81		3.36	0.91		3.65	0.78		3.71	0.76	
3.65	0.74		3.50	0.90		3.81	0.81		3.96	0.64	
3.88	0.68		3.46	0.93		3.93	0.76		4.17	0.50	
① < ②, ④, ⑤; ③ < ⑤									① < ④, ⑤; ③ < ④, ⑤		
		.024			.064			.001			.154
3.17	0.41		3.33	0.52		3.50	0.84		3.67	0.82	
3.32	0.76		3.26	0.89		3.53	0.75		3.68	0.72	
3.42	0.82		3.36	0.90		3.66	0.76		3.74	0.77	
3.51	0.81		3.46	0.94		3.78	0.75		3.82	0.71	
④ > ②						④ > ②					
		.000			.000			.032			.066
3.31	0.85		3.24	0.97		3.60	0.77		3.75	0.78	
3.40	0.82		3.41	0.87		3.65	0.78		3.70	0.77	
3.42	0.80		3.34	0.88		3.62	0.77		3.67	0.78	
3.38	0.81		3.32	0.92		3.69	0.70		3.73	0.74	
3.51	0.80		3.44	0.89		3.69	0.80		3.81	0.73	
3.60	0.73		3.56	0.83		3.79	0.71		3.85	0.64	
⑥ > ①			⑥ > ①								
		.000			.000			.000			.000
3.44	0.97		3.48	1.09		3.81	0.74		4.07	0.87	
3.32	0.82		3.34	0.97		3.61	0.76		3.73	0.76	
3.34	0.83		3.26	0.94		3.57	0.78		3.67	0.79	
3.34	0.80		3.30	0.88		3.60	0.75		3.68	0.76	
3.57	0.78		3.45	0.87		3.76	0.70		3.81	0.71	
3.61	0.76		3.60	0.86		3.86	0.79		3.92	0.66	
⑥ > ②, ③, ④			⑥ > ③, ④			⑥ > ③, ④			⑥ > ③, ④		

thinking strategies, whereas junior administrators tend to opt for evasive strategies and to seek support (Chen, Hsu, Yin, Lin, & Chang, 2012; Gellis & Kim, 2004; Shirey, McDaniel, Ebright, Fisher, & Doebbeling, 2010). Therefore, it is imperative to provide adequate leadership and management training for junior nursing administrators to support their adaptation and problem-solving abilities (Dehghani et al., 2016; Lin et al., 2013).

Conclusions/Implications for Practice

Participants in this study earned an average work environment satisfaction score of 3.59, indicating that there remains

TABLE 4.
Correlations Between Intention to Stay and Work Environment Satisfaction (N = 1,748)

Domain	*M*	*SD*	Stay (*n* = 1,630) *M*	Stay (*n* = 1,630) *SD*	Not Stay(*n* = 118) *M*	Not Stay(*n* = 118) *SD*	*p*	*OR*	95% CI
1. Safe practice environment	3.83	0.70	3.86	0.69	3.45	0.81	< .001	0.46	[0.36, 0.59]
2. Quality and quantity of staff	3.61	0.51	3.65	0.80	3.18	0.84	< .001	0.51	[0.41, 0.63]
3. Workload, salary, and welfare	3.45	0.87	3.49	0.85	2.87	0.94	< .001	0.46	[0.36, 0.57]
4. Professional specialization and team collaboration	3.62	0.77	3.65	0.75	3.10	0.90	< .001	0.42	[0.36, 0.53]
5. Work simplification	3.43	0.81	3.47	0.78	2.82	0.96	< .001	0.38	[0.30, 0.48]
6. Informatics	3.38	0.91	3.42	0.89	2.78	0.95	< .001	0.48	[0.39, 0.58]
7. Personal growth and professional development	3.67	0.76	3.71	0.73	3.06	0.94	< .001	0.37	[0.30, 0.47]
8. Support and caring	3.75	0.75	3.80	0.71	3.07	0.88	< .001	0.31	[0.25, 0.40]
Total	3.59	0.61	3.63	0.68	3.04	0.70	< .001	0.20	[0.15, 0.28]

Note. CI = confidence interval.

significant room for improvement in practice environments and work conditions in hospitals in Taiwan. The eight domains of nursing work environment quality may all be used to predict nursing administrator retention. The informatics domain received the lowest level of satisfaction and thus warrants special attention. In addition, time spent in administrative positions was found to correlate significantly with retention. The domain of support and caring is particularly indicative of intention to stay among junior administrators. Therefore, nursing departments should increase their focus on developing strategies to assist and encourage junior administrators to strengthen the career prospects and satisfaction of these individuals.

TABLE 5.
The Effects on Intention to Stay of Duration in Administrative Positions and Work Environment Satisfaction (N = 1,748)

Item	*p*	*OR*	95% CI
Duration in administrative positions (years)			
< 1	.074	0.58	[0.26, 1.07]
1–3	.334	1.52	[0.65, 3.58]
4–6	.520	0.78	[0.36, 1.67]
7–9	.168	0.57	[0.26, 1.26]
10–14	.681	0.84	[0.37, 1.92]
1. Safe practice environment	.850	1.03	[0.75, 1.43]
2. Quality and quantity of staff	.687	1.06	[0.78, 1.44]
3. Workload, salary, and welfare	.384	1.14	[0.85, 1.55]
4. Professional specialization and team collaboration	.370	1.17	[0.83, 1.64]
5. Work simplification	.404	1.17	[0.81, 1.70]
6. Informatics	.613	1.08	[0.80, 1.45]
7. Personal growth and professional development	.312	1.22	[0.83, 1.77]
8. Support and caring	< .001	1.98	[1.40, 2.81]

Note. CI = confidence interval.

Acknowledgments

This study was funded by the Ministry of Health and Welfare, Taiwan. We would like to acknowledge the assistance from TUNA, local nurses associations, and participating hospitals in organizing the workshops. We are especially grateful to all of the survey respondents who made this study possible.

References

Aiken, L. H., Sloane, D. M., Bruyneel, L., Van den Heede, K., Griffiths, P., Busse, R., ... Sermeus, W. (2014). Nurse staffing and education and hospital mortality in nine European countries: A retrospective observational study. *The Lancet, 383*(9931), 1824–1830. https://doi.org/10.1016/S0140-6736(13)62631-8

Balouch, R., & Hassan, F. (2014). Determinants of job satisfaction and its impact on employee performance and turnover intentions. *International Journal of Learning & Development, 4*(2), 120–140. https://doi.org/10.5296/ijld.v4i2.6094

Chang, H. L., & Lin, C. F. (2016). Taiwanese registered nurses' reasons for failure to practice. *International Journal of Nursing & Clinical Practices, 3,* Article ID 3. https://doi.org/10.15344/2394-4978/2016/176

Chang, H. L., Lu, M. S., & Lin, C. F. (2010). Factors related to new nursing staff turnover rates. *The Journal of Health Science,*

12(3), 161–172. (Original work published in Chinese)

Chen, H. C. (2009). International connection: The current and development of nursing informatics in Taiwan. *The Journal of Nursing, 56*(3), 5–11. https://doi.org/10.6224/JN.58.3.21 (Original work published in Chinese)

Chen, Y. C. (2011). Reformation of the nursing administration and management system. *The Journal of Nursing, 58*(3), 21–26. (Original work published in Chinese)

Chen, Y. C., Hsu, M. Y., Yin, Y. C., Lin, L. Y., & Chang, S. C. (2012). An exploration of hospital nurse manager job stress and job stress coping strategies. *Journal of Nursing and Healthcare Research, 8*(2), 94–105. https://doi.org/10.6225/JNHR.08.2.94 (Original work published in Chinese)

Dehghani, K., Nasiriani, K., & Salimi, T. (2016). Requirements for nurse supervisor training: A qualitative content analysis. *Iranian Journal of Nursing and Midwifery Research, 21*(1), 63–70. https://doi.org/10.4103/1735-9066.174760

Force, M. V. (2005). The relationship between effective nurse managers and nursing retention. *The Journal of Nursing Administration, 35*(7–8), 336–341. https://doi.org/10.1188/05.ONF.765-772

Friese, C. R. (2005). Nurse practice environments and outcomes: Implication for oncology nursing. *Oncology Nursing Forum, 32*(4), 765–772.

Gao, F. L. (2015). *Exploring the correlation between acceptance and effectiveness of nursing records computerization information system among nursing staff—The case of a mental hospital* (Unpublished master's thesis). Department of Health Care Administration, Chang Jung Christian University, Tainan City, Taiwan, ROC. https://doi.org/10.6833/CJCU.2015.00013 (Original work published in Chinese)

Gellis, Z. D., & Kim, J. C. (2004). Predictors of depressive mood, occupational stress, and propensity to leave in older and younger mental health case managers. *Community Mental Health Journal, 40*(5), 407–421. https://doi.org/10.1023/B:COMH.0000040655.09817.e8

Holden, J. (2006). How can we improve the nursing work environment? *MCN: The American Journal of Maternal/Child Nursing, 31*(1), 34–38.

Holston-Okae, B. L. (2017). *Employee turnover intentions in the hospitality industry* (Unpublished doctoral dissertation). College of Management and Technology, Walden University, Minneapolis, Minnesota, USA.

Huang, C. I., & Lu, M. S. (2015). Linking transformational, transactional and authentic leadership to nurses' retention. *Yuan Yuan Nursing, 9*(1), 5–11. https://doi.org/10.6530/YYN/2015.5.01 (Original work published in Chinese)

Huang, C. I., Yu, C., & Yu, C. C. (2016). An exploration of working conditions and flexible system for hospital nurses. *The Journal of Nursing, 63*(2), 80–90. https://doi.org/10.6224/JN.63.2.80 (Original work published in Chinese)

Hung, C. Y. (2012). *The nursing professionals' adoption process of nursing e-learning information system: The construction of e-management model of continuing nursing education* (Unpublished master's thesis). Yuan Ze University, Taoyuan City, Taiwan, ROC. (Original work published in Chinese)

International Council of Nurses. (2007). *Positive practice environments: Quality workplaces = quality patient care—Information and action tool kit.* Retrieved from https://www.twna.org.tw/frontend/un16_commission/webPages_4/IND/1.pdf

Kaur, A., Kaur, S., Kalia, R., & Kumar, P. (2010). A study on "nursing manpower requirement in neo-natal intensive care unit": PGIMER, Chandigarh. *Nursing and Midwifery Research Journal, 6*(1), 1–13.

Kramer, M., & Schmalenberg, C. (2005). Revising the essentials of magnetism tool: There is more to adequate staffing than numbers. *The Journal of Nursing Administration, 35*(48), 188–198.

Lin, C. F., Huang, C. I., Kao, C. C., & Lu, M. S. (2013). The nursing shortage and nursing retention strategies in Taiwan. *The Journal of Nursing, 60*(3), 88–93. https://doi.org/10.6224/JN.60.3.88 (Original work published in Chinese)

Lin, C. F., Lu, M. S., & Huang, H. Y. (2016). The psychometric properties and the development of the indicators of quality nursing work environments in Taiwan. *The Journal of Nursing Research, 24*(1), 9–20. https://doi.org/10.1097/jnr.0000000000000106

Lin, S. J., & Huang, L. H. (2014). Centennial retrospective on the evolution and development of the nursing practice environment in Taiwan. *The Journal of Nursing, 61*(4, Suppl.), 35–45. https://doi.org/10.6224/JN.61.4S.35 (Original work published in Chinese)

Ma, S. C., Wang, H. H., & Chen, J. Y. (2011). Concept analysis of workplace bullying. *The Journal of Nursing, 58*(4), 81–86. (Original work published in Chinese)

Markey, R., Ravenswood, K., & Webber, D. J. (2012). The impact of the quality of the work environment on employees' intention to quit. *Economics Working Paper Series, 1220*, 1–35. Retrieved from https://www2.uwe.ac.uk/faculties/BBS/BUS/Research/economics2012/1221.pdf

Schmalenberg, C., & Kramer, M. (2008). Essentials of a productive nurse work environment. *Nursing Research, 57*(1), 2–13. https://doi.org/10.1097/01.NNR.0000280657.04008.2a

Shirey, M. R., McDaniel, A. M., Ebright, P. R., Fisher, M. L., & Doebbeling, B. N. (2010). Understanding nurse manager stress and work complexity: Factors that make a difference. *The Journal of Nursing Administration, 40*(2), 82–91. https://doi.org/10.1097/NNA.0b013e3181cb9f88

Warshawsky, N. E., Wiggins, A. T., & Rayens, M. K. (2016). The influence of the practice environment on nurse managers' job satisfaction and intent to leave. *The Journal of Nursing Administration, 46*(10), 501–507. https://doi.org/10.1097/NNA.0000000000000393

Wu, W. R., & Hung, C. H. (2009). Change management and implementing a nursing information system. *The Kaohsiung Journal of Nursing, 26*(1), 91–98. (Original work published in Chinese)

Yildirim, A., & Yildirim, D. (2007). Mobbing in the workplace by peers and managers: Mobbing experienced by nurses working in healthcare facilities in Turkey and its effect on nurses. *Journal of Clinical Nursing, 16*(8), 1444–1453. https://doi.org/10.1111/j.1365-27022006.01814.x

9

The Related Factors of Nurses' Participation and Perceived Benefits and Barriers in Health Policy Making

Masoumeh BARZEGAR SAFARI[1] • Mohammadkarim BAHADORI[2*] • Khalil ALIMOHAMMADZADEH[3]

ABSTRACT

Background: Nurses play a critical role in providing good health services.

Purpose: The aim of this study was to examine the factors related to the participation of nurses in the provision of health services and the perceived benefits and barriers to their participation in health policy making.

Methods: A cross-sectional descriptive study was conducted in several hospitals affiliated with the Iran University of Medical Sciences during the first half of 2018 on a sample size of 220 people. A standard, self-management questionnaire was used to collect the data, and SPSS 21.0 software was used for data analysis. None of the demographic characteristics were found to be significantly associated with nurse participation in or the perceived barriers and benefits to health policy making.

Results: The results of this study show that the participants were involved only moderately in health policy making. "Providing written reports on problems or receiving consultation from a related official" was the performance item most frequently cited by the participants in terms of involvement, whereas "Disappointment in work procedures" was the most frequently cited barrier item affecting involvement.

Conclusions/Implications for Practice: Despite the importance of the nursing role in health polices, this study indicates that nurses participate at only a moderate level in health policy-making activities. Providing more information to nurses regarding health policies, enhancing nurses' image of their job and their perceptions about the importance of their participation in the health policy, increasing partnerships with nurses at the upper levels of health services management, and supporting nursing professional organizations in the field of health policy are potential strategies for encouraging greater nursing participation in health policy making.

KEY WORDS:
nurse, health policy, participation, barriers, benefits.

Introduction

Historically, healthcare systems invest most heavily on illness-related care. This emphasis on illness instead of health has given rise to the notion of medical priority and produces substandard economic and health outcomes (Peters, 2002). The mission of a healthcare system is to ensure societal health, which is only fulfilled through the favorable provision of services. The only way to achieve this is to make provisions for the constituent elements of service delivery. As a critical component of health service delivery in all countries, nurses contribute to public health policies as key actors (Clarke , Swider, & Bigley, 2013). Nurses are the largest group of healthcare workers involved in healthcare service delivery (Lewinski & Simmons, 2018). Moreover, the more than 35 million people estimated to work as nurses worldwide make nurses the largest workforce in the health system (Shariff, 2014). Given the rapid development and transformation of healthcare systems, it is incumbent upon nurses to advance in line with these changes. To this end, nurses must be involved in formulating health policies rather than merely implementing these policies (Shariff, 2015).

Health policies are basically policies that are directly associated with the governmental health sector in any country (Shariff, 2014). These policies involve areas such as healthcare services, costs, and healthcare quality and access. Quality provision, accessibility, and cost-effectiveness improve the quality of life and welfare of society (Heydari et al., 2013). The participation of nurses in the development of health policies ensures safe, effective, accessible, and low-cost services (Jivraj Shariff, 2015). Health policies affect the nursing profession and healthcare (Shariff, 2015).

Discussions about health policies and health-policy reforms have focused increasingly on the need for greater participation by nurses and midwives. This need was first identified formally in 2000 and gained a significantly higher

[1]MSc, Nurse, Health Economics Policy Research Center, Tehran Medical Sciences Branch, Islamic Azad University, Tehran, Iran • [2]PhD, Professor, Health Management Research Center, Baqiyatallah University of Medical Sciences, Tehran, Iran • [3]PhD, MD, Associate Professor, Department of Healthcare Management, School of Management and Social Sciences, North Tehran Branch, Islamic Azad University, Health Economics policy Research Center, Tehran Medical Sciences Islamic Azad University, Tehran, Iran.

profile through its inclusion in the 2002 World Health Organization (WHO) Report. Political participation includes involvement in political development processes, including identification of policy areas and policy formulation, implementation, evaluation, and modification (AbuAlRub & Foudeh, 2017).

Despite receiving encouragement to participate, nurses are notably absent from health policy reforms in comparison with other health-affiliated professions and groups (Ditlopo, Blaauw, Penn-Kekana, & Rispel, 2014). The central role of nurses in health service delivery helps explain their commitment to change policies from ethical and professional standpoints (Sayers & DiGiacomo, 2010; Shariff, 2014; Whitehead, 2003). The presence of nurses alongside patients during major life events such as births, illnesses, and recovery has indeed put them in an optimal position to provide health policy information (AbuAlRub & Foudeh, 2017). With their knowledge and experience acquired in the work environment, nurses enjoy a unique position in the health team that allows them to contribute to health policies by enabling effective strategies (Etowa et al., 2016). These characteristics increase the need for greater nursing involvement (AbuAlRub & Foudeh, 2017). Studies point to limited nursing participation in health policy development activities (Shariff, 2015). This may be attributed to the unheard voice of this hardworking group (Cheraghi , Ghiyasvandian, & Aarabi, 2015); the lack of nursing involvement at the higher levels of the healthcare system (Shariff, 2014); the lack of a proper understanding of the reasons or benefits of participation (AbuAlRub & Foudeh, 2017); the lack of knowledge, skill, support, time, negative perceptions of the nursing profession in society; and the lack of authority and available structural resources (Shariff, 2014). Many nurses attempt to play a political role that allows them to influence the activities of health policies directly (Whitehead, 2003). To exert influence in the world of politics, nursing leaders need to have certain characteristics that enable them to develop health policies effectively (Jivraj Shariff, 2015). In Iran, nurses engage in health policy activities through governmental and nongovernmental organizations. Governmental organizations include the Deputy of Nursing in the Ministry of Health and the national Board of Nursing. Nongovernmental organizations include the Iranian Nursing Organization, Iranian Nursing Association, Iranian Nursing Scientific Association, and Iranian Cardiac Nursing Association (Esmaeili, Dehghan-Nayeri, & Negarandeh, 2013). Unfortunately, despite the struggle over the past three decades by Iranian nurses to increase their participation in the policy-making process, their position in this process remains unclear (Cheraghi et al., 2015). All of the studies addressing the participation of Iranian nurses in health policy activities have been qualitative, with no related quantitative studies published. This study was conducted in 2018 with the aim of examining the involvement of Iranian nurses in health policy activities and studying the involvement-related benefits, barriers, and health outcomes. The questions asked in this study included: (a) What is the level of involvement of Iranian nurses in health policy activities? (b) What are the perceived benefits of involvement in health policy activities? (c) What are the perceived barriers to participation in health policy activities?

Methods

Design

This was a descriptive cross-sectional study conducted in several hospitals affiliated to Iran University of Medical Sciences during the first half of 2018.

Statistical Population

The statistical population consisted of 530 nurses working in six hospitals, including Shohadaye Haftome Tir, Lolagar, Shohadaye Yaftabad, Shahid Fahmideh, Hazrat Fatemeh (in Robat Karim), and Imam Sajjad. Two hundred twenty nurses were selected from the statistical population using the Krejcie and Morgan table and enrolled as participants. Cluster and stratified sampling was used, with hospitals used as clusters and hospital units used as stratum. The six hospitals were selected randomly from among the hospitals in the Iran University of Medical of Sciences hospital network, and samples were identified in each of the selected hospitals based on the population of each. The inclusion criteria included having at least a bachelor's degree in nursing and 2 years of work experience.

Data Collection Instrument

Data were collected using a standard self-management questionnaire that was developed in 2000 by Eden et al. (as cited in Juma, Edwards, & Spitzer, 2014), modified by Salvador (Lewinski & Simmons, 2018) in 2010, and used by AbuAlRub in 2016 (AbuAlRub & Foudeh, 2017). This questionnaire comprises four sections, as follows: (a) Demographic information; (b) Participation in health policies, which refers to any activity the purpose or impact of which involves governmental activities that influence the formulation or implementation of public health policies or are indirectly linked to related policy decision-makers. This section includes a 17-item checklist that is scored on a 5-point Likert scale ranging from 1 = *no involvement* to 5 = *strong involvement*; (c) Perceived barriers by nurses, which involves factors that personally prevent activities, with positive outcomes measured using a 19-item checklist scored on a nominal scale of 1 = *yes* and 0 = *no*; (4) Perceived benefits by participants that deals with the perceived positive outcomes from the result of activities and includes 17 items on a nominal scale of 1 = *yes* and 0 = *no*. Participation by participants was assessed as low level of involvement (1–2), moderate level of involvement (3), and high level of involvement (4–5). The total score for participation was based on the mean of the answers to the questions, whereas the total scores of the perceived barriers and benefits were based on the sum of positive answers (Salvador, 2010).

The WHO guidelines were used for the translation and cultural adaptation of the questionnaire into Persian (WHO, n.d.). This process included the following four steps: (1) Forward translation: In this step, the English version was translated into Persian by a translator who was completely familiar with the nursing field, concepts, and terminology and whose mother language was Persian. (2) Expert panel: The translation was reviewed by an expert committee, including a translator and a research team. This committee examined the translation thoroughly based on criteria such as grammar, use of proper equivalents, proper placement of parts of speech, precision, comprehensibility, and lack of ambiguous terms. The result of this process produced a complete translated version of the questionnaire. (3) Back translation: Using the same approach as outlined in Step 1, the Persian questionnaire was translated back into English by an independent translator whose mother tongue is English and who had no prior knowledge of the questionnaire. The back-translated English questionnaire was then compared and discussed with the original version in terms of conceptual equivalence in two sessions that were attended by the translators and the research team to verify its equivalence. (4) Pretesting and cognitive interviews: The Persian version was distributed to 30 participants as a pilot test to determine clarity and accuracy of meaning. These participants provided their feedback. After conducting the test, all of the findings were reexamined by the committee, and the Persian questionnaire was modified and finalized. A Cronbach's alpha of .77 was obtained for the questionnaire at this stage. The validity and reliability of the questionnaire were evaluated using content validity and Cronbach's alpha, respectively. After development, the questionnaire was sent to a group of nursing and health management professors to seek their opinions regarding content validity. Five of the six professors verified that the questionnaire provided good validity. The content validity ratio and the final Cronbach's alpha of the questionnaire were .83 and 85%, respectively.

Data Collection Method

At the beginning of the research implementation, the researcher in charge of data collection visited the hospital administrators and matrons of the selected hospitals to make the necessary arrangements. The process was followed by holding a brief briefing session with the managers of the nursing departments on the research subject. The opinions of the participating nurses were then collected via the questionnaires. Data collection lasted for a period of 3 weeks. The person in charge of the data collection distributed and collected the questionnaires.

Data Analysis

Descriptive statistics were used to analyze the descriptive data. Because the data were not normal, nonparametric Mann–Whitney and Kruskal–Wallis tests were used to examine the associations between the demographic characteristics and participation and the perceived barriers and benefits. Data were analyzed using SPSS Version 21.0 (IBM, Inc., Armonk, NY, USA).

Ethical Considerations

The following fundamental principles were taken into account as ethical considerations in this research. The study was verified by the ethics committee of Islamic Azad University, Tehran Medical Branch (code: IR.IAU.TMU.REC.1396.05); letters of introduction were offered upon visiting different hospitals and departments; the aim of the study and method by which the findings would be used were clearly explained to the participants during the data collection process; participation in the study and responding to the questionnaire items were completely voluntary; participants could stop cooperating with the researcher at any stage of the research; the questionnaires were distributed to all of the participants in a completely anonymous manner in order to observe ethical principles, maintain the dignity of the personnel, and observe information confidentiality; reports were not presented on an individual or case-by-case basis; and findings were analyzed in a completely anonymous and cumulative manner.

Results

Two hundred twenty nurses participated in this study, with 166 (76.1%) women and 52 (23.9%) men. Mean age and work experience were 33.54 ± 4.60 and 8.93 ± 3.53 years, respectively. Most participants were married (52.7%), held a bachelor's degree (92.2%), and worked rotating shift works (83.2%).

The nursing performance in health policy-making participation is shown in Table 1. "Providing written reports of the problems or receiving consultation from a related official" and "Verifying or studying related legal affairs to health policies" were, respectively, the performance items most and least frequently cited by the participants.

The perceived barriers to participation in health policy making by nurses is shown in Table 2. "Disappointment with work procedures" and "Lack of any barriers" were, respectively, the barrier items most and least frequently cited by the participants.

The perceived benefits of participation in health policy making by nurses is shown in Table 3. "Resolution of nursing challenges by nurses" and "Helping those incapable of creating changes" were, respectively, the benefit items most and least frequently cited by the participants.

The associations between the demographic characteristics and participation and perceived barriers and benefits are shown in Table 4. No significant association was identified between any of the demographic characteristics and participation, perceived barriers, or perceived benefits.

Discussion

The results of this study show that the most frequent health policy activities that the participants were involved was "Providing written reports of the problems or receiving

TABLE 1.
Nursing Participation in Health Policy Making

No.	Activity Type	Mean	*SD*
1.	Objection to or disagreement with a health policy-related issue	2.50	1.02
2.	Providing written reports of the problems or receiving consultation from a related official	3.29	1.16
3.	Presenting a plan on the health policy law to higher authorities	2.05	1.09
4.	Contributing to the selection of most competent individuals for related positions	2.44	1.12
5.	Membership in nursing associations and nursing political organizations	2.19	1.09
6.	Communicating information on health policies to applicants or other professions	2.14	0.89
7.	Offering and publishing critiques on health policies in academic conferences	2.30	1.24
8.	Participating in various elections of the nursing system	3.14	1.16
9.	Establishing contact with a related official to health policies	2.75	1.02
10.	Verifying or studying related legal affairs to health policies	1.79	0.92
11.	Campaign advertising in health-related issues for candidates	2.09	1.11
12.	Giving speeches on health policy-related issues in nursing conferences	2.53	1.14
13.	Running for a health policy-related position	2.30	1.06
14.	Using mass media to shed light on health policies	2.94	1.21
15.	Other activities (e.g. discussing certain health policy-making issues in daily reports, sending e-mails to the Ministry of Health and Medical Education with regard to health policy making, and discussing health policy making in nursing associations)	2.82	1.05
16.	Cooperating with a committee or group to develop health policies	2.78	1.05
17.	Investing in a health-related electoral campaign or policy making	2.06	1.29
18.	Participation	2.75	0.94

consultation from a related official." This finding is at odds with previous studies of Jordanian and U.S. nurses, which found voting for a candidate and making health policy proposals to be the most frequent health policy activities in which nurses were involved (AbuAlRub & Foudeh, 2017; Vandenhouten, Malakar, Kubsch, Block, & Gallagher-Lepak, 2011).

Furthermore, the results of this study indicate that Iranian nurses are only moderately involved in health policy making. This differs from the results of AbuAIRub and Foudeh (2017), who found that Jordanian nurses had a low level of involvement in health policy. In another study conducted on South African nurses, the results found a suboptimal level of involvement among the vast majority of nurses, which supports the findings of this study (Ditlopo et al., 2014). Similar to many other countries, the role of Iranian nurses in developing political processes is limited to the implementation of approved policies (Shariff, 2015). Given that an adequate understanding of health issues, laws, and policies is a prerequisite for being involved in health policy activities, another reason for limited nursing participation may be a lack of sufficient understanding of this issue (AbuAlRub & Foudeh, 2017). The primarily unheard voice of the nursing community is yet another factor that may account the persistently low level of nursing participation in health policy making (Cheraghi et al., 2015).

The results of this study show that the most frequently perceived benefits to nurses being involved in health policies were "Resolution of nursing challenges by nurses," followed by "Nursing independence" and "Personal satisfaction of feeling of service" (building self-confidence in nurses). These findings differ from those of Oden, Price, Alteneder, Boardley, and Ubokudom, (2000), who reported "Improving the health of the public" and "Making a difference in others' lives" as the most frequently cited perceived benefits (Oden et al., 2000). Nursing involvement may also be supported by educational programs, standing as candidates for political and administrative positions and finding sponsors for other candidates (AbuAlRub & Foudeh, 2017). Based on the findings of previous studies, the involvement of nurses in the health policy development process is positively associated with gaining experience and participating in political development, having a model to follow, receiving training and acquiring knowledge about health systems and political development processes, having a political orientation, conducting research, providing support through professional organizations, and developing managerial skills (Shariff, 2014). International nursing associations have proposed coordinating nursing activities, maintaining union with the profession, and developing a powerful leadership as ways of increasing nursing involvement and have thus made related investments in academic structures to expand the effective involvement of nurses in the development of global health policies (Gimbel, Kohler, Mitchell, & Emami, 2017). The Institute of Medicine

TABLE 2.
Perceived Barriers to Participation in Health Policy Making by Nurses

No.	Activity Type	Frequency	Percentage
1.	Disappointment in the work procedure	111	50.45
2.	Lack of external support	107	48.64
3.	Lack of time	103	46.82
4.	Lack of access to key figures	103	46.82
5.	Diverging values or attitudes of policy makers	99	45.00
6.	limitations in adopting individual viewpoints	88	40.00
7.	lack of financial support or other resources	78	35.45
8.	Other barriers (nursing shortage, workload, or resistance to the implementation of certain policies)	76	34.55
9.	Lack of political knowledge	71	32.27
10.	Lack of any change with my participation	59	26.82
11.	Unclear path to gaining necessary information in this regard	59	26.82
12.	Unclear nature of the efficacy of political activity	54	24.55
13.	Individual opposition to contradictory viewpoints	53	24.09
14.	Disagreement by others	49	22.27
15.	Lack of change through political activity	35	15.91
16.	Personal priorities	32	14.55
17.	Lack of relevance to the field of nursing	21	9.55
18.	Lack of proper understanding of creating changes	16	7.27
19.	Lack of any barriers	13	5.91

TABLE 3.
Perceived Benefits of Participation in Health Policy Making by Nurses

No.	Activity Type	Frequency	Percentage
1.	Resolution of nursing challenges by nurses	124	56.36
2.	Nursing independence	115	52.27
3.	Personal satisfaction of feeling of service (building self-confidence in nurses)	109	49.55
4.	Developing the capacity for participation in political activity across all nursing specialties	103	46.82
5.	Sense of fulfilling professional obligations	88	40.00
6.	Realizing individual potentials for initiative	84	36.18
7.	Professional progress	75	34.09
8.	Progress in the job or health policy making issues	74	33.64
9.	Public health promotion in society	72	32.73
10.	Other benefits (e.g., enhanced healthcare quality, safety, risk prevention, and nursing empowerment)	66	30.00
11.	Creating opportunity for new skill building	65	29.55
12.	Communicating with others	59	26.82
13.	Ability to impact the health of numerous people	45	20.45
14.	Lack of any benefit	43	20.55
15.	Contributing to the implementation of individual work plans	30	13.64
16.	Creating changes in people's lives	25	11.36
17.	Helping those incapable of creating changes	23	10.45

TABLE 4.

Associations Between Demographic Characteristics and Participation and Perceived Barriers and Benefits

Variable	Participation (*M* ± *SD*)	Perceived Barriers (*M* ± *SD*)	Perceived Benefits (*M* ± *SD*)
Marital status			
Single	2.70 ± 0.91	5.62 ± 4.52	5.62 ± 5.05
Married	2.82 ± 0.95	5.56 ± 4.09	5.32 ± 4.56
Mann–Whitney test	4117	5845	5970
Z	−1.079	−0.278	−0.009
p	.28	.78	.99
Gender			
Male	2.84 ± 0.72	5.30 ± 4.79	5.73 ± 5.15
Female	2.73 ± 1.00	5.70 ± 4.13	5.40 ± 4.69
Mann–Whitney test	3036.5	3859	4222
Z	−0.773	−1.160	−0.242
p	.44	.24	.80
Work shift			
Fixed	2.85 ± 1.00	6.02 ± 4.69	5.38 ± 4.76
Rotating	2.73 ± 0.93	5.04 ± 4.20	5.37 ± 4.79
Mann–Whitney test	2391	3191	3206
Z	−0.807	−0.554	−0.519
p	.42	.58	.60
Education			
Bachelor's degrees	2.78 ± 0.95	5.54 ± 4.29	5.41 ± 4.75
Master's and PhD degrees	2.67 ± 0.54	5.37 ± 4.09	5.06 ± 4.71
Mann–Whitney test	4117	5845	5970
Z	−1.079	−0.278	−0.993
p	.67	.94	.88
Age group (years)			
< 30	2.63 ± 0.90	5.08 ± 3.81	4.63 ± 4.23
30–40	2.77 ± 0.93	5.83 ± 4.45	5.81 ± 4.88
> 40	3.32 ± 1.12	5.64 ± 4.82	5.58 ± 4.28
χ^2	5.045	0.844	2.947
df	2	2	2
p	.80	.65	.22
Work experience (years)			
≤ 5	2.61 ± 0.96	5.76 ± 4.98	4.69 ± 4.55
6–10	2.76 ± 0.92	5.53 ± 3.93	5.59 ± 4.63
11–20	2.85 ± 0.97	5.53 ± 4.50	5.27 ± 5.24
χ^2	2.408	0.192	1.665
df	2	2	2
p	.30	.90	.43

underlined the need for health policy education in health specialization programs in its 2003 report (Heiman, Smith, McKool, Mitchell, & Roth, 2015).

On the other hand, the most frequently perceived barriers to involvement by Iranian nurses found in this study were "Disappointment in work procedures," followed by "Lack of external support" and "Lack of time." These findings are consistent with the results of AbuAIRub and Foudeh (2017) and Oden et al. (2000). In another study, understanding the existing clinical concerns and responsibilities; inadequate time to formulate, implement, or modify policies; lack of a proper understanding of the reasons for and benefits of involvement; and an incorrect understanding of professional boundaries that excludes political development were identified as the most important barriers to the involvement of nurses and midwives in political development (Etowa et al., 2016). Furthermore, other studies have identified lack of supportive organizational structures, inadequate political and policy development skills, insufficient time, lack of resources, and insufficient involvement in policy formulation committees as key barriers to involvement (Akunja, Kaseje, Obago, & Ochieng, 2012; Cramer, 2002; Kunaviktikul et al., 2010; Richter et al., 2013). Proper management, political authority, and education have also been determined as important factors contributing to the positive resolution of barriers to nursing involvement in the design of health policy making (AbuAlRub & Foudeh, 2017). In Iran, nurses are more involved in caring for patients, and in recent years, the process of hospital accreditation has been increasingly long and burdensome on all hospital employees. This has further contributed to nurses in Iran having little time available for involvement in health policy activities.

The results of this study indicate no significant association between any of the demographic characteristics and nurses' participation, perceived barriers, and perceived benefits. AbuAlRub and Foudeh (2017) found that holding the position of staff nurse was associated with a lower level of participation in health policy. In addition, Vandenhouten and colleagues found that psychological engagement, resources, and recruitment networks explained 55% of the variance in the political participation of nurses (Vandenhouten et al., 2011).

The researchers emphasize the use of research as valid documents for understanding the political trend of nurses, despite evidence indicating that they lack adequate support for producing documents. In low- and average-income countries, nurses tend not to receive sufficient training and lack access to the instructors and resources necessary to undertake research. Thus, there is a great need to increase the research capacity of nurses to enhance their skills in understanding, developing, and utilizing politically beneficial knowledge (Juma et al., 2014). Limitations to political involvement in low- and average-income countries arise from the perceived sociocultural issues involved in the nursing profession (Etowa et al., 2016). Moreover, academic cooperation with national, regional, and international nursing and nonnursing organizations has been shown to be an effective way of promoting nursing commitment to global health research and policies (Gimbel et al., 2017).

Conclusions

Nurses are in a position to significantly assist policy makers and improve the policy-making process. They should play an important role in health policy activities, particularly in light of their large representation on hospital staff rosters. Despite the importance of the nursing role, this study found only moderate involvement by the participants in health policy making. Several strategies are thus proposed to increase nursing involvement. These strategies include defining and promoting a specific career path for nurses as health policy experts, identifying nurses' positions in health and health policy, providing more information to nurses regarding health policies and related laws, promoting a positive perception of the nursing profession among nurses, creating an understanding of the significance of nursing participation in health policy making among nurses, increasing nursing involvement through the appointment of nurses to high levels of health service management, supporting nursing professional organizations such as the Nursing Organization of the Islamic Republic of Iran to increase the involvement of nurses in health policy making, increasing nursing knowledge and skills by holding retraining workshops with the aim of teaching health policy-making knowledge and skills, and developing incentives for nurses to provide constructive and insightful health policy-making suggestions.

Acknowledgment

This article was derived from a medical-surgical nursing master's thesis written at Islamic Azad University, Tehran Medical Branch. The researchers express their gratitude to all colleagues and individuals who helped with this research.

Author Contributions

Study conception and design: MB, KA
Data collection: MBS
Data analysis and interpretation: MBS
Drafting of the article: MB, MBS
Critical revision of the article: MB

References

AbuAlRub, R. F., & Foudeh, F. N. (2017). Jordanian Nurses' involvement in health policy: Perceived benefits and barriers. *International Nursing Review, 64*(1), 13–21. https://doi.org/10.1111/inr.12249

Akunja, E., Kaseje, D. C. O., Obago, I., & Ochieng, B. M. (2012). Involvement of hub nurses in HIV policy development: Case study of Nyanza Province, Kenya. *Research on Humanities and Social Sciences, 2*(6), 124–134.

Cheraghi, M. A., Ghiyasvandian, S., & Aarabi, A. (2015). Iranian nurses' status in policymaking for nursing in health system: A qualitative content analysis. *The Open Nursing Journal, 9*, 15–24. https://doi.org/10.2174/1874434601509010015

Clarke, P. N., Swider, S., & Bigley, M. B. (2013). Nursing leadership and health policy: A dialogue with nurse leaders. *Nursing Science Quarterly, 26*(2), 136–142. https://doi.org/10.1177/0894318413477146

Cramer, M. E. (2002). Factors influencing organized political participation in nursing. *Policy, Politics & Nursing Practice, 3* (2), 97–107. https://doi.org/10.1177/152715440200300203

Ditlopo, P., Blaauw, D., Penn-Kekana, L., & Rispel, L. C. (2014). Contestations and complexities of nurses' participation in policy-making in South Africa. *Global Health Action, 7*(1), 25327. https://doi.org/10.3402/gha.v7.25327

Esmaeili, M., Dehghan-Nayeri, N., & Negarandeh, R. (2013). Factors impacting membership and non-membership in nursing associations: A qualitative study. *Nursing & Health Sciences, 15*(3), 265–272. https://doi.org/10.1111/nhs.12012

Etowa, J., Vukic, A., Aston, M., Boadu, N. Y., Helwig, M., Macdonald, D., ... George, A. N. (2016). Experiences of midwives and nurses in policy development in low- and middle-income countries: A systematic review protocol. *JBI Database of Systematic Reviews and Implementation Reports, 14*(11), 72–82. https://doi.org/10.11124/JBISRIR-2016-003191

Gimbel, S., Kohler, P., Mitchell, P., & Emami, A. (2017). Creating academic structures to promote nursing's role in global health policy. *International Nursing Review, 64*(1), 117–125. https://doi.org/10.1111/inr.12338

Heiman, H. J., Smith, L. L., McKool, M., Mitchell, D. N., & Roth Bayer, C. (2015). Health policy training: A review of the literature. *International Journal of Environmental Research and Public Health, 13*(1), 20. https://doi.org/10.3390/ijerph13010020

Heydari, A., Mazloum, S. R., Moonaghil, H. K., Mojallil, M., Hosseini Shahidi, L., & Namdar Areshtanab, H. (2013). Educational challenges ahead of nursing from the perspective of faculty members of Mashhad University of Medical Sciences. *Journal of Advances in Medical Education & Professionalism, 1*(4), 125–128.

Jivraj Shariff, N. (2015). A Delphi survey of leadership attributes necessary for national nurse leaders' participation in health policy development: An east African perspective. *BMC Nursing, 14,* 13. https://doi.org/10.1186/s12912-015-0063-0

Juma, P. A., Edwards, N., & Spitzer, D. (2014). Kenyan nurses involvement in national policy development processes. *Nursing Research & Practice, 2014,* 236573–236510. https://doi.org/10.1155/2014/236573

Kunaviktikul, W., Nantsupawat, R., Sngounsiritham, U., Akkadechanunt, T., Chitpakdee, B., Wichaikhum, O. A., ... Chaowalaksakun, P. (2010). Knowledge and involvement of nurses regarding health policy development in Thailand. *Nursing & Health Sciences, 12*(2), 221–227. https://doi.org/10.1111/j.1442-2018.2010.00523.x

Lewinski, A. A., & Simmons, L. A. (2018). Nurse knowledge and engagement in health policy making: Findings from a pilot study. *Journal of Continuing Education in Nursing, 49*(9), 407–415. https://doi.org/10.3928/00220124-20180813-06

Oden, L. S., Price, J. H., Alteneder, R., Boardley, D., & Ubokudom, S. E. (2000). Public policy involvement by nurse practitioners. *Journal of Community Health, 25*(2), 139–155. https://doi.org/10.1023/a:1005181724388

Peters, R. M. (2002). Nurse administrator's role in health policy: Teaching the elephant to dance. *Nursing Administration Quarterly, 26*(4), 1–8. https://doi.org/10.1097/00006216-200207000-00004

Richter, M. S., Mill, J., Muller, C. E., Kahwa, E., Etowa, J., Dawkins, P., & Hepburn, C. (2013). Nurses' engagement in AIDS policy development. *International Nursing Review, 60*(1), 52–58. https://doi.org/10.1111/j.1466-7657.2012.01010.x

Salvador, D. L. (2010). *Registered nurses perceptions and practices related to health policy* (Unpublished doctoral thesis). The University of Toledo, Ohio, USA.

Sayers, J. M., & DiGiacomo, M. (2010). The nurse educator role in Australian hospitals: Implications for health policy. *Collegian, 17*(2), 77–84. https://doi.org/10.1016/j.colegn.2010.04.005

Shariff, N. J. (2014). Factors that act as facilitators and barriers to nurse leaders' participation in health policy development. *BMC Nursing, 13,* 20. https://doi.org/10.1186/1472-6955-13-20

Shariff, N. J. (2015). Empowerment model for nurse leaders' participation in health policy development: An east African perspective. *BMC Nursing, 14,* 31. https://doi.org/10.1186/s12912-015-0078-6

Vandenhouten, C. L., Malakar, C. L., Kubsch, S., Block, D. E., & Gallagher-Lepak, S. (2011). Political participation of registered nurses. *Policy, Politics & Nursing Practice, 12*(3), 159–167. https://doi.org/10.1177/1527154411425189

Whitehead, D. (2003). The health-promoting nurse as a health policy career expert and entrepreneur. *Nurse Education Today, 23*(8), 585–592. https://doi.org/10.1016/s0260-6917(03)00097-2

World Health Organization. (n.d.). *Process of translation and adaptation of instruments.* http://www.who.int/substance_abuse/research_tools/translation/en/

10

Nursing Students' Perceptions of Nursing Metaparadigms: A Phenomenological Study

Ayse DELIKTAS[1] • Oznur KORUKCU[2]* • Ruveyde AYDIN[1] • Kamile KABUKCUOGLU[3]

ABSTRACT

Background: The paradigm is a vital concept steering the development of a scientific discipline. Paradigms that shape the education, research, and practice steps of a discipline are defined as metaparadigms.

Purpose: The purpose of this study was to explore the perception of nursing students regarding metaparadigms in nursing at Akdeniz University in Antalya, Turkey.

Methods: This was designed as a descriptive phenomenological study, and data were collected from 13 fourth-year students who were chosen via a purposeful sampling method and interviewed face-to-face using a semistructured format. Data were analyzed using the data analysis steps of Giorgi, who is an expert in descriptive phenomenological studies.

Results: Most of the participants in this study associated nursing with humanism. Some of the participants stated that a fundamental building block of the nursing profession is conscience, whereas others stated that nursing is a way to touch people's lives and is now regarded as a professional practice. It has been reported that students have difficulties identifying metaparadigms in nursing and that they believe that human beings have the potential to widen their horizons with wisdom and social skills. According to the participants, the health metaparadigm refers to the harmony between human beings and their environment and to the autonomy of the individual. Moreover, the participants emphasized the well-being of individuals.

Conclusions/Implications for Practice: The participants in this study characterized humans with well-being, transcendence, adaptation and interaction skills with their environment, and harmony beyond physiological mechanisms, which was considered to be promising for the perception of future nurses. It is recommended for nursing educators to enable their students to raise their professional awareness and to internalize professional values.

Key Words:
health, nursing, metaparadigm, paradigm, students.

Introduction

Paradigm is a vital concept in the philosophy of science that has far-reaching influence on contemporary empirical studies (Fawcett, 2000). Kuhn (2017) defined paradigm to identify study models that shape scientific activities and the progress of scientific knowledge (Smith & Parker, 2015). Kuhn argued that scientific paradigms determine the study questions, interview methodology, data collection methods, and interpretation of study results. Paradigms shape individual behaviors, influences of social phenomena, and attitudes of professional groups. Therefore, paradigms serve as a guide for professional education, philosophy, morals, and ethical principles (Özkan & Akduran, 2014).

Metaparadigms, or dominant paradigms, map out general parameters of a scientific discipline and focus on scientific efforts. Metaparadigms may include several concrete and specific paradigms for researchers (Meleis, 2011). Clarifying metaparadigms and their fundamental thesis statements facilitates a deeper understanding of the attitudes of professionals and provides a better appreciation of the scope of scientific studies (Kim, 2000).

Nursing metaparadigms were first classified by Fawcett (1978) into the following categories: person, environment, health, and nursing. The human factor metaparadigm refers to individuals in a definite culture, family, and society. The environment metaparadigm characterizes all regional, national, and global cultural, social, political, and economic conditions related to human health. The health metaparadigm defines processes of life and death. The person metaparadigm describes the nursing profession, nursing practices, and nursing objectives and results (Bahramnezhad, Shiri, Asgari, & Afshar, 2015; Fawcett, 2000). In addition to these four metaparadigms, different versions of the nursing metaparadigm have been offered. For instance, Watson considered nursing care to be the core indicator of nursing practice and suggested nursing care as the fifth metaparadigm (Watson, 2008).

In recent years, the conceptual framework of nursing has been used to design nursing curricula. Conceptual frameworks

[1]*MSc, RN, Research Assistant, Faculty of Nursing, Department of Obstetrics & Gynaecological Nursing, Akdeniz University, Turkey.* • [2]*PhD, RN, Associate Professor, Faculty of Nursing, Department of Obstetrics & Gynaecological Nursing, Akdeniz University, Turkey.* • [3]*PhD, RN, Professor, Faculty of Nursing, Department of Obstetrics & Gynaecological Nursing, Akdeniz University, Turkey.*

are also regarded as models to construct nursing values and concepts (Alligood, 2014). It is utterly important for the professional development of nursing students that they integrate their clinical experiences into theoretical knowledge. An insight into nursing metaparadigms will certainly enable nursing students to cope with the challenges that face them in developing their professional identity (Lee & Fawcett, 2013).

In a recent study, Fawcett (2000) taught "Transition to Professional Nursing" to nursing students and analyzed their feedback with regard to nursing metaparadigms. The participants noted that raising awareness toward nursing paradigms provided a framework for the nursing profession and an intellectual recognition of the fundamentals of nursing while reducing burnout (Fawcett, 2000). A participant further stated that nurses were still a member of a professional group, even when they ignored the significance of nursing paradigms (Lee & Fawcett, 2013). In the same study, another student, on the other hand, admitted that "I have never heard of nursing paradigms before. But now it makes me feel even more dedicated to my professional duties when I think over my nursing philosophy and nursing experiences."

Nurses' perceptions of nursing metaparadigms and their awareness of professional concepts will eventually influence their professional development (Fawcett, 2000). Awareness of professional identities and values is established during professional education. Therefore, it is of utmost importance to investigate nursing students' perceptions of fundamental nursing values and metaparadigms. Accordingly, this study aims to analyze nursing students' perceptions of the four basic nursing metaparadigms (person, human factor, health/illness, and environment).

Methods

Research Design

This study was designed as a descriptive, phenomenological study. The main point of phenomenological studies is to unveil participants' personal experiences and perceptions of concepts (Creswell, 2014). Researchers use descriptive approaches to attempt to describe very carefully the experiences being lived through, and once raw data have been obtained, a thorough phenomenological psychological analysis of the data takes place within the perspective of the phenomenological psychological reduction (Giorgi, 2012). Students are provided with metaphors to signify person and health/illness metaparadigms, which help exemplify the unknown with known examples so that sophisticated ideas may be conveyed and identified more easily, eventually enabling the participants to symbolize their experiences with a single image (Schmitt, 2005).

Participants

The study sample included fourth-year students at Akdeniz University Nursing Faculty in the 2016–2017 academic year. Purposeful sampling was used to recruit participants. The inclusion criteria of this study were as follows: attending the nursing school as a fourth-year student and being interested in nursing philosophy, being an active member of the Turkish Student Nurses Association, and having completed taking History and Deontology of Nursing and Fundamentals of Nursing courses.

In the Turkish nursing education system, metaparadigms are taught only in History and Deontology of Nursing and Fundamentals of Nursing courses. Thus, students in these courses tend to be more aware of these metaparadigms. Otherwise, eligible students who did not successfully pass these courses were excluded from participation.

The sample size in qualitative studies is determined by data saturation, which is marked by repetitive input from newly added participants (Morse, 2015). Data saturation was reached in this study after 13 participants had been interviewed. The participants included only two male students.

Data Collection

The participants were interviewed in the meeting hall of the department using an in-depth interview method, which is the most frequently used data collection tool in phenomenological studies (Creswell, 2014).

A personal information form and a semistructured questionnaire, both designed by the researchers, were used in the interviews. The researchers consulted with the experts while designing the semistructured questionnaire. All of the interviews were audio recorded. The interview room was set up for the interviews, and a notice was put at the door. The purpose of the research was explained to the participants by the researchers before their interview session. As suggested by Moustakas (1994), the researchers began the interview with an ice-breaking question like "Would you like to talk about concepts that are significant for nursing practice?" to test their awareness of metaparadigms and to encourage participants' participation in the interview. Afterward, the interview continued with main items and subitems, if necessary, to help the participants express their perceptions and opinions (Table 1). The interview lasted approximately 35–45 minutes.

Rigor and Trustworthiness

Lincoln and Guba (1985) proposed that certain criteria, including credibility, transferability, dependability, and confirmability, must be sought in qualitative studies to test reliability and validity. Rigor and trustworthiness were achieved through individual interviews using a semistructured interview form to ensure that the participants were asked a similar range of questions. The researchers, who interviewed the participants and who were not teachers of the participants, were doctoral candidates who held master of science degrees in nursing, had training in qualitative research, and had published more than 10 nursing articles each. Data were coded by two independent researchers (a professor and an assistant professor who were experts in nursing education and qualitative research). For validity, all interview data were transcribed without adding any comments for dependability criterion, and data coding was carried out by two researchers individually. During the coding process, researchers

TABLE 1.
Research Questions

Main questions/ Sub-questions
1. What would you say about nurses?
• What are the basic qualities of nurses?
• If you were to associate nurses with a person or an object, what would it be?
2. What would you say about environment?
• Would you please define environment?
• Would you like to talk about the positive effects of environment on individuals?
• Would you like to talk about the negative effects of environment on individuals?
3. What would you say about health and diseases?
• Would you please define health?
• Would you please define disease?
• What do you think about the influences of health and diseases on individuals?
• If you were to associate diseases with a person or an object, what would it be?
4. What would you say about human beings?
5. What would you say about care?
• Which qualities should proper care incorporate in your opinion?
• What are the distinctive characteristics of nursing care (like caregivers, mechanics, or maids)?
• Please discuss the effects of nursing care on yourself that you provide as a nurse.

exchanged and discussed their opinions regarding the compliance of codes obtained from data that were repeated. For confirmability (verifiability), a comprehensive interview form and the final version of thematization were evaluated by an expert person.

Data Collection

Study data were collected using a 6-item personal information form that gathered information on the descriptive characteristics of the participants and a 15-item semi-structured interview form that gathered information on the participant's perception of nursing metaparadigms (Table 1). The suitability of the questions in the semi-structured interview form was assessed by a professor and a doctor working in the field of nursing education. Individual, in-depth interviews were conducted with three students to test the validity and reliability of the semi-structured interview form. The researcher rearranged interview questions according to the results of the pilot study. The question "Do you think that your life changed after you encountered nursing paradigms?" was asked to start the interview.

Data Analysis

The interviews were recorded on camera and with a voice recorder. The author analysed the data obtained from the study through interview outputs using a written solution and then determined the themes. The study data were analysed in four basic steps, as suggested by Giorgi (2012) for descriptive phenomenological studies. According to this approach a phenomenological attitude, i.e., looking at objects from the perspective of how they are experienced, allows a search for the essence of the phenomenon using free, imaginative variation to reveal why the object makes a specific example of the phenomenon. The procedure consists of the following steps: (a) total impression—from chaos to themes; (b) identifying and sorting meaning units—from themes to codes; (c) condensation—from code to meaning; (d) synthesizing—from condensation to descriptions and concepts (Giorgi 2012; Malterud, 2012).

Ethical Considerations

Ethical approval was obtained from the ethical committee of the Akdeniz University Clinical Studies Board of Ethics, confirming that this study follows international standards and the principles adopted in the World Medical Association Declaration of Helsinki (approval No. 15, August, 2017). The Declaration of Helsinki was signed by all researchers. Before commencing the study, the researchers obtained permission from the dean of the Faculty of Nursing. The contact information for the students who met the inclusion criteria was obtained. Oral and written consent was obtained after the students who were targeted for participation were informed about the study. Before each interview session, the participants were informed that interviews would be recorded by camera and voice recorder. Furthermore, they were notified that their voice recordings would not be used for any purpose other than the study. Then, the permission of the participants was obtained. The participants were informed that they were free to leave the room and quit the interview anytime they wished and that their decision to participate or not carried no risk to them.

Results

The age of participants ranged from 20–23 years old; a majority were females (n = 11); and most stated having a moderate interest in philosophy (n = 9).

The perceptions and opinions of student nurses regarding the four basic metaparadigms of nursing were thematically grouped and analysed (Table 2).

Theme 1. "Person" Metaparadigm from the Perspective of Participants

The thoughts of participants about the person metaparadigm were investigated under five sub-themes, including: person as a wise being, person as a potentially self-transcendent being, person in interaction with his/her environment, person as a socially adaptable being, and person with management skills.

1. Person as a wise being

The student nurses defined person in a variety of ways. One participant expressed that it was difficult to define what a person is, as humans cannot be easily generalized. However, she said, the most distinguishing characteristic of personhood is the ability to think.

> *Human beings are difficult to define and impossible to stereotype. Even the most basic physiological needs may vary from individual to individual. Some sleep for long hours, some less; some eat a lot, some only a little; some show their love easily, some can't . . . I believe words are not enough to define human beings. Because each human being is a distinct world and needs individual attention. But, I believe their most distinguishing characteristics is their ability to think.* (S6)

One of the participants remarked that a person is special for his/her cognitive skills:

TABLE 2.

Metaphors That Nursing Students Associated With Nursing and Disease Metaparadigms and Their Explanations

Metaphor	Frequency	Explanation
Nurse		
Land	2	I think a nurse is like land. Nurses give you more than they get from you.
Mother	3	Nurses are like mothers because mothers are protective, we ask everything from our mothers, we expect them to do everything for us. Without our mothers, the balance at home is disrupted. In the same way, without nurses, the balance at the hospital is disrupted.
Air	1	Nurses are like air for patients. Patients can't live without air and they can't live without nurses.
Seeds	1	Nurses are like seeds. When you educate yourself, you grow like a tree. Otherwise, you rot like a seed under the ground.
Robots	1	Nurses are like robots because they never stop like a machine. They are versatile, quite mechanical.
Angel	2	They are the emblem of kindness, they help everyone around.
Fascicules	1	When I think of nurses as inanimate objects, I think of fascicules. Not as thick as an encyclopaedia, but they have everything that you need.
Blanket	1	Nurses embrace and protect patients like a blanket.
Tree roots	1	Nurses are at the roots of a hospital. Like a tree root, everything grows from them.
Disease		
Sparkle	1	Diseases are like sparkles, they can start with a little thing and then grow into a volcano and destroy everything.
Atom bomb	1	Diseases are atom bombs, like two very small substances colliding and emitting a great amount of energy. Diseases may seem very insignificant at first but later they become important.
Broken radio	1	Diseases are like broken radios. When the radio is broken, we can't listen to the songs we like, which irritates us.
War	2	Diseases are like wars. You either defeat them or be defeated and fall. They are just like wars. You either die or survive, leaving your family alone which affects everyone.
Scales	1	Disease are like scales. You can strike a balance between things on your own. You may not prevent diseases, you can get sick but again it's up to you to maintain that balance.
Learning process	1	For me, you have two ways with diseases. You can learn about them and do your best to cope with them or just burst out with anguish and let it go. For me, coping is a better option. I think disease is a lesson, a learning process.
Rabies	1	Because it spreads, one little insignificant disease affects all body functions.
Rotten apple	2	A ripe apple is red, shining red. This is our healthy body. But a rotten apple is brown inside, worms live inside the apple. This is what a disease does to the human body.
Bump	1	When everything is going well, everything is kind of smooth. I associate diseases with bumps that will make us stumble.
Stone	1	Diseases are like stones on the street that make us stumble down. They unsettle things in our life when everything seems to be OK.
Monster	1	I would associate diseases with a monster, which is there but actually doesn't exist. It nestles down waiting for a moment of weakness.

> *I think what makes human beings special is their ability to think. Human beings, with the help of their thinking skills, can make their own decisions, make their own choices, and face the consequences of their decisions.* (S3)

Another participant expressed that people can only exist as social beings due to their ability to think:

> *I think the best part of being a person is having the ability to think. With that ability, a person can create, perform scientific research, and produce art. People exist as social beings to the extent of their thinking ability. Isn't this what distinguishes them from other living beings?* (S8)

Another student thought that the ability to think and reason is the greatest gift for humanity:

> *I think the potential to think and reason is the greatest gift for humanity. A thinking human being has the ability to make decisions, make their own choices, and face the consequences of their decisions. Thinking is the only humane way for an individual to lead a free life endowed with fraternity and civil rights.* (S9)

2. Person as a potentially self-transcendent being

A participant expressed the belief that people are not machines but potentially self-transcendent beings:

> *A person is not only a machine composed merely of eyes, heart, veins, and muscles. A person is their emotions, spirit, and a sum of pieces. What is more, people are extraordinary creatures who transcend themselves with aging, proving their potential to go beyond and their ability to widen their horizon.* (S10)

Another participant posited that people have, in fact, an ability to go beyond their potential but that they may also be full of remorse when they are unable to fulfil their potential:

> *People are amazing and they can do whatever they want when they want it deep in their heart. They have hobbies and skills. They listen to music, play musical instruments, paint, do all kind of sports, and dance. They find hobbies to enjoy their time among their daily routines. But there are also a lot of people who don't care about themselves, live their life in stress, and don't appreciate what life brings to them.* (S11)

3. Person in interactions with his / her environment

Most participants defined people as social beings and stated that people should interact with their social environment:

> *People are social beings, and they should interact with their environment for a happy life. I think that you can't be happy if you are all alone and isolated from others and the environment. People must be in a relationship with their friends, family members, other people, and even other living beings.* (S12)

4. Person as a socially adaptable being

One of the participants identified people in the context of their ability to adapt to changing conditions. Regardless of their material conditions, people can adapt to new conditions:

> *I believe that a characteristic of people is being able to adapt to different conditions. People are so amazing that they can eventually adapt to new conditions despite having difficulties at first. For example, someone who lost his/her whole family or who became disabled for the rest of his/her life after an accident, life can be difficult at first. Sometimes it takes years to get used to their new life, or they might even receive psychological support. But, in the end, they learn how to deal with their new life. Because they have no other option but to learn how to struggle with changes in their lives.* (S7)

5. Person with management skills

Some participants agreed that one peculiar quality of personhood is having management skills, although these may cause some problems at times:

> *Although it may occasionally create problems, I believe that one of the most significant characteristics of a person is the ability to manage other people. Indeed, they manage not only other people but also themselves.* (S1)

Another stated that:

> *I believe that people are capable of educating each other, with the potential to develop and grow and manage their environment and other people.* (S13)

Theme 2. "Health/Illness" Metaparadigm from the Perspective of Participants

The perceptions of the participants regarding the health/illness metaparadigm were categorized into the sub-themes of stability/instability, well-being/deterioration in well-being, and independence/dependence. The participants were also asked what metaphors they would use for the illness meta-paradigm and their answers were sparkle, atom bomb, broken radio, war, scales, rotten apple, learning process, rabies, monster, and bumper (Table 2).

1. Stability/instability

Some participants associated health and illness with stability, defined health as the harmony between human beings and their environment, and defined illness as the disturbance of well-being:

> *I think that the human body works in harmony. Illness is the disturbance of this harmony. For instance, mothers maintain harmony in the house. When they get sick, all harmony is disrupted and things go wrong. In the same way, when there is a health problem in the human body, things go wrong and all systems are negatively affected.* (S11)

Another student compared human health to wheel alignment on cars. S/he stated that the slightest instability disrupts balance in the human body and eventually causes illnesses.

> *The human body is like a machine, and health is a state of balance. People are healthy to the extent that they maintain that balance. Even if the smallest part of the human body doesn't work in harmony with other parts, it causes instability in human health.* (S13)

2. Well-being/ deterioration in well-being

A majority of participants identified health and illness with well-being. They defined health as well-being of the body and soul, and interpreted illness as a deterioration in well-being:

> *Health means feeling well. I think you are healthy as long as you feel well. I mean, you are healthy when your body works normally. For instance, if a person with high blood pressure feels well, they are healthy. I believe that being diagnosed with high blood pressure doesn't make one a sick person.* (S7)

Another student who characterized health with well-being stated that:

> *In Turkish culture, when people ask how you feel, people answer "I am good, I am healthy" instead of just saying "I am feeling well". I mean, health is equal to feeling well in our culture. People are healthy as much as they feel well, I think.* (S1)

3. Independence/dependence

One of the participants defined health as the capacity to cover one's own needs independently and illness as being dependent on others:

> *Health is the capacity to cover one's own needs, whereas illness is not. In other words, we can't say one is healthy if they need help from other people to cover their needs.* (S5)

Theme 3. "Environment" Metaparadigm from the Perspective of Students

Most participants defined environment as almost everything that is around a person:

> *I can't find a word to define environment. Everything, abstract or concrete, is your environment. Having my hand on that desk now, the heat of the weather I feel, having eye contact with you at this very moment - all are components of our environment ... When I talk to my friends, what they make me feel is abstract. Feeling comfortable or anxious here and now is an example of such feelings.* (S4)

Another participant associated environment with happiness:

> *Any place where people feel happy or unhappy and in which they interact is their environment.* (S9)

While some students referred to environment as physical environment, others defined the social environment and psychological environment. The main theme of environment was examined under three sub-themes: physical environment, psychological environment, and social environment.

1. Physical environment

Some participants in the study stressed the healing effect of environment and they underlined certain qualities of environment such as warmth, light, comfort, cleanliness, and silence to have a healing effect:

> *A room should be well-lighted with enough windows. The walls may be painted in colours. Each clinic has a certain order of its own. For instance, rooms in paediatric clinics must have balloons and ornaments. The physical environment should make people feel good.* (S3)

2. Psychological environment

Some participants mentioned several qualities of environment that have a healing effect, including being kind, sincere, good-humoured, and trustworthy.

One participant stated that:

> *When one talks about environment, it is not only furniture and rooms, of course. Psychological environment is also important. Family life, friends, nurses, ... these are all your environment. A nurse should provide quality care, be good-humoured, and ask patients how they feel, which is very precious for a patient. This is what comprises a patient's psychological environment.* (S2)

3. Social environment

Some participants approached the environment from a social perspective:

One's environments isn't only made of mechanical components. I mean, air, water, sun, or houses ... They don't define one's environment. People around you are your social environment. Nurses, in a hospital environment, are a part of patient's social environment. Nurses affect patients and patients affect nurses in turn. (S13)

The social environment for a patient should be warm and sincere. People around the patient should be good-humoured. For example, patients must feel like they are at home rather than in a hospital room. We, the nurses, must work to ensure this. (S8)

Theme 4. Nursing Paradigm from the Perspective of Participants

The participants associated the nursing metaparadigm with humanism, touching the lives of individuals and professional identity. Moreover, when they were asked "If you were to associate nurses with a person or an object, what would it be?", their answers included land, air, seed, robots, angels, fascicules, blanket, and tree roots (Table 2).

1. Humanism

A majority of participants identified nursing with humanism. One participant who believes that one should learn to love themselves before they serve others stated that:

I think humanism is at the heart of nursing. A good nurse should love himself/herself in order to love other people. How can you expect a person to help other people heal if s/he doesn't love him/herself in the first place? (S1)

Another expressed that the humanism factor is frequently emphasized in their courses and said that becoming a good nurse is only possible by loving people:

In all our courses and practices in the department, we are reminded of the significance of a humanistic approach before teaching the theory of nursing. Humanism is basically loving and understanding people. I learned in the Ethics of Nursing course that the first and foremost human right is the right to live and that my duty is to ensure that my patients' lives take a humane course to the last moment. I believe that the secret of success in nursing lies in humanism. (S2)

Furthermore, some participants pointed out that conscience should be one of the key components of nursing.

I think students should be taught the merits of conscience. I believe that people without mercy in their heart can't help other people. A good nurse is also a good person and, in my humble opinion, only people with a conscience can be good people. As the number of nurses with a conscience and with mercy in their hearts increases, the nursing profession will no longer be limited to giving injections, aspirating patients, and checking blood pressure. (S3)

2. Touching the lives of people

One of the participants stated that nurses should touch patients not only with their hands or eyes but also with their hearts, and defined nursing as a way of touching people's lives:

Nursing is touching people's lives. The nursing profession is based on patient care, which is indeed very precious in itself. I think nursing is the ability to touch people's lives not with your hands or eyes but with your heart. Any individual can provide care for sick people but it is a special skill to take care of a person in need with your whole heart. That is what makes nursing a special and meaningful profession - touching a patient's life with your heart. (S4)

Another participant stated:

I love nursing. We are asked to take care of two patients during our clinical practice. I meet two new families every week and become a part of these families. I touch their lives and they touch mine. I think that is the best part of nursing - getting involved in new lives. (S5)

3. Professional identity

Some participants associated nursing with professional identity. A student who defied the angel stereotype highlighted that:

I am mad at people who define nurses as angels without wings, as sacred, as a sacrifice, as white angels ... Hearing such clichés disinclines me in my professional ambitions. It makes me sad when people only identify nurses as white angels, when nurses actually strive to provide a quality of care that is exactly what their patients need. People must understand what a professional means and demand quality care. (S6)

Another participant stated the belief that nursing should be based on professional principles:

Like any other service business, nursing should be based on professional practice. I can't think of any nursing care without professional principles. I believe that there is need for a professional practice to maintain mutual respect between nurses and patients and their relatives and to provide quality care. (S7)

Discussion

Paradigms are indispensable for the development of the nursing profession on a scientific basis (Mc Evan & Will, 2006). Therefore, nursing students who will carry the nursing profession into the future are expected to raise awareness of the metaparadigms of nursing and build up their own nursing philosophy upon these paradigms. It is obvious that providing students with the fundamental principles of nursing and special skills to define nursing care requires more than only teaching them the theory of nursing (Mc Evan & Will, 2006).

Undergraduate nursing students take theoretical and practical courses for four years (total 240 ECTS credits) in the university where this study was conducted. In their first year in the department, they are taught basic principles of nursing in the Fundamentals of Nursing I course. Besides, they are also given the fundamentals of effective communication and of the nursing profession in the Interpersonal Relations course. In their second semester in the first year, students establish close contact with patients, first in labs and then in clinical practice in the Fundamentals of Nursing II course. Furthermore, the students are offered elective theoretical courses such as the History and Deontology of Nursing, Professional Communication, Ethics of Medical Care, and Communication Skills. In their eighth semester, students have a chance to put theoretical education into practice under the supervision of their mentor nurses and clinical lecturers. It is of utmost importance to enable nursing students to define the nursing profession on their own and to develop their own perspectives on nursing values before graduation.

A humanistic approach has a far-reaching influence on an individual's attitudes and behaviours (RØnnow-Rasmussen, 2008). Moreover, a humanistic approach brings out a humble and merciful attitude (Pembroke, 2006). Nurses who cherish their patients will certainly enjoy their jobs and have a successful professional career (de Vries, 2004; Stickley & Freshwater, 2002). In this study, participants widely agreed that nurses should love people before helping them. In addition, Watson (2007), suggested that nursing care is based on universal humanistic values. In this study, the participants expressed that humanism is a vital aspect of nursing and that humanism is, at its core, loving people. Furthermore, it is noteworthy that the participants believed that nurses should first and foremost touch their patients not with their hands or eyes but with their hearts. It encouraging that the student nurses in this study regarded professional identity, humanism, and mercy as the fundamental values of nursing.

The primary focus of nursing is the human factor (Rodgers, 2005). Therefore, it is necessary to understand people and their needs in order to provide the best care possible (Mc Evan & Will, 2006). Leininger (1997) emphasized the necessity of care to maintain health and individuality and added that care was different from treatment. The fundamental values of nursing should be integrated into the nursing curricula in both theoretical courses and clinical practices (Rodgers, 2005). The health metaparadigm plays a crucial role in nursing education and practice and has been widely institutionalized. In a study on the perceptions of nursing students toward health metaparadigm conducted in Sweden, it was found that students associated health with physical and mental well-being and that they considered that individuals were primarily responsible for promoting their health. In addition, these students believed that promoting health is also deeply related with maintaining a balance between diet, activities, work, and leisure. Furthermore, having healthy relations with family and friends is a prerequisite for having good health. A student in the study also stated that individuals may feel healthy despite having relatively bad health (Skär & Söderberg, 2016).

Hernandez (2009) carried out a similar study and asked nursing students to write down their opinions toward the person, health, human, and environment metaparadigms after having participated in a course on nursing theory. They were also asked to work in study groups and to reflect on their own nursing philosophy through case studies. The assessment of case studies illustrated that these studies provided students with a critical perspective and helped them better grasp the core of nursing theories. Consequently, it was suggested that teaching nursing metaparadigms enhanced the acquisition of professional values.

Nursing practice is not only putting theory of nursing into practice but also a professional field in which new ideas are produced and tested to develop nursing knowledge (McEvan & Will, 2006). In addition, metaparadigms pave the way for students to develop a critical perspective and to become a professional member of an academic discipline. Thus, nursing education should be designed holistically to include nursing paradigms to assist nursing students understand the basic needs and experiences of individuals (Eriksson, 2007).

Thus, student nurses should raise awareness toward nursing values from the onset of undergraduate education. Nursing students, consciously or unconsciously, develop their own nursing definitions throughout theoretical and practical education. Therefore, nursing educators should design programs that pave the way for professional nursing education by encouraging the more active participation of nursing students.

Conclusions and Implications for Practice

This study found that nursing students focused not only on the physical but also on the emotional, spiritual, social, and environmental aspects of nursing metaparadigms. Most of the students in the study associated nursing with humanism. Previous studies have also reported that students have difficulties in identifying nursing metaparadigms and that they believe that humans have the potential to widen their horizons with wisdom and social skills. In this study, most of the participants were aware of the meaning of nursing and their perceptions toward nursing paradigms were in line with mainstream nursing theories. However, it is quite challenging for nursing students to connect nursing paradigms with nursing practice, which eventually causes discrepancies between theory and practice. Therefore, nursing students should be encouraged to internalize metaparadigms through courses or study groups in order to successfully comprehend the significance of metaparadigms and establish strong ties between nursing theory and practice. Thus, nursing students may acquire a professional identity, consciously or unconsciously, during their professional education. Nursing educators are recommended to develop professional education programs and to promote the active participation of the students.

Limitations

The limitations of this study include the non-generalizable nature of qualitative studies and the inclusion of participants from one nursing school only. Furthermore, the participants did not confirm the correctness of their information after transcription and thematisation and only two male nursing students joined this study as participants.

References

Alligood, M. R. (2014). *Nursing theorists and their work* (8th ed.). St. Louis, MO: Elsevier.

Bahramnezhad, F., Shiri, M., Asgari, P., & Afshar, P. F. (2015). A review of the nursing paradigm. *Open Journal of Nursing, 5*(1), Article ID 53094. https://doi.org/10.4236/ojn.2015.51003

Creswell, J. W., & Creswell, J. D. (2014). *Research design: Qualitative, quantitative, and mixed methods approaches* (4th ed.). London, England: Sage.

de Vries, K. (2004). Humility and its practice in nursing. *Nursing Ethics, 11*(6), 577–586. https://doi.org/10.1191/0969733004ne740oa

Eriksson, K. (2007). Becoming through suffering—The path to health and holiness. *International Journal for Human Caring, 11*(2), 8–16. https://doi.org/10.20467/1091-5710.11.2.8

Fawcett, J. (1978). The "what of theory development. In National League for Nursing (Ed.), *Theory development: What, why, how?* (pp. 17–38). New York, NY: National League for Nursing.

Fawcett, J. (2000). *Analysis and evaluation of contemporary nursing knowledge: Nursing models and theories.* Philadelphia, PA: F. A. Davis.

Giorgi, A. (2012). The descriptive phenomenological psychological method. *Journal of Phenomenological Psychology, 43*(1), 3–12. https://doi.org/10.1163/156916212X632934

Kim, H. S. (2000). An integrative framework for conceptualizing clients: A proposal for a nursing perspective in the new century. *Nursing Science Quarterly, 13*(1), 37–40. https://doi.org/10.1177/08943180022107258

Kuhn, T. S. (2017). *Structure of scientific revolutions.* (N. Kuyas, Trans.). Ankara, Turkey: Alan. (Original work published 1982; in Turkish)

Hernandez, C. A. (2009). Student articulation of a nursing philosophical statement: An assignment to enhance critical thinking skills and promote learning. *Journal of Nursing Education, 48*(6), 343–349. https://doi.org/10.3928/01484834-20090515-08

Leininger, M. (1997). Transcultural nursing research to transform nursing education and practice: 40 years. *Journal of Nursing Scholarship, 29*(4), 341–348. https://doi.org/10.1111/j.1547-5069.1997.tb01053.x

Lee, R. C., & Fawcett, J. (2013). The influence of the metaparadigm of nursing on professional identity development among RN-BSN students. *Nursing Science Quarterly, 26*(1), 96–98. https://doi.org/10.1177/0894318412466734

Lincoln, Y. S., & Guba, E. G. (1985). *Naturalistic inquiry.* Beverly Hills, CA: Sage.

McEvan, M., & Will, E. (2006). *Theoretical basis for nursing.* Philadelphia, PA: Lippincott.

Malterud, K. (2012). Systematic text condensation: A strategy for qualitative analysis. *Scandinavian Journal of Public Health, 40*(8), 795–805. https://doi.org/10.1177/1403494812465030

Meleis, A. I. (2011). *Theoretical nursing: Development and progress* (5th ed.). Philadelphia, PA: Lippincott Williams & Wilkins.

Moustakas, C. (1994). *Phenomenological research methods* (1st ed.). Thousand Oaks, CA: Sage.

Morse, J. M. (2015). Analytic strategies and sample size. *Qualitative Health Research, 25*(10), 1317–1318. https://doi.org/10.1177/1049732315602867

Özkan, H. A., & Akduran, F. (2014). Importance of paradigms in nursing. *Journal of Education and Research in Nursing, 11*(2), 3–5. (Original work published in Turkish)

Pembroke, N. (2006). Marcelian charm in nursing practice: The unity of agape and eros as the foundation of an ethic of care. *Nursing Philosophy, 7*(4), 266–274. https://doi.org/10.1111/j.1466-769X.2006.00285.x

R⊘nnow-Rasmussen, T. R. (2008). Love, value and supervenience. *International Journal of Philosophical Studies, 16*(4), 495–508. https://doi.org/10.1080/09672550802335838

Rodgers, B. L. (2005). *Developing nursing knowledge: Philosophical traditions and influences* (1st ed.). Philadelphia, PA: Lippincott Williams & Wilkins.

Skär, L., & Söderberg, S. (2016). Swedish nursing students' perceptions of the concept of health: A phenomenographic study. *Health Education Journal, 75*(4), 385–395. https://doi.org/10.1177/0017896915591370

Schmitt, R. (2005). Systematic metaphor analysis as a method of qualitative research. *The Qualitative Report, 10*(2), 358–394. Retrieved from https://nsuworks.nova.edu/tqr/vol10/iss2/10

Smith, M. C., & Parker, M. E. (2015). *Nursing theories and nursing practice* (4th ed.). Philadelphia, PA: F. A. Davis.

Stickley, T., & Freshwater, D. (2002). The art of loving and the therapeutic relationship. *Nursing Inquiry, 9*(4), 250–256. https://doi.org/10.1046/j.1440-1800.2002.00155.x

Watson, J. (2007). Watson's theory of human caring and subjective living experiences: Carative factors/caritas processes as a disciplinary guide to the professional nursing practice. *Texto & Contexto-Enfermagem, 16*(1), 129–135. https://doi.org/10.1590/S0104-07072007000100016

Watson, J. (2008). *Nursing: The philosophy and science of caring* (Revised ed.). Louisville, CO: University Press of Colorado.

11

Predictors of Caregiver Burden in Caregivers of Bedridden Patients

Aysun BEKDEMİR[1] • Nesrin İLHAN[2]*

ABSTRACT

Background: Caregivers are at risk of experiencing caregiver burden. It is therefore important to determine the caregiver burden of caregivers who provide care to bedridden patients and related factors.

Purpose: The aim of this study was to determine the caregiver burden of caregivers who provide care to bedridden patients and the factors that impact this burden.

Methods: This cross-sectional study was executed at a state hospital in Istanbul, Turkey, on bedridden patients registered in the home healthcare unit and their caregivers. During study period, the researchers made 312 visits to patients and their caregivers. A sociodemographic questionnaire, the Burden Interview, and the Katz Index of Independence in Activities of Daily Living were used to collect data. Descriptive statistics, an independent sample *t* test, one-way analysis of variance, and stepwise multiple regression analysis were used for data analysis.

Results: The participants reported a moderate level of caregiver burden. Existing caregiver health problems, caregiver employment status, the ability of the caregiver to maintain his or her own good health, type of home, and the degree of patient dependence in terms of activities of daily living were each found to be significant predictors of caregiver burden.

Conclusions/Implications of Practice: The support provided to caregivers by home healthcare units is important in terms of protecting the physical, mental, and social health conditions of caregivers and preventing the exacerbation of caregiver burden.

KEY WORDS:
caregiving, caregiver burden, caregiver health, home care, nurse.

Introduction

Bedridden patients are patients who stay in bed for short or long periods for various reasons, including chronic illnesses, old age, and disability. Bedridden patients cannot perform self-care and medical care partially or completely and need the help of others. Bedridden patients are usually cared for by family members, paid caregivers, and/or health professionals (Handicap International, n.d.; Vieira et al., 2015).

Family caregivers are defined as relatives and friends who provide care free of charge to individuals with chronic or debilitating conditions (Collins & Swartz, 2011; Sanuade & Boatemaa, 2015). Family members play important roles in the care of the sick and those unable to take care of their own needs (Adelman, Tmanova, Delgado, Dion, & Lachs, 2014; Chiou, Chang, Chen, & Wang, 2009). Providing care adversely affects the health and quality of life of the caregiver (Bauer & Sousa-Poza, 2015; Jeong, Myong, & Koo, 2015; Rha, Park, Song, Lee, & Lee, 2015). Caregivers are likely to spend less time with their family and friends, experience increased levels of emotional stress, and neglect self-care activities such as getting a good night's sleep, exercising, and healthy eating (Collins & Swartz, 2011).

Caregivers are at risk of caregiver burden (Chang, Chiou, & Chen, 2010; Chiou et al., 2009; Roopchand-Martin & Creary-Yan, 2014). Caregiver burden is defined as a multidimensional response to perceived stress and negative assessments that derive from providing care to a sick person (Kim, Chang, Rose, & Kim, 2012). The risk factors that have been identified in the literature as affecting caregiving burden include being female, having a lower level of education, living in the same house with the care recipient, providing care for long hours, having depression, being socially isolated, being under financial stress, and having no choice but to be a caregiver (Adelman et al., 2014). Caregiver burden threatens the physical, psychological, emotional, and functional health of caregivers (Bauer & Sousa-Poza, 2015; Etters, Goodall, & Harrison, 2008; Ma, Lu, Xiong, Yao, & Yang, 2014). Moreover, caregiver burden is known to be a significant predictor of quality of life (Jeong et al., 2015; Rha et al., 2015).

Researchers have found that caregiver burden is affected by many factors related to providing care. The health of both caregivers and care recipients impact strongly on caregiver burden (Rha et al., 2015; Sanuade & Boatemaa, 2015). The health of persons receiving care and their degree of dependence affect caregiver burden (Abdollahpour, Noroozian, Nedjat, & Majdzadeh, 2012; Conde-Sala, Garre-Olmo, Turró-Garriga,

[1]*MSc, Specialist Nurse, Home Health Services Coordination Center, Üsküdar State Hospital, Istanbul, Turkey* • [2]*PhD, Assistant Professor, Faculty of Health Sciences, Department of Nursing, Bezmialem Vakif University, Istanbul, Turkey.*

Vilalta-Franch, & López-Pousa, 2010; Zaybak, Güneş, Günay İsmagloğlu, & Ülker, 2012). Furthermore, caregiver burden affects the level of well-being of the caregiver and, as a consequence, reduces the caregiver's ability to provide good care (Collins & Swartz, 2011; Sanuade & Boatemaa, 2015). Chang et al. (2010) found that the mental health and caregiver burden of care providers were related to the health problems experienced by caregivers. Women make up the large majority of caregivers in family settings (Jeong et al., 2015; Rha et al., 2015; Yıkılkan, Aypak, & Görpelioğlu, 2014). Whereas some research has identified gender as a significant predictor of caregiver burden (Brodaty et al., 2014; Etters et al., 2008; Sousa et al., 2016), some have found no correlation between gender and caregiver burden (Orak & Sezgin, 2015; Roopchand-Martin & Creary-Yan, 2014; Sanuade & Boatemaa, 2015). Chiou et al. (2009) reported that caregivers with poor social support and family functions have a higher level of caregiver burden and that perceived social support is a better indicator of caregiver burden than the social support actually received. Furthermore, studies have shown that living in the same house with a patient (Adelman et al., 2014; Conde-Sala et al., 2010) and having a direct role in that patient's physical care (Sanuade & Boatemaa, 2015) increase caregiver burden.

Professional healthcare providers have an important impact on the health and well-being of caregivers (Yıkılkan et al., 2014). Nurses may engage in training primary caregivers and support caregivers by aiding in care-related activities. Thus, nurses have an important role to play in lessening the caregiver burden of care providers (Schulz & Sherwood, 2008). Nurses are best positioned to make early diagnoses of caregiver burden and to help caregivers avoid/minimize the adverse effects of caregiving (Etters et al., 2008). Nurses should observe caregivers during their home visits and evaluate them in terms of caregiver burden risk (Etters et al., 2008; Yıkılkan et al., 2014). When caregiver burden is identified, the perceptions of caregivers regarding the burden that they are taking on may be eased with appropriate interventions (Etters et al., 2008). Thus, for all of the above-stated reasons, it is important to identify caregiver burden and its related factors, to ensure that caregivers receive support, and to develop, organize, and implement caregiver-burden prevention programs. Therefore, the purpose of this study was to determine the caregiver burden of individuals who provide care to bedridden patients and the factors that impact this burden. This study is significant in that it was conducted in Turkey with a large sample and because many factors affecting caregiver burden were examined as variables. The study sought answers to the following research questions:

- What is the relationship between the sociodemographic characteristics of caregivers and their caregiver burden?
- What is the relationship between the way caregivers provide care and their caregiver burden?
- What is the relationship between the degree of dependency of bedridden patients and the caregiver burden of their caregivers?
- Are caregiving-related factors predictive of caregiver burden?

Methods

Design and Data Collection

This study used a cross-sectional design and was executed at a state hospital in Istanbul, Turkey, between January and April 2014. The participants were bedridden patients who were registered in the hospital's home healthcare unit and their caregivers.

Participants

Home healthcare services in Turkey are given by the Ministry of Health, municipalities and private organizations. Home healthcare units of Ministry of Health work in affiliation with the hospitals. Individuals who require services from these units at home are provided examination, testing, treatment, medical care, rehabilitation, and social and psychological support services during home visits. The costs of these services are covered by the social security administration. This study targeted the caregivers of bedridden patients registered in the home healthcare unit of a state hospital in Anatolian Istanbul (N = 4,500). The formula that was used to determine the necessary sample size on the basis of a finite population determined that a minimum sample size of 251 bedridden patients and caregivers was required (Sümbüloğlu & Sümbüloğlu, 2002).

$$n = \frac{Nt^2pq}{d^2(N-1)+t^2pq} = \frac{4500\times(2.58)^2\times0.12\times0.88}{(0.05)^2\times(4500-1)+(2.58)^2\times0.12\times0.88} = \frac{2992}{2.5} = 251$$

Abbreviations used in the formula:

N = Number of individuals in the target population
n = Number of individuals to be sampled
p = Frequency of occurrence of the event to be investigated (probability)
q = Frequency of nonoccurrence of the events to be investigated (1 p)
t = Theoretical value in the t table at a certain degree of freedom and at the determined error level
d = The desired deviation according to the occurrence frequency of an event
N = 4,500 (number of patients registered at home health units in 2013)
p = .12 (the proportion of disabled in Turkey; Turkish Statistical Institute, 2002)
q = 0.88
d = 0.05
t = 2.58 (when t = 0.01 in the case of α = .01)

The study was conducted on 312 bedridden patients and their caregivers who met the criteria for inclusion. The criteria for inclusion included being responsible for the care of a bedridden patient, providing care for at least 1 month, willing to participate in this research, aged 18 years or older, able to read and write, and able to understand and answer questions. The questionnaires were filled out during face-to-face interviews that were conducted with the participants during a home visit by the researcher. Patient information was obtained from patients and caregivers. Questionnaires with missing data were excluded from the study.

Ethical Considerations

Verbal and written permission was obtained from the institution in advance. The university's ethics committee granted its approval for this study (September 9, 2013, No. 47). The purpose of this study was explained to the patients and their caregivers, and their written and verbal consent was obtained.

Measures

Demographic variables

The descriptive characteristics of the caregivers (gender, age, educational status, civil status, type of residence, employment status, and income status), their personal health situation, their ability to attend to their own health, their relationship to the patient, the duration that they had been caring for their patient, the areas of caregiving, and the patient's gender, age, and educational status were collected using a standard questionnaire.

Caregiver burden

The caregiver burden of the caregivers was measured using the Zarit Burden Interview (BI). In 1980, Zarit, Reever, and Bach-Peterson developed BI as a scale to evaluate the level of stress experienced in providing care to the sick and older adults. The scale questionnaire, which may be filled out either by the caregiver or a researcher, consists of 22 statements on the effect of caregiving on the respondent caregiver's life. Each of the statements is answered using a Likert-type scale, with scores ranging from 0 to 4 (*never*, *rarely*, *sometimes*, *frequently*, and *always*). Studies have indicated an internal consistency coefficient of .87–.94 for the scale and a test–retest reliability of .71. The total possible scores for the BI range from 0 to 88, with 0–20 indicating "no burden," 21–40 indicating "mild burden," 41–60 indicating "moderate burden," and 61–88 indicating "severe burden." The scale items generally address the social and emotional domains, with a higher total score associated with a greater burden experienced (Zarit et al., 1980). İnci and Erdem (2008), who carried out the validity and reliability studies for the Turkish version of this scale, found a Cronbach's alpha value of .95. The Cronbach's alpha value for the BI found in this study was .90.

Functional status

The dependency status of participants was assessed using the Katz ADL was used as Katz Index of Independence in Activities of Daily Living. In 1963, Katz, Ford, Moskowitz, Jackson, and Jaffe developed Katz ADL as a tool to assess basic ADL, and Yardımcı (1995) completed the Turkish translation of the index. The index contains six headings, including bathing, dressing, toileting, transferring, continence, and feeding. Each heading has three possible responses: "*dependent*," "*partially dependent*," and "*independent*," which are assigned scores of 1, 2, and 3, respectively. ADL index score totals are assessed as follows: 0–6 = dependent, 7–12 = partial dependence, and 13–18 = independent. The ADL Cronbach's alpha value for this scale found in this study was .92.

Data Analysis

The study data were analyzed using SPSS 16.0 (SPSS, Inc., Chicago, IL, USA). Descriptive statistics (numbers, percentages, means, and standard deviations) were used in the analysis. The one-sample Kolmogorov–Smirnov test was used to assess normal distribution, and the p value was found to be > .05. As the data displayed normal distribution, parametric tests were employed in the advanced analysis. The parametric tests used included the independent sample t test for two independent variables and the one-way analysis of variance for more than two independent variables. Stepwise multiple regression analysis was used to determine the factors affecting caregiver burden. The Durbin–Watson statistic was used to measure autocorrelation. The Durbin–Watson statistic was found to be 2.086. Tolerance was found to be between .85 and .99, and the variance inflation factor was 1.00–1.17. Tolerance and variance inflation factor values were both found to be within acceptable limits. The results were found to be within the 95% confidence interval, and significance was assessed as $p < .05$.

Results

Sample Characteristics

Two thirds (65.1%) of the caregiver participants were women, 57.4% were 36–55 years old, and 60.6% had received over 8 years of training. In addition, 72.8% were married, 30.4% were employed, 64.1% earned an income that was roughly equal to their expenditures, and a large majority (80.1%) lived in apartment residences. Slightly over two fifths (42.6%) self-reported as having some kind of health problem, and 57.1% stated that they did not tend to their health needs. It was found that 71.8% were taking care of their parent or sibling, 56.7% had been a caregiver for 2 years or more, and 85.9% said they tended to every need of their patient. In terms of care recipients, 56.7% were women, the large majority (82.4%) were older than 65 years, and 79.5% had an education of 8 years or less (Table 1). The ADL item mean scores of the care recipients varied between 1.16 ± 0.47 and 1.52 ± 0.70, and their ADL total mean score was 7.64 ± 2.94 (Table 2).

Factors Associated With the Burden of Caregiving

The BI total mean score in this study was 43.56 ± 15.05. The BI mean score of the female caregivers was significantly higher than that of the male caregivers ($p < .01$). The BI mean score of the caregivers who were 56 years old or more was significantly higher than those of caregivers in the other age

TABLE 1.

Comparison of the Burden Interview Mean Scores of Caregivers According to Various Personal Characteristics (N = 312)

Variable	Burden Interview *n*	*%*	*M*	*SD*	*F/t*	*p*	Post Hoc Test
Gender					*t* = 2.709	.007**	
Women	203	65.1	45.24	12.86			
Men	109	34.9	40.44	18.11			
Education (years)					*t* = 1.620	.106	
≤ 8	123	39.4	45.26	15.81			
> 8	189	60.6	42.44	14.47			
Age (years)					12.861	< .001***	③ > ①, ②
① 20–35	53	16.9	38.68	12.52			
② 36–55	179	57.4	41.97	15.19			
③ 56 and above	80	25.6	50.36	14.15			
Marital status					*t* = −0.444	.657	
Married	227	72.8	43.79	14.66			
Single	85	17.0	42.94	16.14			
Employment status					*t* = −5.629	< .001***	
Employed	95	30.4	36.64	14.86			
Unemployed	217	69.6	46.59	14.14			
Family income status					1.992	.138	
Income less than expenditures	56	17.9	47.02	15.50			
Income equal to expenditures	200	64.1	42.51	14.87			
Income more than expenditures	56	17.9	43.88	14.99			
Type of home					8.207	< .001***	①, ② > ③
① Squatter home	23	7.4	47.57	16.83			
② Apartment	250	80.1	44.55	14.96			
③ Private home	39	12.5	34.87	11.43			
Health problems					*t* = 6.694	< .001***	
Yes	133	42.6	49.76	15.04			
No	179	57.4	38.96	13.34			
Ability to tend to own health					*t* = 3.447	< .001***	
Yes	134	42.9	40.23	14.69			
No	178	57.1	46.06	14.88			
Relation to care recipient					1.100	.334	
Caring for spouse or child	62	18.9	45.95	13.77			
Caring for parent or sibling	224	71.8	43.13	15.40			
Distant relative	26	8.3	41.58	14.84			
Caregiving duration					2.698	.046*	④ > ③
① 1–6 months	29	9.3	39.79	12.81			
② 7–12 months	44	14.1	43.75	15.70			
③ 1–2 years	62	19.9	39.97	14.41			
④ 2 years and more	177	56.7	45.39	15.23			
Areas of caregiving					4.295	.014*	③ > ①, ②
① Financial support	8	2.6	32.25	10.74			
② Psychological support	36	11.5	39.28	15.27			
③ All needs	268	85.9	44.47	14.94			

(continues)

TABLE 1.

Comparison of the Burden Interview Mean Scores of Caregivers According to Various Personal Characteristics (N = 312), Continued

Variable	Burden Interview *n*	*%*	*M*	*SD*	*F/t*	*p*	Post Hoc Test
Patients' gender					*t* = 1.030	.304	
Female	177	56.7	44.33	15.45			
Male	135	43.3	42.56	14.51			
Patients' age (years)					*t* = −0.383	.702	
< 65	55	17.6	42.85	15.27			
≥ 65	257	82.4	43.71	15.27			
Patients' educational status (years)					*t* = −2.04	.042	
< 8	248	79.5	42.68	14.85			
≥ 8 years and over	64	20.5	46.96	15.46			

**p* < .05. ***p* < .01. ****p* < .001.

groups ($p < .001$). The BI mean score of the unemployed caregivers was significantly higher than that of the employed caregivers ($p < .001$). The BI mean score of caregivers living in squatters' homes and apartments was significantly higher than that of caregivers living in private homes ($p < .001$). The BI mean score of caregivers who had health problems was significantly higher than that of caregivers with no health problems ($p < .001$).

Those caregivers who did not tend to their health needs had a BI mean score significantly higher than that of caregivers who did take care of their health needs ($p < .001$). Caregivers who had been tending to their patients for 2 years or more had a BI mean score significantly higher than that of caregivers who had been tending to their patients for 1–2 years ($p < .05$). The BI mean score of caregivers who tended to all of the patients' needs was significantly higher than that of caregivers who provided only financial or psychological support ($p < .05$). The BI mean scores did not display any statistically significant differences based on the level of education, marital status, or family income level of the caregivers or on their relationship to the care recipient ($p > .05$). The BI mean score of the caregivers of patients with a level of education over 8 years was significantly higher than that of caregivers of patients with a level of education of 8 years or less

TABLE 2.

Patients' ADL and BI Mean Scores

Scale	Minimum	Maximum	*M*	*SD*
BI	0	82	43.56	15.05
ADL				
Bathing	1	3	1.16	0.47
Dressing	1	3	1.26	0.55
Toileting	1	3	1.21	0.54
Transferring	1	3	1.20	0.53
Continence	1	3	1.29	0.58
Feeding	1	3	1.52	0.70
Total points	6	18	7.64	2.94

Note. ADL = Activities of Daily Living; BI = Burden Interview.

TABLE 3.

Comparison of Caregivers' BI Mean Scores According to Patients' ADL

ADL	BI *n*	*%*	*M*	*SD*	*F*	*p*
Bathing					2.841	.060
Dependent	277	88.8	42.87	14.94		
Partially dependent	21	6.7	50.43	15.97		
Independent	14	4.5	46.86	13.90		
Dressing					7.168	.001***
Dependent	247	79.2	42.01	14.90		
Partially dependent	48	15.4	50.69	14.32		
Independent	17	5.4	45.94	13.92		
Toileting					2.712	.068
Dependent	265	84.9	42.80	15.17		
Partially dependent	27	8.7	49.59	14.13		
Independent	20	6.4	45.55	13.20		
Transferring					0.856	.426
Dependent	269	86.2	43.13	15.43		
Partially dependent	23	7.4	46.91	11.68		
Independent	20	6.4	45.55	13.19		
Continence					4.760	.009**
Dependent	245	78.5	42.22	15.07		
Partially dependent	45	14.4	49.11	15.46		
Independent	22	7.1	47.14	10.75		
Feeding					7.272	.001***
Dependent	190	60.9	41.05	14.64		
Partially dependent	83	26.6	48.10	15.23		
Independent	39	12.5	46.15	14.34		

Note. BI = Burden Interview; ADL = activities of daily living.
**p* < .05. ***p* < .01. ****p* < .001.

($p < .05$). No statistically significant differences were found between the BI mean scores of caregivers categorized, respectively, by care recipient gender and age ($p > .05$; Table 1).

In comparing the BI mean scores of patients according to their ADL, the BI mean scores for caregivers of patients who were partially dependent on the caregiver for dressing, continence, and feeding issues were significantly higher than the mean scores for those caregivers who were caring for completely dependent patients ($p < .01$). No statistically significant differences were found between the BI mean scores of caregivers based on the bathing, toileting, and transfer dependency needs of patients ($p > .05$; Table 3).

Determinants of the Burden of Caregiving

A stepwise multiple regression analysis was performed to determine the predictors of the burden of caregiving. In the univariate analysis, the variables that had a significant effect on the burden of caregiving were considered as independent variables. Thus, gender, age, employment status, the health problems of the caregiver, the ability of the caregiver to tend to personal health, type of home, duration of care, the areas of care, and the patient ADL score were adopted as the independent variables. It was determined that gender, age, duration of care, and the areas of care of caregivers were not significant predictors of caregiver burden. However, significant relationships were found between burden of caregiving and the caregivers' health problems, employment status, ability to tend to personal health, type of home, and ADL ($R^2 = .25, p < .001$), with 25% of the total variance explained by these variables. The order of significance for the variables ranged from the caregiver's health problems ($\beta = .257$, $p < .001$) to employment status ($\beta = -.225$, $p < .001$), type of home ($\beta = -.182$, $p < .001$), ability to tend to personal health ($\beta = -.170$. $p < .001$), and the dependency of the patient in ADL ($\beta = .147, p < .001$; Table 4).

The burden of the caregivers in this study was found to be higher in those who had health problems, who were unable to manage their own health, who were not employed, who lived in a squatter home or in an apartment, and who were less dependent on their patients.

Discussion

The aim of this study was to determine the caregiver burden of individuals who were caring for bedridden patients and the factors that impact this burden. This study was conducted on a sample of bedridden patients who were receiving services from a home healthcare unit and their caregivers. It was determined that the caregivers experienced a moderate level of caregiver burden. Using univariate analysis, a significant relationship was found between caregiver burden and the caregiver's gender, age, employment status, type of home, health problems, ability to tend to personal health, and duration of caregiving and the areas where caregiving was needed as well as the patient's dependency in terms of ADL. Multiple regression analysis showed that caregiver health problems, their employment status, their ability to tend to their own health, their type of home, and the degree of dependence of patients in terms of ADL were each significant predictors of caregiving burden.

The caregiver burden scores for caregivers with health problems were higher than those of caregivers who had no health problems, indicating that caregiver burden increases when caregivers have personal health problems. One study pointed to correlations between health problems and the mental health of caregivers and caregiver burden (Chang et al., 2010). Half of the caregivers in one prior study had at least one chronic health problem (Collins & Swartz, 2011). Caregiving creates a physical and mental burden that adversely affects the health of caregivers (Bauer & Sousa-Poza, 2015; Etters et al., 2008; Kim et al., 2012), and poor personal health disrupts personal quality of life (Jeong et al., 2015). Furthermore, poor caregiver health lowers the quality of care given, increases caregivers' formal demands for healthcare (Bauer & Sousa-Poza, 2015; Collins & Swartz, 2011), and increases healthcare costs (Bauer & Sousa-Poza, 2015). It is important that caregivers are supported by home healthcare units so that they do not feel alone and helpless, do not develop health issues, and do not experience a deterioration in their existing health problems.

The caregiver burden of caregivers who do not tend to their own health is higher than that of caregivers who

TABLE 4.
Caregiver Burden Predictors According to Results of Multiple Regression Analysis

	Burden Interview			
Variable	*B*	β	*t*	*p*
Constant	47.800		20.220	< .001
Caregiver's health problems	7.822	.257	4.816	< .001
Employment status	−7.341	−.225	−4.274	< .001
Ability of caregiver to tend to own health	−5.162	−.170	−3.427	< .001
Type of home	−8.269	−.182	−3.581	< .001
Activities of daily living	0.751	.147	2.964	.003

Note. $R^2 = .254$, adjusted $R^2 = .242$, $F = 20.84$.

do. Paying appropriate attention to personal health reduces caregiver burden. The health of caregivers is known to impact caregiver burden strongly (Rha et al., 2015). Chiou et al. (2009) observed that caregivers with a low level of social and functional family support experienced higher levels of caregiver burden. The fact that caregivers allocate time to deal with their own health problems indicates that they receive social support from friends and family when needed. The literature supports that social support reduces the caregiver burden and increases the quality of life of caregivers who provide care for patients with chronic diseases (Atagün, Balaban, Atagün, Elagöz, & Özpolat, 2011).

This study found that the caregiving burden of unemployed caregivers was higher than that of their employed counterparts, indicating that outside employment reduces caregiver burden. A prior study reported that the caregiver burden of employed caregivers is of a lower level compared with that of unemployed caregivers (Sanuade & Boatemaa, 2015). Another study found that self-employed caregivers had lower caregiver burden scores (Roopchand-Martin & Creary-Yan, 2014). As caregivers who hold jobs outside the home cannot serve as primary, full-time caregivers, their caregiving time is shorter than that of caregivers who are not employed, which may explain why employed caregivers have a lower caregiver burden. Chiou et al. (2009) found that caregiver burden increases as the duration of caregiving. In Yeşil, Uslusoy, and Korkmaz (2016), no difference was found in caregiver burden based on employment status.

The caregiver burden of caregivers who live in squatter houses or apartments was shown to be higher than those who live in private houses, indicating that living in a private house reduces caregiver burden. This result indicates that physical circumstances may affect caregiver burden. Istanbul is one of Turkey's most densely populated and most expensive cities. Accordingly, it is likely that people who live in private homes in Istanbul are of a relatively high socioeconomic status. As caregivers at higher economic levels care for their patients in more comfortable physical conditions and are more likely to employ outside help, their caregiver burden may subsequently be less.

Caregivers of patients with higher levels of education were found to have higher burdens of care than those of patients with low levels of education. As patients with higher levels of education have higher life expectancies, they likely have greater expectations from their caregivers. This may increase the burden of care of their caregivers.

This study found that patients were most commonly dependent on their caregivers for bathing and least dependent for feeding, with results showing that the degree of patient dependency was a significant predictor of caregiving burden. As patient dependency lessened, caregiver burden increased. Concurrently, the caregiver burden of individuals caring for patients who were partially dependent because of continence or feeding issues was higher than the burden of those caring for dependent patients. This outcome suggests that the caregivers of partially dependent patients may not have been able to accept the additional dependency-related burdens. As patient dependency increases, caregivers tend to feel that the patients actually do need them and therefore accept the situation, leading to lower levels of perceived caregiver burden. In a study by Taşdelen and Ateş (2012), as patient dependency grew in terms of ADL, the caregiver's emotional burden lessened, which is consistent with the results of this study. However, contrary to the results of this study, other studies have shown that caregiving burden increases as patient dependency rises (Abdollahpour et al., 2012; Kim et al., 2012; Zaybak et al., 2012). It is important that further qualitative studies be conducted to discover the reasons for these outcomes, so that appropriate interventions may be designed to lessen the burden of caregiving.

Women comprised a large majority of caregivers in this study. Other studies have also found that most caregivers are women (Rha et al., 2015; Unver, Basak, Tosun, Aslan, & Akbayrak, 2016; Yeşil et al., 2016). Whereas the univariate analysis revealed a higher level of caregiver burden in female caregivers compared with male caregivers, the multiple regression analysis did not reveal a significant relationship between gender and caregiver burden. Similar to the results of this study, other studies have not detected any significant relationship between gender and caregiver burden (Orak & Sezgin, 2015; Roopchand-Martin & Creary-Yan, 2014; Sanuade & Boatemaa, 2015). However, other studies still have pointed to female caregivers having greater levels of caregiver burden than their male counterparts (Sanuade & Boatemaa, 2015; Sousa et al., 2016; Unver et al., 2016). These results reveal that the burden of caregiving in women may be affected not only by gender but also by normal responsibilities such as housework and childcare, by personal characteristics, by employment status, and by other relevant factors.

Although the burden of caregiving was found to be higher in caregivers aged 56 years and above, age was found not to be a significant determinant of this burden. Similarly, other studies have shown age not to significantly impact the burden of caregiving (Abdollahpour et al., 2012; Roopchand-Martin & Creary-Yan, 2014). Despite this, it is still believed that the older a caregiver is, the higher the caregiving burden may be because of age-related health problems and physical limitations.

It was found that caregivers with 2 or more years of caregiving experience had a higher level of caregiver burden than those with durations of care of 1–6 months and 1–2 years. Similar to the results of this study, Çetinkaya and Karadakovan (2012) found that longer caregiving durations were positively associated with higher caregiver burden. In a study by Yıkılkan et al. (2014), caregivers who cared for their patients for more than 3 years had higher levels of depression and anxiety than caregivers with shorter caregiving durations. Regression analysis showed that duration of caregiving was not a significant predictor of the burden of caregiving. This finding is an important outcome, as it shows that caregiver burden is associated with more than only the duration of the caregiving. It may be that long-term caregiving results in higher caregiver burden because of the increases in frequency and severity of physical, mental, and social problems.

In this study, the caregiver burden of caregivers who were required to meet all of the needs of their patients was higher than that of caregivers who met only the financial needs or provided psychological support to their care recipients. Multiple regression analysis found no significant relationship between areas of care and caregiver burden. Mollaoğlu, Özkan Tuncay, and Kars Fertelli (2011) found that those caregivers who met all of the needs of their patients had a higher level of caregiver burden. Moreover, Sanuade and Boatemaa (2015) found that caregivers who provided only financial support and caregivers who received outside financial and physical support had lower levels of caregiver burden. Caregivers who provide patients with only financial or psychological support are not primary caregivers. In these types of cases, the main caregiver is usually another member of the family, and the caregiver's burden is less compared with those who must meet all of their patients' needs.

The cross-sectional approach used in this study limits its generalizability to similar populations only. In addition, the self-report nature of data collection potentially limits the accuracy and generalization of results. The relatively large sample size is a strength of this study. Future studies should consider more complex variables dealing with caregiving as predictive variables (e.g., caregiver-perceived social support, coping strategies, daily care hours, having help available at home, number of caregivers). Furthermore, in line with the results of this study, it is recommended that experimental studies be carried out to evaluate the effectiveness of nursing interventions that are carried out to reduce the caregiver burden of individuals who provide care to bedridden patients.

Conclusions

The caregivers in this group reported a moderate overall level of caregiver burden. Furthermore, the health status, employment status, ability to tend to personal health matters, and type of home of the caregiver and the degree of dependence of the patient in terms of ADL were all found to be significant predictors of caregiver burden.

References

Abdollahpour, I., Noroozian, M., Nedjat, S., & Majdzadeh, R. (2012). Caregiver burden and its determinants among the family members of patients with dementia in Iran. *International Journal of Preventive Medicine, 3*(8), 544–551.

Adelman, R. D., Tmanova, L. L., Delgado, D., Dion, S., & Lachs, M. S. (2014). Caregiver burden: A clinical review. *JAMA, 311*(10), 1052–1060. https://doi.org/10.1001/jama.2014.304

Atagün, M. İ., Balaban, Ö. D., Atagün, Z., Elagöz, M., & Özpolat, A. Y. (2011). Caregiver burden in chronic diseases. *Current Approaches in Psychiatry, 3*(3), 513–552. https://doi.org/10.5455/cap.20110323 (Original work published in Turkish)

Bauer, J. M., & Sousa-Poza, A. (2015). Impacts of informal caregiving on caregiver employment, health, and family. *Journal of Population Ageing, 8*(3), 113–145. https://doi.org/10.1007/s12062-015-9116-0

Brodaty, H., Woodward, M., Boundy, K., Ames, D., Balshaw, R., & PRIME Study Group. (2014). Prevalence and predictors of burden in caregivers of people with dementia. *The American Journal of Geriatric Psychiatry, 22*(8), 756–765. https://doi.org/10.1016/j.jagp.2013.05.004

Çetinkaya, F., & Karadakovan, A. (2012). Investigation of care burden in dementia patient caregivers. *Turkish Journal of Geriatrics, 15*(2), 171–178. (Original work published in Turkish)

Chang, H. Y., Chiou, C. J., & Chen, N. S. (2010). Impact of mental health and caregiver burden on family caregivers' physical health. *Archives of Gerontology and Geriatrics, 50*(3), 267–271. https://doi.org/10.1016/j.archger.2009.04.006

Chiou, C. J., Chang, H. Y., Chen, I. P., & Wang, H. H. (2009). Social support and caregiving circumstances as predictors of caregiver burden in Taiwan. *Archives of Gerontology and Geriatrics, 48*(3), 419–424. https://doi.org/10.1016/j.archger.2008.04.001

Collins, L. G., & Swartz, K. (2011). Caregiver care. *American Family Physician, 83*(11), 1309–1317.

Conde-Sala, J. L., Garre-Olmo, J., Turró-Garriga, O., Vilalta-Franch, J., & López-Pousa, S. (2010). Differential features of burden between spouse and adult–child caregivers of patients with Alzheimer's disease: An exploratory comparative design. *International Journal of Nursing Studies, 47*(10), 1262–1273. https://doi.org/10.1016/j.ijnurstu.2010.03.001

Etters, L., Goodall, D., & Harrison, B. E. (2008). Caregiver burden among dementia patient caregivers: A review of the literature. *Journal of the American Academy of Nurse Practitioners, 20*(8), 423–428. https://doi.org/10.1111/j.1745-7599.2008.00342.x

Handicap International. (n.d.). *Training material—PT protocol for bedridden patients.* Retrieved from https://static.aminer.org/pdf/PDF/000/355/038/therapy_of_bedridden_patients.pdf

İnci, F. H., & Erdem, M. E. (2008). Validity and reliability of the burden interview and its adaptation to Turkish. *Atatürk University School of Nursing Journal, 11*(4), 85–94. (Original work published in Turkish)

Jeong, Y. G., Myong, J. P., & Koo, J. W. (2015). The modifying role of caregiver burden on predictors of quality of life of caregivers of hospitalized chronic stroke patients. *Disability and Health Journal, 8*(4), 619–625. https://doi.org/10.1016/j.dhjo.2015.05.005

Katz, S., Ford, A. B., Moskowitz, R. W., Jackson, B. A., & Jaffe, M. W. (1963). Studies of illness in the aged. The index of ADL: A standardized measure of biological and psychosocial function. *JAMA, 185*(12), 914–919. https://doi.org/10.1001/jama.1963.03060120024016

Kim, H., Chang, M., Rose, K., & Kim, S. (2012). Predictors of caregiver burden in caregivers of individuals with dementia. *Journal of Advanced Nursing, 68*(4), 846–855. https://doi.org/10.1111/j.1365-2648.2011.05787.x

Ma, H. P., Lu, H. J., Xiong, X. Y., Yao, J. Y., & Yang, Z. (2014). The investigation of care burden and coping style in caregivers of spinal cord injury patients. *International Journal of Nursing Sciences, 1*(2), 185–190. https://doi.org/10.1016/j.ijnss.2014.05.010

Mollaoğlu, M., Özkan Tuncay, F., & Kars Fertelli, T. (2011). Care burden of care givers of stroke patients and related factors. *Dokuz Eylul University Faculty of Nursing Electronic Journal, 4*(3), 125–130. Retrieved from http://acikerisim.deu.edu.tr/xmlui/bitstream/handle/12345/4595/125-130_mollaoglu.pdf?sequence=1&isAllowed=y (Original work published in Turkish)

Orak, O. S., & Sezgin, S. (2015). Caregiver burden in family members of cancer patients. *Journal of Psychiatric Nursing, 6*(1), 33–39. https://doi.org/10.5505/phd.2015.02986 (Original work published in Turkish)

Rha, S. Y., Park, Y., Song, S. K., Lee, C. E., & Lee, J. (2015). Caregiving burden and the quality of life of family caregivers of cancer patients: The relationship and correlates. *European Journal of Oncology Nursing, 19*(4), 376–382. https://doi.org/10.1016/j.ejon.2015.01.004

Roopchand-Martin, S., & Creary-Yan, S. (2014). Level of caregiver burden in Jamaican stroke caregivers and relationship between selected sociodemographic variables. *The West Indian Medical Journal, 63*(6), 605–609. https://doi.org/10.7727/wimj.2013.060

Sanuade, O. A., & Boatemaa, S. (2015). Caregiver profiles and determinants of caregiving burden in Ghana. *Public Health, 129*(7), 941–947. https://.doi.org/10.1016/j.puhe.2015.05.016

Schulz, R., & Sherwood, P. R. (2008). Physical and mental health effects of family caregiving. *American Journal of Nursing, 108*(9, Suppl.), 23–27. https://doi.org/10.1097/01.NAJ.0000336406.45248.4c

Sousa, M. F. B., Santos, R. L., Turro-Garriga, O., Dias, R., Dourado, M. C. N., & Conde-Sala, J. L. (2016). Factors associated with caregiver burden: Comparative study between Brazilian and Spanish caregivers of patients with Alzheimer's disease (AD). *International Psychogeriatrics, 28*(8), 1363–1374. https://doi.org/10.1017/S1041610216000508

Sümbüloğlu, K., & Sümbüloğlu, V. (2002). *Biostatistics* (10th ed., p. 264). Ankara, Turkey: Hatipoğlu Publication. (Original work published in Turkish)

Taşdelen, P., & Ateş, M. (2012). The needs of home care patients and the burdens of their caregivers. *Journal of Education and Research in Nursing, 9*(3), 22–39. (Original work published in Turkish)

Turkish Statistical Institute. (2002). *The proportion of disability.* Retrieved from http://www.tuik.gov.tr/PreTablo.do?alt_id=1017

Unver, V., Basak, T., Tosun, N., Aslan, O., & Akbayrak, N. (2016). Care burden and self-efficacy levels of family caregivers of elderly people in Turkey. *Holistic Nursing Practice, 30*(3), 166–173. https://doi.org/10.1097/HNP.0000000000000148

Vieira, H. F., Bezerra, A. L. D., Sobreira, M. V. S., Ankilma, J. B. S., Feitosa, D. N. A., & Paraíba, F. S. M. C. (2015). Nursing care patient bedridden in household: A systematic review. *FIEP Bulletin, 85*, 253–257. https://doi.org/10.16887/85.a2.60

Yardımcı, A. E. (1995). *The correlation of the health problems of the elderly teachers who live in Istanbul with their daily life activities and instrumental activities of daily life* (Unpublished master's thesis), University of Istanbul, Turkey. (Original work published in Turkish)

Yeşil, T., Uslusoy, E. Ç., & Korkmaz, M. (2016). Examining of the life quality and care burden of those who are looking after the patients suffering from chronic diseases. *Gümüşhane University Journal of Health Sciences, 5*(4), 54–66. (Original work published in Turkish)

Yıkılkan, H., Aypak, C., & Görpelioğlu, S. (2014). Depression, anxiety and quality of life in caregivers of long-term home care patients. *Archives of Psychiatric Nursing, 28*(3), 193–196. https://doi.org/10.1016/j.apnu.2014.01.001

Zarit, S. H., Reever, K. E., & Bach-Peterson, J. (1980). Relatives of the impaired elderly: Correlates of feelings of burden. *Gerontologist, 20*(6), 649–655. https://doi.org/10.1093/geront/20.6.649

Zaybak, A., Güneş, Ü., Günay İsmagloğlu, E., & Ülker, E. (2012). The determination of burden care of caregivers for bedridden patients. *Journal of Anatolia Nursing and Health Sciences, 15*(1), 48–54. (Original work published in Turkish)

12

Satisfaction with the Quality Nursing Work Environment Among Psychiatric Nurses Working in Acute Care General Hospitals

Chiou-Fen LIN[1] • Fu-Chih LAI[2] • Way-Ren HUANG[3] • Chung-I HUANG[4] • Chia-Jung HSIEH[5]*

ABSTRACT

Background: The objective of this study was to investigate the impact on patient care quality of a positive, high-quality environment that is tailored to the practice of nursing. This study enabled nurses to show their professional skills and knowledge, which may help enhance job satisfaction. To date, little research has been done to assess the relationship between the nursing work environment and the job satisfaction of psychiatric nurses employed in acute wards of general hospitals.

Purpose: This study was designed to explain the relationship between job satisfaction and the perceived indicators of a quality nursing work environment (QNWE) after adjusting for demographic characteristics and work characteristics.

Methods: A cross-sectional correlational design was employed, and a stratified random sample of 185 psychiatric nurses (99% response rate) working in acute wards in Taiwan was surveyed in 2013. Nurses were asked to complete a self-administered questionnaire that included measures of perceived QNWE and job satisfaction and demographic variables.

Results: A statistically significant, positive relationship was found between perceived indicators of QNWE and job satisfaction ($r = .813$, $p < .001$). In the hierarchical multiple linear regression model, for the subdimensions of QNWE, the variables "perceived indicators of professional specialization and teamwork" and "support and caring" showed a significant and positive association with job satisfaction, after adjusting for personal demographic characteristics.

Conclusions/Implications for Practice: Job satisfaction is related to the perception of nurses regarding their work environment. Therefore, nursing managers should improve workplace satisfaction by supporting and caring for nurses and creating better career development and teamwork opportunities for nurses through job training and planning.

Key Words:
job satisfaction, nursing work environment, psychiatric nurse, organizational support, teamwork.

Introduction

Nurses are a critical part of the healthcare system and make up the largest segment of the healthcare workforce. However, shortages and high rates of turnover have become issues affecting the nursing profession in many countries (Marć, Bartosiewicz, Burzyńska, Chmiel, & Januszewicz, 2019). Although the reasons for these shortages are varied and complex, key reasons include unhealthy work environments and poor organizational climates, which characterize many workplaces today (International Council of Nurses, 2007). In recent decades, many countries have restructured, reorganized, and reengineered their healthcare systems, and as a result, positive work environments for healthcare delivery have become an important and powerful factor affecting nurses in clinical practice (Hinno, Partanen, Vehviläinen-Julkunen, & Aaviksoo, 2009). A positive environment for nursing practice leads to higher quality patient care (Ward, 2011), may enable nurses to show their professional skills and knowledge (Currie, Harvey, West, McKenna, & Keeney, 2005), and may foster self-actualization in nurses (Burtson & Stichler, 2010). A further effect of a positive environment is an improved sense of job satisfaction (Lu, Barriball, Zhang, & While, 2012). Finally, a positive work environment may help increase employee retention in a current workplace (Al-Hamdan, Manojlovich, & Tanima, 2017). Previous studies have found a negative relationship between job satisfaction and intent to leave (Alsaraireh, Quinn Griffin, Ziehm, & Fitzpatrick, 2014; Baum & Kagan, 2015). In addition, job satisfaction has been found to mediate the relationship between organizational commitment and intent to leave. Thus, for nurses, job satisfaction is associated with greater organizational commitment, reducing the percentage of nurses expressing intent to leave

[1]*PhD, RN, Professor, School of Nursing, Taipei Medical University, and Nursing Consultant, Department of Nursing, Shuang Ho Hospital, Taipei Medical University* • [2]*PhD, RN, Associate Professor, College of Nursing, Taipei Medical University* • [3]*PhD, RN, Postdoctoral Research Fellow, Operations Center for Industry Collaboration, National Tsing Hua University* • [4]*PhD, Deputy Director, Center for Management and Development, and Adjunct Assistant Professor, School of Health Care Administration, Taipei Medical University* • [5]*PhD, RN, Associate Professor, School of Nursing, College of Nursing, National Taipei University of Nursing and Health Sciences.*

the current workplace (Shacklock, Brunetto, Teo, & Farr-Wharton, 2014).

A positive work environment has been defined as a work setting in which nurses are able to achieve organizational goals and to derive personal satisfaction from their work (Lin, Lu, & Huang, 2016). Managerial strategies designed to reduce the negative effects of organizational complexity on employee productivity, work quality, and retention have emerged in a variety of industries and settings. Recent research has focused on "Magnet hospitals" because of their reputation for good work environments, success in attracting and retaining qualified nurses, and improved patient outcomes (Friese, Xia, Ghaferi, Birkmeyer, & Banerjee, 2015). In the Magnet Recognition Program of the American Nurses Credentialing Center, which identifies hospitals that epitomize nursing excellence, using a win-win strategy for nursing and hospitals was highlighted as an effective approach to achieving collaboration among healthcare institutions (Centrella-Nigro et al., 2015); in other words, nursing managers must be able to create work situations that are assertive and cooperative with each other. Interest is growing regarding the perceptions of nurses toward their work and work environment to address current and potential future nursing workforce-related problems (Friese et al., 2015). As a result, understanding nurses' perceptions of their work and work environment is critical to effective management. It is important to note associations among burnout, job satisfaction, and work environment (Khamisa, Oldenburg, Peltzer, & Ilic, 2015). Research findings have linked burnout in nurses to several specific work environment factors, including high workload, poor collegial support, sense of coherence, and overall work-environment quality (Hanrahan, Aiken, McClaine, & Hanlon, 2010; Levert, Lucas, & Ortlepp, 2000). Moreover, prolonged exposure to stressful work environments diminishes job satisfaction (Khamisa et al., 2015).

Background

The qualities of a positive nursing environment identified in previous studies include the leadership attributes of nursing administrators (e.g., vision and responsiveness), professional attributes of staff nurses, and support provided for professional practice, including regard for nurse autonomy and control over practice, ability to establish and maintain nurse–patient and collaborative nurse–physician relationships, and nurses' perceptions of empowerment (Budge, Carryer, & Wood, 2003; Harwood et al., 2007, Kieft, de Brouwer, Francke, & Delnoij, 2014). Schmalenberg and Kramer (2008) identified eight key indicators of a quality work environment and provided guidance on how to improve the unit-work environment. Furthermore, the research team involved in this study previously developed a list of indicators for a quality nursing work environment (QNWE), with eight dimensions and 65 items that are associated with the indicator data collected by the American Nurses Association (Lin et al., 2016). Nurses working in QNWEs are encouraged to provide patients with excellent nursing care (International Council of Nurses, 2007). Although a QNWE increases job satisfaction for nurses (Lu et al., 2012), empirical evidence indicates the need for continued improvement. However, nurses in different countries may hold different perceptions of what constitutes quality in the work environment (Lu et al., 2012).

Previous studies have investigated the essential qualities for nurses in the hospital environment, and other work has investigated important aspects of a healthy work environment and nurses' work experiences (Budge et al., 2003; Milisen, Abraham, Siebens, Darras, & Dierckx de Casterle, 2006). However, few studies have concentrated on the perceptions of psychiatric nurses regarding their work environment (Gardner, Thomas-Hawkins, Fogg, & Latham, 2007). Although the psychiatric nursing shortage persists and the number of individuals with mental health issues and psychiatric disorders increases, empirical data on psychiatric nurses' perceptions regarding the quality of nursing work environments in acute inpatient care are scarce. Psychiatric nursing is a stressful occupation, with potential effects on the health and job satisfaction of care providers (Alsaraireh et al., 2014). One qualitative study indicated that job satisfaction in the psychiatric workplace might influence the retention rate of nurses who work in mental health services (Ward & Cowman, 2007).

Minimal research has assessed the relationships among elements in the nursing work environment and job satisfaction in psychiatric nurses employed in acute wards. Moreover, to the knowledge of the investigative team, the correlation between perceived QNWE and job satisfaction adjusted for personal characteristics among psychiatric nurses in Taiwan is a topic rarely considered in the literature. Therefore, this study was designed to fill a gap in understanding regarding psychiatric nursing in Taiwan and provide critical information to human resource managers.

The aims of this study were as follows: (a) to explore the perceived QNWE from the perspective of psychiatric nurses using a nationwide survey, (b) to compare the differences in perceived indicators of QNWE between two groups of nurses with different levels of job satisfaction, and (c) to explain the relationship between job satisfaction and the perceived indicators of QNWE after adjusting for demographic and work characteristics. The researchers hypothesized that the perceived indicators of QNWE affect the job satisfaction of psychiatric nurses after adjusting for the demographic characteristics of age, gender, marital status, and level of nursing education.

Methods

Sample

This study used a correlational cross-sectional design. The formulation of 95% with a minimum effect size of 0.15 for 11 predicting factors, p values at .05 significance, and a sample size of 178 were calculated based on a power analysis for partial correlation and linear multiple regression analyses. This study included 185 participants, with an initial distribution of 188 surveys (response rate: 99%), representing

14.21% of the entire population of registered nurses working in the acute psychiatric care wards of general hospitals in Taiwan. Approximately 48.25% of registered nurses in Taiwan work in acute psychiatric care (Ping, Hsieh, & Chou, 2008).

Inclusion criteria used in this study were a nursing license, full-time employment in an acute psychiatric ward at a hospital for at least 6 months, and age between 20 and 60 years. Exclusion criteria included student nurses, nurse assistants, and qualified nurses working in specialized care settings in a community rehabilitation center.

Data Collection

The Taiwan Nurses Association used a stratified random sampling method to conduct a nationwide survey under the authority of the Taiwan Ministry of Health and Welfare. Stratified random sampling ensured that a representative sample of psychiatric nurses in all hospitals was obtained. The research team constructed the study framework using existing healthcare delivery systems guidance and the accreditation policy of the National Ministry of Health and Welfare (Wu, Majeed, & Kuo, 2010). Study participants were selected in three steps. First, stratified random sampling was conducted to select the hospitals by tier. Next, a second round of stratified random sampling selected acute psychiatric wards. Finally, after obtaining permission from the selected hospitals, survey questionnaires were distributed to participants, who placed the completed forms in self-addressed, stamped envelopes to be returned to the researchers by the designated representative at each hospital. Four academic medical centers, nine metropolitan hospitals, and 12 district hospitals participated in this survey. The target population consisted of registered nurses employed by acute care institutions, principally because this sector of the nursing profession has been the most severely affected by the nursing shortage. The target population was chosen from a multistate sample and selected to represent specific nursing and demographic characteristics.

Ethical Considerations

Ethics approval was obtained from both the university and the hospitals involved in this study (TMU-JIRB No. 20130738). All respondents received written and verbal information regarding the study's aims and its contents. Study participation was voluntary. Completed research packets were collected daily and secured in a locked file. Data were analyzed anonymously, and the results were not traceable to individual participants.

Data Analysis

All of the data were analyzed using IBM SPSS Statistics v.19.0 (IBM, Inc., Armonk, NY, USA). Descriptive analyses included frequencies and percentages for categorical variables and means and standard deviations. For continuous variables, two independent sample *t* tests were used for normally distributed data to compare the differences between the two groups. Analysis of the Spearman rank order correlation was utilized to examine the relationships between job satisfaction and the QNWE total score and QNWE subscores. The significant factors were included in hierarchical multiple linear regression to further ascertain their associations with job satisfaction, after adjusting for demographic characteristics and work experience. Statistical significance was defined as $p < .05$, with the probability of a Type I error of .05.

Measures

The three instruments included in the self-administered questionnaire respectively measured the perceived indicators of QNWE, job satisfaction, and demographics.

Indicators of a quality nursing work environment

The indicators of QNWE, developed by the Taiwan Union of Nurses Association, were designed to measure nurses' perceptions of their working environment (Lin et al., 2016). The Cronbach's alpha value for the entire scale was .90. Validity was examined based on expert review of content validity and content validity indices, with the latter ranging from .83 to 1 for all dimensions. In addition, exploratory factor analysis was used for factor extraction. Principal component analysis was used to find the initial factor solution and factor rotation and to check for varimax. After the exploratory factor analysis, the final version of the QNWE metric included eight dimensions and 65 items, with 77.57% of the total variance explained. The reliability estimate for the QNWE metric was .91. The eight dimensions encompassed by the QNWE were as follows: a safe practice environment (16 items), quality and quantity of staff (four items), salary and welfare (seven items), professional specialization and teamwork cooperation (seven items), work simplification (five items), informatics (five items), career development (nine items), and support and caring (12 items). The indicators for each item were selected based on their suitability using a 5-point Likert scale, with scores ranging from 1 = *totally unqualified* to 5 = *fully qualified*. A higher score on the scale indicated greater perceived nursing work environment quality (Lin et al., 2016). The reliability of the QNWE metric possessed excellent internal consistency in this study, with a Cronbach's alpha value of .93.

Job satisfaction

Job satisfaction focuses on the feelings that people have with regard to their work environment. A single item, based on a prior study (Yoder, 1995), was used to assess the job satisfaction of the participants in this study. This item was scored on a 5-point scale, ranging from 1 = *very dissatisfied* to 5 = *very satisfied*. The average value for job satisfaction was used to divide the participants into two groups, including the "satisfied" group (score range: 3–5) and the "dissatisfied" group (score range: 1–2).

Demographic variables

The first section of the questionnaire included a demographic datasheet and questions pertaining to hospital tier (academic medical hospital, regional hospital, and district hospital), hospital geographic area, administrative position (years in nursing work and job title) at the current hospital, and length of professional nursing experience (10 years was used as the cutoff point). Personal characteristics such as age, gender, marital status, and nursing education were considered.

Results

Participant Characteristics, Perceived Quality of Nursing Work Environment, and Job Satisfaction

One hundred eighty-five questionnaires were collected. Most participants were female (90.8%), more than half (57.3%) were over 31 years old, and most worked at regional hospitals (63.3%) and held the job title of registered nurse (83.2%; Table 1).

The mean score for job satisfaction was 3.04 ± 1.04. Most respondents (73.0%) reported satisfaction with their jobs, and 27.0% reported dissatisfaction.

Perceived QNWE levels were found to be statistically different across hospital tiers ($F = 4.53$, $p < .05$), with post hoc results revealing that nurses in academic medical centers had statistically higher QNWE scores than in the other two tiers. Furthermore, a difference analysis of participants across the three hospital tiers also indicated a significant difference in the QNWE subscale (Table 2). Registered nurses reported the lowest QNWE levels, whereas managers reported the highest QNWE levels, based on mean scores ($t = 2.84$, $p < .01$). The results of the descriptive analyses included means and standard deviations of job satisfaction among different sociodemographic variables. However, a significant difference in job satisfaction was found based on marital status ($t = 3.15$, $p < .01$) and years of nursing experience ($t = 2.75$, $p < .01$); participants with

TABLE 1.
Demographic Characteristics of Participants and Differences Among Variables (N = 185)

			QNWE				Job Satisfaction			
Variable	*n*	%	*M*	*SD*	*t*	*p*	*M*	*SD*	*t*	*p*
Demographic characteristics										
Gender					−1.68	.095			−1.39	.168
Male	17	9.2	2.92	0.58			2.71	0.99		
Female	168	90.8	3.25	0.80			3.07	1.04		
Age (years)					−0.24	.807			−1.87	.063
≤ 30	79	42.7	3.20	0.70			2.87	1.03		
≥ 31	106	57.3	3.23	0.84			3.16	1.03		
Highest nursing education					1.06	.292			1.25	.210
Bachelor's degree and above	124	67.0	3.26	0.74			3.10	0.99		
Diploma degree and below	61	33.0	3.14	0.87			2.90	1.14		
Marital status					2.01*	.046			3.15**	.002
Married	73	39.5	3.36	0.82			3.33	1.00		
Single[a]	112	60.5	3.13	0.75			2.85	1.02		
Job status										
Work experience in nursing					−1.48	.140			2.75**	.007
≤ 10 years	104	56.2	3.15	0.74			2.86	0.99		
> 10 years	81	43.8	3.31	0.83			3.27	1.05		
Hospital tier					4.53*	.012			2.53	.080
Academic medical center	18	9.7	3.69	0.71			3.56	1.15		
Regional hospital	117	63.3	3.12	0.78			2.97	1.00		
District hospital	50	27.0	3.29	0.77			3.00	1.05		
Hospital geographic area					0.77	.464			0.97	.380
Northern	137	74.1	3.16	0.80			3.03	1.06		
Central	4	2.2	3.53	0.93			3.75	0.96		
Southern	44	23.8	3.29	0.72			3.00	0.96		
Job title					2.84**	.005			3.48**	.001
Manager	31	16.8	3.58	0.68			3.61	0.88		
Registered nurse	154	83.2	3.15	0.78			2.92	1.03		

Note. QNWE = quality nursing work environment.
[a]Includes never married, widowed, divorced, and separated.
*$p < .05$. ** $p < .01$. *** $p < .001$.

TABLE 2.
Difference Analysis of the Participants at Three Hospital Tiers for Job Satisfaction and Quality Nursing Work Environment Subscale

	Academic Medical Center		Regional Hospital		District Hospital			
Item/Dimension	Mean	*SD*	Mean	*SD*	Mean	*SD*	*F*	*p*
Job satisfaction	3.56	1.15	2.97	1.00	3.00	1.05	2.53	.08
Quality nursing work environment	3.73	0.69	3.12	0.78	3.29	0.77	4.53	.01
Safe practice environment	4.13	0.59	3.47	0.86	3.81	0.86	6.34	< .01
Quality and quantity of staff	3.97	0.70	3.35	0.86	3.05	0.79	8.49	< .01
Salary and welfare	3.20	1.06	2.76	1.01	2.92	1.09	1.55	.21
Professional specialization and teamwork	3.59	0.66	3.23	0.91	3.31	0.84	1.41	.25
Work simplification	3.04	1.37	2.99	1.07	3.13	1.07	0.27	.76
Informatics	4.13	0.51	2.90	0.90	3.18	0.99	15.07	< .01
Career development	3.82	0.96	3.12	0.95	3.45	0.98	5.40	.01
Support and caring	3.53	0.99	3.01	0.89	3.18	0.90	2.89	.06

fewer than 10 years of nursing experience reported lower job satisfaction levels. In addition, those with the job title of manager reported higher job satisfaction ($t = 3.48$, $p < .01$; Table 1).

Perceived Quality of Nursing Work Environment and Comparisons With Different Levels of Job Satisfaction

The mean score for overall QNWE was 3.04 ± 1.04 in this study, with safe practice environment receiving the highest (3.63 ± 0.86) and salaries and welfare receiving the lowest (2.85 ± 1.04) mean scores (Table 3).

A detailed analysis of the satisfied and dissatisfied groups showed that the satisfied group scored highly on perceived QNWE ($t = 21.44$, $p < .001$) and on each of the eight QNWE dimensions (Table 3).

Correlation Between Job Satisfaction and Quality Nursing Work Environment Ratings

Bivariate associations between job satisfaction and the terms of perceived QNWE ratings are shown in Table 4. Significant positive correlations were found between job satisfaction and perceived QNWE ($r = .813$, $p < .001$). In addition, significant and positive correlations were found between job satisfaction and the eight dimensions of QNWE.

TABLE 3.
The Rank and Mean (SD) Scores for Quality Nursing Work Environment and Comparisons of Different Job Satisfaction Levels

				Dissatisfaction (n = 50)		Satisfaction (n = 135)			
Item/Dimension	Mean	*SD*	Rank	Mean	*SD*	Mean	*SD*	*t*	*p*
QNWE	3.04	1.04		1.66	0.48	3.55	0.65	21.44	< .001***
1. SE	3.63	0.86	1	2.88	0.86	3.90	0.68	8.84	< .001***
2. QQS	3.33	0.86	2	2.94	0.76	3.47	0.85	3.88	< .001***
3. SW	2.85	1.04	8	1.86	0.64	3.21	0.92	11.27	< .001***
4. PST	3.28	0.87	3	2.44	0.77	3.60	0.68	9.99	< .001***
5. WS	3.03	1.10	7	2.16	0.93	3.36	0.97	7.54	< .001***
6. Info	3.10	0.96	6	2.37	0.74	3.37	0.89	7.07	< .001***
7. CD	3.26	0.98	4	2.26	0.71	3.65	0.77	11.15	< .001***
8. SC	3.21	0.90	5	2.13	0.71	3.47	0.69	11.70	< .001***

Note. QNWE = quality nursing work environment; SE = safe practice environment (16 items); QQS = quality and quantity of staff (four items); SW = salary and welfare (eight items); PST = professional specialization and teamwork (six items); WS = work simplification (five items); Info = informatics (five items); CD = career development (nine items); SC = support and caring (11 items).
***$p < .001$.

TABLE 4.
Correlations Between Job Satisfaction and Quality Nursing Work Environment

Item	Job Satisfaction	QNWE	①	②	③	④	⑤	⑥	⑦	⑧
Job satisfaction	1									
QNWE	.813***	1								
① SE	.633***	.817***	1							
② QQS	.412***	.591***	.496***	1						
③ SW	.758***	.882***	.676***	.407***	1					
④ PST	.732***	.846***	.627***	.392***	.739***	1				
⑤ WS	.620***	.836***	.596***	.374***	.708***	.714***	1			
⑥ Info	.582***	.796***	.631***	.487***	.625***	.565***	.574***	1		
⑦ CD	.794***	.939***	.743***	.438***	.817***	.782***	.768***	.745***	1	
⑧ SC	.842***	.892***	.673***	.387***	.815***	.772***	.716***	.631***	.888***	1

Note. QNWE = quality nursing work environment; SE = safe practice environment (16 items); QQS = quality and quantity of staff (four items); SW = salary and welfare (eight items); PST = professional specialization and teamwork (six items); WS = work simplification (five items); Info = informatics (five items); CD = career development (nine items); SC = support and caring (11 items).
***$p < .001$.

Identifying the Important Factors of Quality Nursing Work Environment Related to Job Satisfaction

To determine the extent to which demographic variables and work experience explained job satisfaction, these variables and the subdimensions of QNWE were used in a hierarchical multiple linear regression analysis that employed job satisfaction as the dependent variable. Subdimensions of QNWE ("professional specialization and teamwork" and "support and caring") showed a significant correlation with job satisfaction levels, after adjusting for demographic characteristics (marital status) and work experience ($t = 2.496$, $\beta = .203$, $B = .170$, $p < .05$; $t = 5.531$, $\beta = .592$, $B = .514$, $p < .001$, respectively). The full regression model explained 72.9% of the overall variance related to job satisfaction ($R^2 = .746$, $p < .001$; Table 5).

Discussion

Participants in this study were a representative sample of psychiatric nurses from acute wards in general hospitals in Taiwan. Overall, both the perceived QNWE and job satisfaction were identified as moderate. To the best knowledge of the research team, this is the first academic examination of the correlation between perceived QNWE and job satisfaction after adjusting for demographic and work characteristics in a Taiwanese psychiatric nurse population within a general hospital setting.

In this study, participants working in academic medical centers reported better working experiences with respect to the set of indicators (safe practice environment, quality and quantity of staff, career development, support and caring) of a QNWE and reported the highest perceptions of their work environment. Wu et al. (2010) found that the characteristics of a medical center may relate to service resources and the quality of working conditions. Medical centers in Taiwan typically have more equipment and a larger workforce available to protect the safety of patients and staff in acute care settings as well as more comprehensive continuing education programs and career advancement opportunities. This finding is similar to results in a study by Ward and Cowman (2007), who found that nurses identified teamwork and the work environment as important factors in psychiatric nursing. The hospital grouping in this study was based on the quality accreditation of the national hospital service network, which was planned according to certain criteria such as service population size, service divisions, distance, and geographical location in the healthcare system. The participants working in academic medical centers perceived a more positive nursing work environment than peers in other hospital settings. It is unclear why nurses of different experience levels have different perceptions of the nursing workforce, although the organizational attributes of the practice environment may affect these perceptions. Hanrahan et al. (2010) stated that nurses in their study perceived a better overall QNWE when factors including strong organizational support by effective managers, strong nurse–physician relationships, and higher psychiatric nurse-to-patient staffing ratios received high ratings. These factors may have a positive effect on the capacity of psychiatric nurses to sustain safe and effective patient care environments. It is important to note that, regardless of hospital type, perceived level of positive practice work environment affected perceived QNWE. For nurses who are dissatisfied and stressed because of an unhealthy environment, a positive practice environment not only affects their perception of services but also contributes to improved patient outcomes (International Council of Nurses, 2007).

The effect of current professional position found in this study, with managers reporting a higher perceived QNWE, aligns with previous research (Spence Laschinger, 2008). It

TABLE 5.

Predictors of Job Satisfaction: Hierarchical Regression Models After Adjusting for Variables

	Model 1[a]		Model 2[b]		Full Model[c]	
Item	β	*p*	β	*p*	β	*p*
Intercept	3.809	< .001	4.451	< .001	−0.471	.306
Marital status						
Married (reference group)						
Single[d]	−0.481	.002	−0.331	.069	−0.058	.577
Work experience in nursing						
≤ 10 years (reference group)						
> 10 years			0.075	.691	0.098	.344
Job title						
Manager (reference group)						
Registered nurse			−0.539	.013	0.008	.950
QNWE						
1. SE					0.027	.727
2. QQS					0.088	.127
3. SW					0.135	.073
4. PST					0.203	.013
5. WS					−0.080	.191
6. Info					−0.014	.835
7. CD					0.116	.323
8. SC					0.592	.000

Note. QNWE = quality nursing work environment; SE = safe practice environment (16 items); QQS = quality and quantity of staff (four items); SW = salary and welfare (eight items); PST = professional specialization and teamwork (six items); WS = work simplification (five items); Info = informatics (five items); CD = career development (nine items); SC = support and caring (11 items).

[a]Adjusted R^2 = .046, df = 183, F = 9.907, p < .001.

[b]Adjusted R^2 = .076, df = 181, F = 3.937, p < .05.

[c]Adjusted R^2 = .729, df = 173, F = 55.656, p < .001.

[d]Includes never married, widowed, divorced, and separated.

is likely that the registered nurse (RN) participants enjoyed greater perceptions of autonomy and control over their practice in a professional capacity. With regard to job satisfaction, married nurses reported higher levels of job satisfaction than their single peers. Moreover, nursing experience influenced job satisfaction, with more experienced nurses reporting higher levels of job satisfaction. These results are consistent with an earlier study by Zheng et al. (2017), in which the authors identified greater resilience in more experienced nurses and higher levels of job satisfaction in older age groups (Zheng et al., 2017). Resilience may be a characteristic worth exploring in future research.

The higher level of job satisfaction among married nurses in this study aligns with the findings of previous research (Alsaraireh et al., 2014). Nurses with less experience were usually younger and burdened with less responsibility, especially in social contexts. Married nurses reported higher job satisfaction than single nurses. These studies highlight the important effect of personal characteristics on the overall job satisfaction of nurses.

Significant differences in job satisfaction were also found by job title, with managers reporting the highest mean score. This finding is consistent with earlier studies (Lu, While, & Barriball, 2008), in which managerial responsibilities were associated with a slightly higher level of job satisfaction. Moreover, as professional commitments are known to influence job satisfaction (Lu et al., 2008), enhancing professional nursing commitments has the potential to benefit both individuals and employers. Another possible explanation is that registered nurses tend to have a more stressful, unpredictable, and emotionally burdensome professional life in acute clinical settings than managers. These findings underscore the importance of taking measures to understand and caring for the perceptions of working conditions. An important component of the retention strategy must address the predictors of job satisfaction and the differences in the implementation of this strategy between RNs and managers in acute wards.

Interestingly, the results of this study revealed a strong and significant correlation (r = .813, p < .001) between perceived QNWE and job satisfaction. These results confirm our underlying assumption. With regard to the perceived QNWE of RNs, higher levels of job satisfaction were reported. These results are consistent with an earlier study by Lu et al. (2008). A systematic review by Lu et al. (2012) found the sources and effects of job satisfaction to be similar across studies despite varying levels of job satisfaction. Hospital nurse job satisfaction levels are closely related to working conditions and organizational environment (Lu et al., 2012). The findings of this study are similar to that investigation.

Starting with this innovative approach, the authors of this study found that perception of support and caring in the work environment affected the overall job satisfaction of psychiatric nurses working in an acute ward environment. This finding emphasizes the importance of taking measures that not only support nurses administratively but also apply a supportive managerial strategy that deals with the predictors of job satisfaction in psychiatric nursing. In addition, it is important to enhance the factors that promote and strengthen job satisfaction such as greater supervisory support, a more flexible work schedule, more responsiveness to staff work and lifestyle needs, stress and relief interventions, and care for nursing staff to optimize their performance (Madathil, Heck, & Schuldberg, 2014).

A further finding in this study that echoes those of earlier studies is the strong and positive correlation between team collaboration (professional specialization and teamwork) and job satisfaction (Roche & Duffield, 2010; Ward, 2011). Moreover, a previous multiple linear regression analysis identified that better "perceptions of professional specialization and teamwork" in the work environment are a significant predictor of job satisfaction in psychiatric nursing environments. However, it is important to develop and maintain a collaborative working relationship with professionals. The roles of psychiatric nurse are evolving, and psychiatric inpatients often present both physical and mental distress because of the side effects of atypical antipsychotic agents and multiple risk factors. Therefore, monitoring both physical signs and mental symptoms has become a common nursing task for psychiatric inpatients, working with complex and integrated physical and psychological problems requires strong nurse–physician workplace collaboration, and close-knit cooperation within the multidisciplinary team is likely to influence job satisfaction and patient care positively (Hanrahan et al., 2010; Zheng et al., 2017). According to another qualitative study, healthcare providers must discuss patient care on the basis of their respective expertise. Thus, problems are solved more rapidly when ideas are freely exchanged (Kieft et al., 2014). As stated by the participants in this study, communication among healthcare workers is necessary to ensure that information does not conflict and treatment is uniform. Moreover, it is important to enhance the organizational sources of job satisfaction such as ward climate, professional practice level, quality of communication and interaction, quality of relationships among colleagues, and managerial support (Lu et al., 2012; Ward, 2011).

Limitations

This study was affected by several limitations. The central limitation was its cross-sectional design. In addition, as the measurements of perceived QNWE were based on self-reported data, their validity may be influenced by recall bias. Furthermore, this study did not investigate family obligations and whether these were understood as obligations to care for children, parents, elderly relatives, and the home. Another limitation of this study is the representativeness of the sample. Because we used stratified random sampling, only four nurses from hospitals in central Taiwan responded, suggesting that it would be more appropriate to use a probability proportional to size (PPS) approach to sampling in the future. Using PPS, the probability of selection in a sampling unit is directly proportional to its size. PPS takes varying sample sizes into account, avoiding underrepresenting subgroups and yielding more accurate results. Therefore, the findings of this study may not be sufficiently representative of the nursing profession as a whole.

Practical Implications

This was the first study to address the relationship between perceived QNWE and job satisfaction after adjusting for personal characteristics in hospital nurses working in acute psychiatric units. The results should be of interest to nursing administrators and healthcare policymakers. The findings indicate that job satisfaction in nurses relates to perceptions regarding work environment. Therefore, nursing managers should work to improve workplace satisfaction, support and care for nurses, and create better career advancement and teamwork opportunities through job training and career planning programs.

Conclusion and Recommendations

The findings of this study corroborate the findings of other recently published articles in the literature regarding a positive relationship between perceptions of nurses regarding work environment and job satisfaction. The findings provide new information regarding nurses who work in the acute psychiatric wards of general hospital services. Perceived QNWE has implications for nurse job satisfaction in psychiatric nursing. The dimensions of perceived professional specialization, teamwork, support, and care in the workplace were identified as the primary predictors of satisfaction in psychiatric nurses.

One recommendation supported by study results is to address the relationship between perceived QNWE and job satisfaction after adjusting for personal characteristics by conducting a nationwide survey of nurses working in acute psychiatric units. This initiative would acknowledge the often-challenging work environment in these units while taking action at the managerial level to improve the dimensions that promote and strengthen job satisfaction. The result may be expected to enhance the organizational resources that were associated with greater job satisfaction and fulfillment in this study.

Acknowledgments

This study was supported by grants from the Ministry of Health and Welfare, Executive Yuan of Taiwan, ROC (DOH101-TD-M-113-101009, 2 of 2). We gratefully acknowledge all of the participants for their generous cooperation.

Author Contributions

Study conception and design: CFL, CJH
Data collection: WRH, CIH, FCL
Data analysis and interpretation: CJH
Drafting of the article: CFL, FCL, CJH
Critical revision of the article: WRH, CJH

References

Al-Hamdan, Z., Manojlovich, M., & Tanima, B. (2017). Jordanian nursing work environments, intent to stay, and job satisfaction. *Journal of Nursing Scholarship, 49*(1), 103–110. https://doi.org/10.1111/jnu.12265

Alsaraireh, F., Quinn Griffin, M. T., Ziehm, S. R., & Fitzpatrick, J. J. (2014). Job satisfaction and turnover intention among Jordanian nurses in psychiatric units. *International Journal of Mental Health Nursing, 23*(5), 460–467. https://doi.org/10.1111/inm.12070

Baum, A., & Kagan, I. (2015). Job satisfaction and intent to leave among psychiatric nurses: Closed versus open wards. *Archives of Psychiatric Nursing, 29*(4), 213–216. https://doi.org/10.1016/j.apnu.2015.03.004

Budge, C., Carryer, J., & Wood, S. (2003). Health correlates of autonomy, control and professional relationships in the nursing work environment. *Journal of Advanced Nursing, 42*(3), 260–268. https://doi.org/10.1046/j.1365-2648.2003.02615.x

Burtson, P. L., & Stichler, J. F. (2010). Nursing work environment and nurse caring: Relationship among motivational factors. *Journal of Advanced Nursing, 66*(8), 1819–1831. https://doi.org/10.1111/j.1365-2648.2010.05336.x

Centrella-Nigro, A. M., Faber, K., Wiklinski, B., Bognar, L., Flynn, D. L., & LaForgia, M. (2015). Effective collaboration among magnet hospitals: A win-win for nurses and institutions. *The American Journal of Nursing, 115*(7), 50–54. https://doi.org/10.1097/01.NAJ.0000467279.13447.ea

Currie, V., Harvey, G., West, E., McKenna, H., & Keeney, S. (2005). Relationship between quality of care, staffing levels, skill mix and nurse autonomy: Literature review. *Journal of Advanced Nursing, 51*(1), 73–82. https://doi.org/10.1111/j.1365-2648.2005.03462.x

Friese, C. R., Xia, R., Ghaferi, A., Birkmeyer, J. D., & Banerjee, M. (2015). Hospitals in 'magnet' program show better patient outcomes on mortality measures compared to non-'magnet' hospitals. *Health Affairs, 34*(6), 986–992. https://doi.org/10.1377/hlthaff.2014.0793

Gardner, J. K., Thomas-Hawkins, C., Fogg, I., & Latham, C. E. (2007). The relationships between nurses' perceptions of the hemodialysis unit work environment and nurse turnover, patient satisfaction, and hospitalization. *Nephrology Nursing Journal, 34*(3), 271–281.

Hanrahan, N. P., Aiken, L. H., McClaine, L., & Hanlon, A. L. (2010). Relationship between psychiatric nurse work environments and nurse burnout in acute care general hospitals. *Issues in Mental Health Nursing, 31*(3), 198–207. https://doi.org/10.3109/01612840903200068

Harwood, L., Ridley, J., Lawrence-Murphy, J. A., White, S., Spence-Laschinger, H. K., Bevan, J., & O'Brien, K. (2007). Nurses' perceptions of the impact of a renal nursing professional practice model on nursing outcomes, characteristics of practice environments and empowerment—Part II. *CANNT Journal = Journal ACITN, 17*(2), 35–43.

Hinno, S., Partanen, P., Vehviläinen-Julkunen, K., & Aaviksoo, A. (2009). Nurses' perceptions of the organizational attributes of their practice environment in acute care hospitals. *Journal of Nursing Management, 17*(8), 965–974. https://doi.org/10.1111/j.1365-2834.2009.01008.x

International Council of Nurses. (2007). *Positive practice environments: Quality workplaces = quality patient care—Information and action tool kit.* Geneva, Switzerland: Author. Retrieved from https://www.twna.org.tw/frontend/un16_commission/webPages_4/IND/1.pdf

Khamisa, N., Oldenburg, B., Peltzer, K., & Ilic, D. (2015). Work related stress, burnout, job satisfaction and general health of nurses. *International Journal of Environmental Research and Public Health, 12*(1), 652–666. https://doi.org/10.3390/ijerph120100652

Kieft, R. A., de Brouwer, B. B., Francke, A. L., & Delnoij, D. M. (2014). How nurses and their work environment affect patient experiences of the quality of care: A qualitative study. *BMC Health Services Research, 14*, 249–259. https://doi.org/10.1186/1472-6963-14-249

Levert, T., Lucas, M., & Ortlepp, K. (2000). Burnout in psychiatric nurses: Contributions of the work environment and a sense of coherence. *South Africa Journal of Psychology, 30*(2), 36–43. https://doi.org/10.1177/008124630003000205

Lin, C. F., Lu, M. S., & Huang, H. Y. (2016). The psychometric properties and the development of the indicators of quality nursing work environments in Taiwan. *The Journal of Nursing Research, 24*(1), 9–20. https://doi.org/10.1097/jnr.0000000000000106

Lu, H., Barriball, K. L., Zhang, X., & While, A. E. (2012). Job satisfaction among hospital nurses revisited: A systematic review. *International Journal of Nursing Studies, 49*(8), 1017–1038. https://doi.org/10.1016/j.ijnurstu.2011.11.009

Lu, H., While, A. E., & Barriball, K. L. (2008). Role perceptions and reported actual role content of hospital nurses in Mainland China. *Journal of Clinical Nursing, 17*(8), 1011–1022. https://doi.org/10.1111/j.1365-2702.2007.01950.x

Madathil, R., Heck, N. C., & Schuldberg, D. (2014). Burnout in psychiatric nursing: Examining the interplay of autonomy, leadership style, and depressive symptoms. *Archives of Psychiatric Nursing, 28*(3), 160–166. https://doi.org/10.1016/j.apnu.2014.01.002

Marć, M., Bartosiewicz, A., Burzyńska, J., Chmiel, Z., & Januszewicz, P. (2019). A nursing shortage—A prospect of global and local policies. *International Nursing Review, 66*(1), 9–16. https://doi.org/10.1111/inr.12473

Milisen, K., Abraham, I., Siebens, K., Darras, E., & Dierckx de Casterlé, B. (2006). Work environment and workforce problems: A cross-sectional questionnaire survey of hospital nurses in Belgium. *International Journal of Nursing Studies, 43*(6), 745–754. https://doi.org/10.1016/j.ijnurstu.2005.10.008

Ping, L. C., Hsieh, C. J., & Chou, K. R. (2008). An analysis of the current manpower situation in mental health nursing. *The Journal of Psychiatric and Mental Health Nursing, 3*(1), 46–51. (Original work published in Chinese)

Roche, M. A., & Duffield, C. M. (2010). A comparison of the nursing practice environment in mental health and medical–surgical settings. *Journal of Nursing Scholarship, 42*(2), 195–206. https://doi.org/10.1111/j.1547-5069.2010.01348.x

Schmalenberg, C., & Kramer, M. (2008). Essentials of a productive nurse work environment. *Nursing Research, 57*(1), 2–13. https://doi.org/10.1097/01.NNR.0000280657.04008.2a

Shacklock, K., Brunetto, Y., Teo, S., & Farr-Wharton, R. (2014). The role of support antecedents in nurses' intentions to quit: The case of Australia. *Journal of Advanced Nursing, 70*(4), 811–822. https://doi.org/10.1111/jan.12239

Spence Laschinger, H. K. (2008). Effect of empowerment on professional practice environments, work satisfaction, and patient care quality: Further testing the nursing work life model. *Journal of Nursing Care Quality, 23*(4), 322–330. https://doi.org/10.1097/01.NCQ.0000318028.67910.6b

Ward, L. (2011). Mental health nursing and stress: Maintaining balance. *International Journal of Mental Health Nursing, 20*(2), 77–85. https://doi.org/10.1111/j.1447-0349.2010.00715.x

Ward, M., & Cowman, S. (2007). Job satisfaction in psychiatric nursing. *Journal of Psychiatric and Mental Health Nursing, 14*(5), 454–461. https://doi.org/10.1111/j.1365-2850.2007.01104.x

Wu, T. Y., Majeed, A., & Kuo, K. N. (2010). An overview of the healthcare system in Taiwan. *London Journal of Primary Care, 3*(2), 115–119. https://doi.org/10.1080/17571472.2010.11493315

Yoder, L. H. (1995). Staff nurses' career development relationships and self-reports of professionalism, job satisfaction, and intent to stay. *Nursing Research, 44*, 290–297.

Zheng, Z., Gangaram, P., Xie, H., Chua, S., Ong, S. B. C., & Koh, S. E. (2017). Job satisfaction and resilience in psychiatric nurses: A study at the Institute of Mental Health, Singapore. *International Journal of Mental Health Nursing, 26*(6), 612–619. https://doi.org/10.1111/inm.12286

13

The Buffering Effect of Perceived Organizational Support on the Relationships Among Workload, Work–Family Interference and Affective Commitment: A Study on Nurses

Ozge TAYFUR EKMEKCI[1*] • Dorela XHAKO[2] • Selin METIN CAMGOZ[3]

ABSTRACT

Background: Minimal research has been conducted to explore the associations among workload, work-to-family conflict, family-to-work conflict, support, and affective commitment.

Purpose: This study was designed to explore the moderating role of perceived organizational support on the mediating effects of work-to-family conflict, family-to-work conflict in perceived workload, and affective commitment linkage.

Methods: The data were collected using a self-report survey from 164 nurses working at two public hospitals. The hypothesized model was tested using PROCESS macro.

Results: Perceived organizational support was found to influence the mediating effect of work-to-family conflict on the linkage between workload and affective commitment, yet not to moderate the mediating effect of family-to-work conflict. The results revealed that workload predicts affective commitment negatively and work-to-family conflict positively. However, perceived organizational support was found to change the effect that workload has on affective commitment. The negative effect of workload on affective commitment was found to be weaker for nurses with adequate organizational support.

Conclusions/Implications for Practice: Perceived organizational support was found to have both main and buffering effects on the emotional attachment of nurses toward their organizations. The findings support the importance of creating supportive work settings to alleviate the adverse effects on nurses of workload and work–family interference.

KEY WORDS:
workload, work–family interference, perceived organizational support, affective commitment.

Introduction

While the growth in the world population and the augmentation of illnesses have increased demands on the nursing profession, healthcare organizations continue to face challenges in retaining qualified nurses. Thus, scholars and practitioners are searching for strategies and policies to enhance the commitment of employees to healthcare organizations. Organizational commitment (OC), a central variable in fostering organizational effectiveness (Wasti, 1999), has been defined as "a psychological state involving employees' decision to remain or not in the same organization" (Meyer & Allen, 1991, p. 67). Among the three subfactors of OC, affective commitment (AC) has gained particular attention, as it relates directly to increased job performance (Reiley & Jacobs, 2019) and reduced absenteeism (Jacobsen & Fjeldbraaten, 2019). AC reflects an "employee's emotional attachment to, identification with, and involvement in the organization" (Meyer et al., 2002, p. 21). Studies conducted on nurses have revealed nurses who are affectively committed to be more likely to remain in their organizations for more years (Chang et al., 2019) and to perceive more professional satisfaction (Barać et al., 2018).

Work overload, a prominent situational factor that affects the OC of employees, reflects an excess in task demands requiring significant amounts of effort (Schulz et al., 1998, p. 91). Work overload may occur because of a shortage of nurses, increases in overtime or patient numbers, or an aging population and may reduce the AC of nurses by stimulating conflicts between work and life spheres. Particularly, the perception of high workload may accelerate work–family interference in terms of both work-to-family conflict (WFC) and family-to-work conflict (FWC), which mainly arise from

[1]*PhD, Associate Professor, Faculty of Economics and Administrative Science, Department of Business Administration, Hacettepe University, Ankara, Turkey* • [2]*MS, Faculty of Economics and Administrative Science, Department of Business Administration, Hacettepe University, Ankara, Turkey* • [3]*PhD, Professor, Faculty of Economics and Administrative Science, Department of Business Administration, Hacettepe University, Ankara, Turkey.*

"the perceptions of insufficient time and energy to successfully perform work and family roles" (Grandey & Cropanzano, 1999, p. 350). Such heightened levels of WFC and FWC may erode an individual's emotional attachment toward their organization (e.g., Yang et al., 2018).

"Perceived organizational support" (POS) is a variable that may significantly and positively influence AC. When employees receive favorable treatment from their organizations, they feel obligated to respond by exercising more effort and committing more to their workplaces. Thus, AC to their organization may increase when nurses perceive increased support from administrators and experience less workload and fewer work–family issues. This study was developed to address the predictive effects of workload and work–family interference (WFC and FWC) and the buffering effect of POS on AC in nurses. In this study, the mediating roles of WFC and FWC on the linkage between workload and commitment and the effects of workload and work–family interference on AC change when nurses perceive organizational support are explored.

This study was conducted using data from Turkey. The status of women in Turkish society has progressed since the founding of the Turkish Republic in 1923. This progress has improved the nursing profession and increased the number of professional women who work as nurses (Bahçecik & Alpar, 2009). Currently, whereas men may work in the nursing profession, women comprise most nurses in Turkey (Bahçecik & Alpar, 2009). In the Turkish healthcare system, nurses in public hospitals are employed as civil servants and thus work either as permanent staff or as annual (temporary) contract employees (S. C. Durmus et al., 2018). Most of the nurses in private hospitals are employed as contract employees. According to the latest Organization for Economic Co-operation and Development (2017) data, Turkey is ranked as one of the worst countries in terms of the nursing ratio, which is approximately 2.1 per 1,000 population. Benligiray and Sonmez (2013) state that the shortage of qualified nurses in Turkey is because primarily of long working hours, work overloading, and inadequate job-training opportunities. Moreover, research has shown most nurses in Turkey are "insensitive" to their organizations, with no or low degrees of commitment (Benligiray & Sonmez, 2013). Excessive workload, day and night shifts, irregular work hours (Yildirim & Aycan, 2008), insufficient salary, and awards seem to result in quitting their job or the profession completely. Therefore, this study may provide important insights to healthcare practitioners in Turkey to help them develop policies to enhance OC and reduce work-to-family interference in nurses.

Theoretical Background

Work overload and affective commitment

The adverse outcomes of work overload, a type of pressure that individuals experience in the workplace, include higher levels of emotional exhaustion (e.g., Sianoja et al., 2018) and lower levels of job satisfaction (e.g., Zeytinoglu et al., 2007). Although the significance and severity of work overload depend on the type of job, it is an important factor affecting the healthcare sector, where direct communication with patients and their relatives is intensive. Although workload accelerates with job intensity and working hours, two individuals working in the same organization and having the same task demands may perceive their workload differently. Therefore, workload should be measured in subjective terms rather than in terms of number of hours worked. Accordingly, a high workload should be defined as reflecting the perception of an individual lacking or having insufficient "personal resources needed to fulfill job-related commitments, obligations, and requirements" (Peterson et al., 1995, p. 430).

Researchers have also argued that employees perceiving high levels of work overload are less satisfied and less committed and tend to quit the organization (Malik et al., 2010). A plausible linkage between AC and workload may be explained using the premises of the psychological contract theory (Rousseau, 1990). Under this theory, when an employee perceives an inconsistency between an employer's words and actions, he or she experiences psychological contract breach. Thus, if employees perceive that their workload exceeds a manageable level, they may experience psychological contract breach. As time passes, these employees lose confidence that their employer is acting in their interests and, more importantly, is dealing with them honestly, which erodes their organizational trust and, subsequently, their emotional bonds with their employer. Drawing upon the tenets of this theory and prior research, perceived workload is presumed in this study to be negatively associated with AC.

Work–family interference, workload, and affective commitment

Work–family interference has been defined as "inter role conflict where the role pressures from the work and family domains are mutually incompatible in some respect" (Greenhaus & Beutell, 1985, p. 77) and rests on the premise that fulfilling the demands of one domain (family or work) makes it more difficult to accomplish the demands of the opposite domain (Netemeyer et al., 1996). These definitions assume a unidimensional meaning of WFC, with work acting unilaterally on family responsibilities. However, recent studies have highlighted that family responsibilities also interfere with work responsibilities. In other words, conflict may originate in the family (FWC) and work (WFC) contexts. WFC occurs when work-related demands interfere with family responsibilities (e.g., childcare, household chores), whereas FWC occurs when family responsibilities impede work activities (Netemeyer et al., 1996). More particularly, individuals who work beyond their scheduled working hours and do not fulfill their home responsibilities may experience WFC. Conversely, FWC occurs when individuals experience an "inter-role conflict in which the general demands of time devoted to, and strain created by the family interfere with performing work-related responsibilities" (Netemeyer et al., 1996, p. 401). Thus, individuals who are absent from work because of household chores tend to experience FWC. The literature indicates that scholars should focus more attention on both WFC and FWC, as each necessitates different interventions (Mesmer-Magnus & Viswesvaran, 2005).

In line with previous studies conducted with nurses (e.g., Asiedu et al., 2018; Ghislieri et al., 2017), perceived workload is presumed to be positively related to both WFC and FWC. Conservation of resources (COR) theory (Hobfoll et al., 2018) and resource drain theory (Edwards & Rothbard, 2000) may help explain the associations among WFC, FWC, and workload. COR theory argues that conflict arises from limited resources (e.g., energy, time) and the desire of individuals to retain and protect these resources. When employees perceive the risk of losing resources that are valuable and meaningful to them, they tend to experience stress, leading to conflict between the roles of work and family (Hobfoll et al., 2018). Resource drain theory argues that, when a significant amount of resources (e.g., energy and time) are spent in one domain (e.g., family), a few resources are left to invest in other domains such as work, resulting in a conflict between these domains (Edwards & Rothbard, 2000). Following this corollary, perceived workload may be expected to positively predict conflicts in both work and life domains.

As with perceived workload, WFC and FWC are assumed to be negatively associated with AC. Experiencing conflict in either work or home domains has been associated with heightened stress levels (Stoeva et al., 2002), which may influence organizational attitudes and reduce the employee's emotional attachment to his or her organization. Considering the premises of COR, psychological contract, and resource drain theories, the workload is assumed in this study to be a distal workplace strain that is expected to affect WFC and FWC and, in turn, act as proximal predictors of AC in nurses. Thus, we assert the following hypotheses:

Hypothesis 1: WFC mediates the relationship between workload and AC.

Hypothesis 2: FWC mediates the relationship between workload and AC.

The moderating effect of perceived organizational support

As part of the social exchange between employees and their organizations, employees express loyalty and dedication by increasing work performance and reducing absenteeism and turnover (Rhoades & Eisenberger, 2002). Employers reciprocate this loyalty and dedication by offering a decent salary and wages and by showing interest and genuine concern for the well-being of their employees (Dawley et al., 2010). POS plays a critical role in this mutually rewarding social exchange in terms of assuring employees that "their organization stands behind them as they perform their jobs and handle stressful conditions" and assuring employers that employees value and respect their organization (George et al., 1993; cited in Dawley et al., 2010, p. 241). Therefore, in line with the reciprocity principle, it is reasonable to expect that "the obligation to exchange caring for caring" acts to enhance employees' AC to the personified organization (Foa & Foa, 1980; cited in Arshadi, 2011, p. 1101). In other words, POS could directly influence nurses' AC toward their organizations.

POS may also positively influence AC by satisfying the affiliation needs of employees (Eisenberger et al., 1986). The satisfaction of socioemotional needs may create a sense of belonging to an organization, which may lead employees to incorporate this sense into their social identity. Multiple studies have elucidated the relationship between POS and AC using the social identity and social exchange theory (Blau, 1964). Meyer and Allen (1991) argued that employers satisfying the needs of their employees through effort and status recognition helps employees create a social identity that bolsters OC. Therefore, POS could positively influence AC and may buffer the effects of WFC, FWC, and workload by reducing perceived stress. For example, if work-related concerns interfere with an employee's home responsibilities, he or she may experience WFC. However, if that employee works for a supportive organization that makes accommodations for home responsibilities, he or she may experience lower workload-related stress and WFC and thus have greater emotional attachment toward their employer. In line with the premises of the norm of reciprocity and social identity theory, we assert the following hypothesis:

Hypothesis 3a: POS moderates the mediated relationship between workload and AC via WFC. The mediated relationship is weaker in individuals who perceive a higher level of organizational support than those with lower levels of POS.

Hypothesis 3b: POS moderates the mediated relationship between workload and AC via FWC. The mediated relationship is weaker in individuals who perceive a higher level of support from their organizations than those with lower levels of POS.

These hypothesized relations are depicted in Figure 1.

Methods

Participants and Procedures

Before collecting the data, ethical approval for this study was received from the Ethics Commission of Hacettepe University (approval number: 35853172/433-3548), and permission was obtained from the authors to use the relevant scales for research purposes. All of the participants read and signed informed consent, which provided a brief description of the study aims and their rights (e.g., voluntary participation, withdrawal rights). No incentives were offered for participation.

Figure 1

Conceptual Model

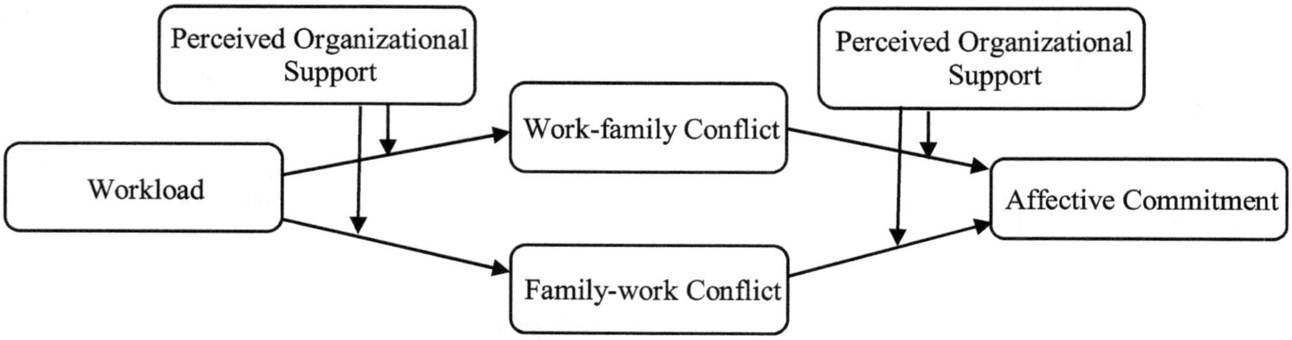

Data were gathered from nurses working at two public hospitals located in Ankara, the capital city of Turkey, in December 2016. Throughout the data collection period, the total number of nurses working at these hospitals was 390. The sample size was determined based on the suggestions of Tabachnick and Fidell (2013) as well as power analysis. The optimal sample size was calculated using the formula $N \geq 104 + m$ (in which m represents the number of independent variables) and was found to be at least 108 participants (Tabachnick & Fidell, 2013). A power analysis was conducted using an alpha of .05, and it was found that 194 participants were required to achieve a power of 0.80. Presuming a maximum attrition rate of 30%, 250 questionnaires were delivered via convenience sampling and 177 were returned (response rate: 71%). Considering the suggestions of Tabachnick and Fidell (p. 63), 13 of the collected questionnaires were excluded because of a large number of missing values (more than 50% missing data). Therefore, the total number of respondents was 164. Women comprised 94.5% of the sample (n = 155), which is representative of the nursing population in Turkey. The age of the participants ranged between 21 and 60 years (mean = 36 years). Most were married (73%, n = 120) and had children (69.5%, n = 114). Most were employed in alternative (nondaytime) working arrangements (67% alternative vs. 33% daytime work) and worked on weekends (79%). Weekly working hours exceeded 40 hours (74%).

Instruments

The questionnaire consisted of five sections, covering demographics (gender, age, marital status, and children), work-related conditions (total number of working hours, weekend working, and working schedule), and study variables (i.e., workload, WFC, FWC, POS, and AC). All of the study variables were measured using a 5-point Likert-type scale ranging from *strongly disagree* (1) to *strongly agree* (5).

Affective commitment scale

AC was measured using the scale of Meyer et al. (1993). Wasti (1999) added two more items to the original scale to create the Turkish version of this scale, which contains eight items (e.g., "I really feel as if this organization's problems are my own"). The Cronbach's alpha for the Turkish version of the AC scale was found to be .77.

Work overload scale

The Turkish version of Peterson et al.'s (1995) 11-item scale, created by Derya (2008), was used to assess the work overload status of the participants. A sample item is "My workload is too heavy." Higher scores indicate higher levels of perceived workload. The internal reliability coefficient of Cronbach's alpha was found to be .84 for this scale.

Work–family conflict and family–work conflict

Work–family interference was measured using the Turkish version of the 10-item scale of Netemeyer et al. (1996), created by Derya (2008). The first set of five items measures WFC, and the second set of five items measures FWC. Scale reliability in this study was found to be .92 for WFC and .93 for FWC.

Perceived organizational support

The short version of the POS scale, developed by Eisenberger et al. (1986), was adopted to measure the perceptions of the participants regarding the support provided by their organizations. The items on this scale were modified by V. Durmus (2011) to better reflect the working environment faced by healthcare workers. The modified Turkish version was utilized in this study. A sample item is "Help is available from the organization when I have a problem." Respondents rate 12 items, with higher scores indicating higher levels of perceived support. The Cronbach's alpha coefficient for this scale was found to be .93.

Results

Preliminary Analysis

A confirmatory factor analysis was conducted to examine whether the scale items measured the study variables adequately.

Table 1

Descriptive Statistics

Variable	*M*	*SD*	1	2	3	4	5	6	7	8	9	10	11
1. Gender	–	–	–										
2. Age	–	–	−.06	–									
3. Marital status	–	–	.03	−.28**	–								
4. Number of children	–	–	.06	.45**	−.59**	–							
5. Working format	–	–	−.01	−.12	.05	−.04	–						
6. Weekend work	–	–	−.07	.10	−.05	.05	−.69**	–					
7. Affective commitment	2.96	0.69	.10	.00	.01	.10	−.22**	.21**	.77				
8. Workload	3.43	0.76	−.05	.09	−.04	−.01	.17*	−.19*	−.23**	.84			
9. Work–family conflict	3.74	0.91	.03	.06	−.10	.05	.21**	−.24**	−.20*	.49**	.92		
10. Family–work conflict	2.66	1.06	−.10	.05	−.11	.08	.05	−.01	−.05	.25**	.33**	.93	
11. Perceived organizational support	2.53	0.80	.16*	−.05	.13	−.01	−.11	.11	.39**	−.32**	−.27**	−.06	.93

In the specified measurement model, all of the scale items were assigned to five study variables. Initial examination of the fit indices suggested a poor fit. After examining the modification indices and factor loadings, one workload item (Item 7: "I can finish my work on time") was excluded because of insignificant factor loading. The revised model yielded an acceptable model fit ($\chi^2(530) = 710.43$, $p < .05$, $\chi^2/df = 1.34$, comparative fit index = .94, Tucker–Lewis index = .94, root mean square error of approximation = .05, squared multiple correlation = .07) using the criteria of Schermelleh-Engel et al. (2003). As all of the item–construct relations were found to be significant, composite scores of WFC (n = 5 items), FWC (n = 5 items), workload (n = 10 items), POS (n = 12 items), and AC (n = 8 items) were created by taking the average of the responses. On the basis of the composite scores, we calculated the means and intercorrelations among the variables. The mean score, correlation coefficients, and scale reliabilities of the instruments are presented in Table 1. The Pearson correlation coefficients provided initial support for the hypotheses, with the results showing a moderate relationship between AC and workload ($r = -.23$, $p < .01$), POS negatively related to WFC ($r = -.27$, $p < .01$), and no significant correlation between demographic variables and AC. For the female participants, the mean score of FWC ($M = 2.63$, $SD = 1.04$) was significantly lower than the mean score of WFC ($M = 3.76$, $SD = 0.90$; $t(155) = -12.55$, $p < .001$).

Testing the Hypotheses

In this study, POS was assumed to moderate the impact of WFC, FWC, and workload on AC. Moreover, the impact of workload on AC was assumed to be mediated by WFC and FWC. The PROCESS macro was used to test the moderated mediation model (Hayes, 2018). As suggested by Hayes (2018), initially, the mediating effect of WFC and FWC on the linkage between workload and AC was tested. Working conditions were added as control variables, and the effects of these control variables were found to be insignificant at

Table 2

Regression Results for Mediation

Path		*b*	*SE*	*t*	*p*
Direct and total effects					
Workload → AC		−.24	.08	−3.09	.001
Workload → WFC		.56	.08	6.74	< .001
Workload → FWC		.36	.11	3.31	.001
WFC → AC		.13	.07	1.84	.060
FWC → AC		−.02	.05	−0.35	.720
	Boot *b*	**Boot β**	***SE***	**Boot LLCI**	**Boot ULCI**
Bootstrap results for indirect effect					
Effect through WFC	.070	.080	.04	−.001	.15
Effect through FWC	−.001	−.001	.02	−.050	.04

Note. AC = affective commitment; WFC = work–family conflict; FWC = family–work conflict; *b* = unstandardized regression estimate; β = standardized regression estimate; Boot LLCI = bootstrapping lower level confidence interval; Boot ULCI = bootstrapping upper level confidence interval.

Table 3

Regression for Conditional Indirect Effects of Workload Through Work–Family Conflict

Predictor	*b*	*SE*	*t*	*p*
Work–family conflict				
Constant	.37	.49	0.93	.35
Working format	.01	.10	0.06	.95
Weekend work	−.30	.24	−1.25	.21
Workload	.51	.10	5.02	< .01**
POS	−.15	.08	−1.76	.08
Workload × POS	.07	.10	0.68	.50
Affective commitment				
Constant	3.03	.43	7.09	< .01**
Working format	−.09	.09	−1.03	.30
Weekend work	.11	.20	0.57	.57
Workload	−.16	.08	−2,22	.03*
Work–family conflict	.16	.06	2.54	.01*
POS	.32	.07	4.79	< .01**
WFC × POS	.01	.09	0.10	.90
POS	**Boot Indirect Effect**	**Boot *SE***	**Boot LLCI**	**Boot ULCI**
Conditional Indirect Effect at Support = *M* ± 1 *SD*				
−1 *SD*	.07	.05	−.01	.20
M	.08	.03	.02	.16
+1 *SD*	.09	.04	.02	.19

Note. "Constant" indicates the expected mean value of dependent variables when the value of independent variables is 0. Working format; 1 = *daytime working* and 2 = *other.* Weekend work: 1 = *yes* and 2 = *no.* AC = affective commitment; POS = perceived organizational support; *B* = unstandardized regression estimate; β = standardized regression estimate; *SE* = standard error of unstandardized estimate; WFC = work–family conflict; Boot LLCI = bootstrapping lower level confidence interval; Boot ULCI = bootstrapping upper level confidence interval.

$^{*}p < .05$. $^{**}p < .01$.

each stage. The regression results for the mediation hypothesis are presented in Table 2, with workload showing a positive effect on WFC ($b = .56$, $t = 6.74$, $p < .001$) and FWC ($b = .36$, $t = 3.31$, $p = .001$). Unexpectedly, the effects of WFC ($b = .13$, $t = 1.84$, $p = .060$) and FWC ($b = -.02$, $t = -0.35$, $p = .720$) on AC were found to be insignificant, although the effect of WFC was nearly significant.

Although the mediating effects of WFC and FWC on workload and AC were found to be insignificant, these mediations may be significant contingent upon the values of POS. Thus, through PROCESS macro, the conditional indirect effect of workload on AC via WFC and FWC was evaluated as a function of POS after controlling for the working format and weekend working. The moderated mediation tests were conducted separately for each WFC and FWC. In Table 3 and Figure 2, the results of the moderated mediation model testing the conditional indirect effect of workload on the AC through WFC for three values of POS are presented (1 *SD* above and below the mean as well as the mean).

As shown in Table 3 and Figure 2, the moderating effects of POS on workload–WFC and WFC–AC linkages were found to be insignificant. However, as argued in Preacher et al.'s (2007) study, the moderated mediation model may still be significant if bootstrap confidence intervals for conditional indirect effects do not contain zero. In this study, bootstrap confidence intervals for conditional indirect effects were found to be [0.02, 0.16] at medium and [0.02, 0.19] at high CI levels of POS. The indirect effects at all values of the moderator are shown in Figure 3, with a 95% confidence interval. As seen, the conditional meditational effects of WFC (i.e., the indirect effect of workload) at medium and high levels of POS were found to be significant, as the values between the lower and upper bounds (i.e., the confidence intervals) did not contain zero. Thus, confirming expectations, POS moderated the indirect effect of workload on AC through WFC only in medium and high levels of POS. Although workload increases WFC, these heightened levels of WFC contribute to AC when nurses believe that they receive adequate support from their organization. In addition to this buffering effect, POS was found to have a relatively strong main effect ($b = .32$, $p < .01$). Accordingly, nurses who perceive high levels of support from their organizations are more likely to have higher emotional attachment toward their organizations (i.e., AC).

Figure 2

Results of Regression Analyses for Moderated Mediation: Work-To-Family Conflict as Mediator

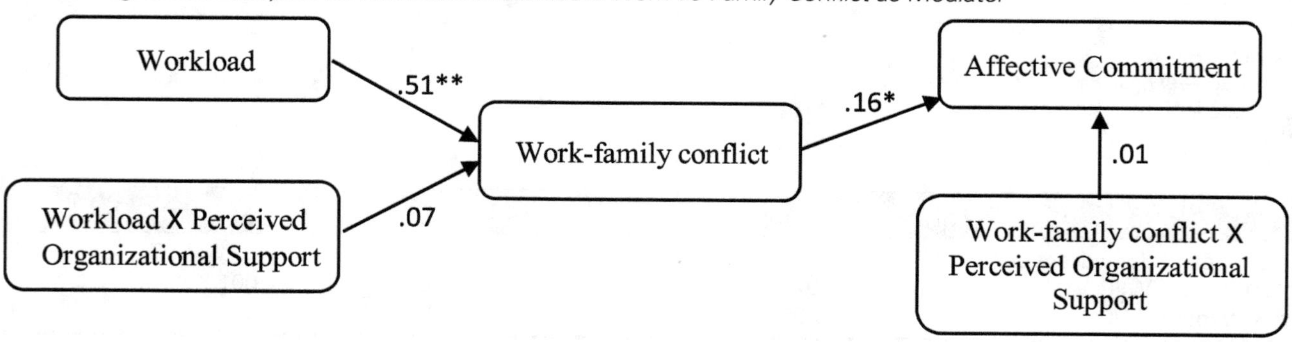

Note. Mediation is significant at meduim and high levels of perceived organizational support.

Figure 3

The Moderated, Indirect Effect of Workload on Affective Commitment Through Work-To-Family Conflict with a 95% Confidence Band

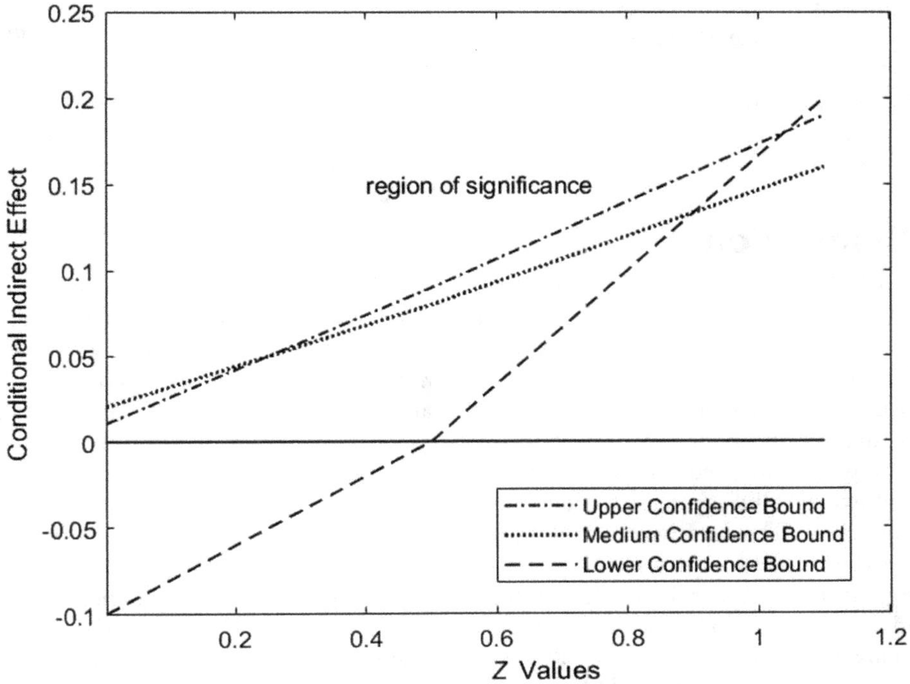

In the second moderated mediation test, we examined the conditional indirect effect of workload on AC via FWC as a function of POS after controlling for the working format and weekend work scheduling. The results of this moderated mediation test are shown in Figure 4. The moderating effects of POS on workload–FWC and FWC–AC linkages were not significant. Besides, bootstrap confidence intervals for conditional indirect effects were insignificant at all levels of POS (low CI [−0.07, 0.06], medium CI [−0.03, 0.06], and high CI [−0.03, 0.10] levels of spousal support). Hence, POS did not moderate the indirect effect of workload on AC through FWC at all levels of POS. Although POS did not have a buffering effect, it was found to have a significant main effect on AC ($b = .34, p < .05$).

In summary, moderated mediation tests were conducted in this study to assess the mediating effects of work–family interference (WFC and FWC, respectively) on the linkage between workload and AC. Then, the moderating effects of POS on two of the hypothesized mediated relationships ([a] workload → WFC → AC; [b] workload → FWC → AC) were explored using the same models. The significance of the findings was tested using bootstrap confidence intervals. The findings of the analyses revealed that neither WFC nor FWC acts as a mediator when POS is not taken into account.

Figure 4

Results of Regression Analyses for Moderated Mediation: Family–Work Conflict as Mediator

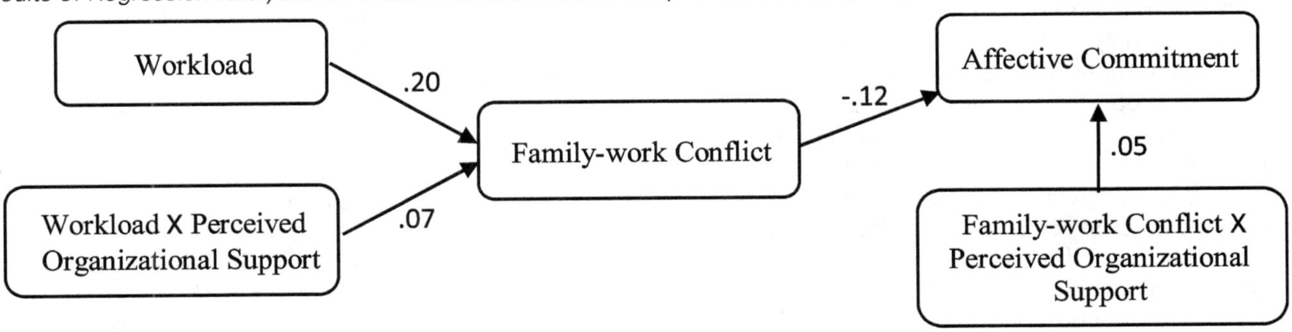

Note. Mediation is not significant at all levels of perceived organizational support.

However, when different levels of POS are considered, the mediating effect of only WFC (but not FWC) was shown to be significant on medium and higher levels of POS. This implies that, even when perceiving a high workload that exacerbates their WFC, nurses with sufficiently high levels of POS may maintain a relatively high level of emotional commitment to their organizations. However, as shown before, POS did not moderate the indirect relationship between workload and AC via FWC.

Discussion

In this study, it was assumed that workload, WFC, and FWC would negatively impact AC and that this negative impact would be decreased by POS. The results support this hypothesis only partially. POS moderated the mediating effect of WFC on the relationship between workload and AC, but not moderated the mediating effect of FWC. Specifically, the results suggest that workload predicts AC negatively and WFC positively. However, POS changes the direction of the workload's effect on AC. The negative effect of workload on AC was found to be weaker for nurses with adequate support from their organizations. Accordingly, the deleterious effect of workload on AC seems to be lessened in nurses who self-perceive as being adequately supported by their organizations, which makes the buffering effect of POS a prominent factor in nurses. In addition to this buffering effect, the main effect of POS on AC is also noteworthy. The effect of POS may be explained in terms of the premises of the norm of reciprocity and social identity theory. POS seems to give nurses the feeling that the organization supports them while they are doing their jobs and coping with problems and strains. These nurses seem to reciprocate this genuine interest and support with increased commitment toward their organizations. Moreover, by fulfilling affiliation and emotional support needs (Eisenberger et al., 1986), POS may produce a strong sense of belonging, thus making organizational membership part of the self-identity of nurses. This sense of belonging seems to increase the affection of nurses toward their organization (i.e., increase AC).

As indicated before, POS may not moderate the mediating effect of FWC on the relationship between workload and AC. This finding may be explained by the conceptualization of POS. In this study, POS measures nurses' perceptions regarding whether they receive direct assistance and advice from their organizations regarding work-related responsibilities or self-development (i.e., instrumental support) and whether they are shown emphatic understanding and genuine concern for their well-being (i.e., emotional support). By improving working conditions for nurses, POS becomes more likely to alleviate conflicts arising from work (WFC), but not conflicts arising from family (FWC). In parallel with this argument, Aycan and Eskin (2005) showed that organizational support was not significantly associated with FWC and was significantly associated with WFC. In particular, the researchers revealed that organizational support is more important in reducing WFC in men, whereas spousal support is more important in reducing FWC in women. As most participants in this study were women, finding a significant moderating effect of POS on the workload–WFC and AC linkage but not on the workload–FWC and AC linkage seems reasonable. Furthermore, as the direct and indirect effects of FWC are less clear than those of WFC, future studies should focus and explore FWC and its effects on multiple outcomes.

Remarkably, the main effects of WFC and FWC on AC were found to be insignificant. This seemingly contradictory finding may be because of the characteristics of the sample. Most (70%) of the participants were employed mothers. Mothers of especially young children may regard WFC and FWC as inherent, even normal in fulfilling parent and employee roles. Expecting work–family interference as natural, nurses in this study may have found coping mechanisms allowing them to separate work and life domains, resulting in their AC being less affected by workload, WFC, and FWC. Furthermore, Casper et al. (2002) argued that, when employees experience conflict in their home or work lives, they sometimes continue to remain in their organization because they have no choice. In other words, there is a possibility that participants experiencing WFC and FWC remain with their organization out of necessity rather than choice. Therefore, we suggest researchers investigate whether WFC and FWC are associated with different forms of commitment such as a continuance or normative commitment.

Remarkably, the women nurses in this study stated that they experienced more WFC than FWC. This finding may be explained by the traditional gender roles and working conditions of nurses in Turkey. Women in Turkey are expected to fulfill their primary roles in families, and their roles in the workplace are in general regarded as secondary. As women have possibly internalized this gender role, it is reasonable to expect them to perceive less FWC and more WFC (Polat et al., 2018). Moreover, because of the shortage of nursing staff and the increasing patient population, nurses in Turkey must deal with high patient-to-nurse ratios (Organization for Economic Co-operation and Development, 2017) and heavy mental workloads (Sönmez et al., 2017). As shown in previous studies on Turkish nurses (e.g., Ekici et al., 2017; Yildirim & Aycan, 2008), heightened levels of objective and subjective workload inevitably interfere with nurses' family lives, resulting in WFC. Future studies should expand the scope of research into the potential effects of FWC and WFC.

This study is affected by several limitations. The first relates to sample characteristics. The sample was mainly composed of nurses working in public hospitals. The working schedule of nurses in private healthcare institutions may differ from the schedule of those in public institutions. Thus, our findings may not be generalizable to all nurses. The second limitation relates to sample size. Although the sample size was adequate to test the hypothesized relations using regression analysis, a larger sample size will contribute to the generalizability of findings.

Despite these limitations, this study showed the importance of organizational support to increasing nurses' AC toward their organization. It seems that showing special consideration to the nurses' well-being and assisting them to resolve work-related problems are very important for nurses to function optimally. Supportive workplaces may be created by giving nurses opportunities to participate in decision making, being fair in the implementations of procedures, providing kindergarten services, and acknowledging their responsibilities at home. Supervisors should give sufficient consideration to the impact of workload and frequency of stressful events, which have been identified to predict WFC in nurses (Nissly, 2004). Moreover, administrators should be sensitive to working schedules that require nurses to work long hours and interfere with their family life. Offering flexibility in work schedules or at least providing nurses opportunities to voice their opinions may be viable solutions. Although it is not always possible to reduce workload, administrators may at least mitigate the negative effects of time-based conflicts by fostering supportive cultures. In other words, supervisors may provide a supportive working environment that permits flexibility in schedules, personal time off, onsite child care, or other family-supportive programs to reduce the conflicts originating from the work and home domains. In doing so, nurses may increase their emotional attachment to their organizations and thus perform better and have better physical and mental health.

Conclusions

This study investigated the mediating roles of WFC and FWC on the relationship between perceived workload and AC and explored whether these mediated relationships are affected by differing levels of POS. This study builds on previous knowledge regarding the linkages among workload, work–family interference, and AC and provides a new understanding of how organizational support alleviates the adverse effects of workload on AC. Utilizing a novel, moderated mediation model in a sample of nurses working at two public hospitals in Turkey, the results highlight the importance of POS on nurses' emotional attachment toward their organizations, making them more resilient to the detrimental effects of workload and work-to-family interference. In Turkey, a developing country with substantial problems with regard to the working conditions of nurses, the findings emphasize the importance of creating a supportive work environment to address and improve the commitment problems of healthcare employees.

Author Contributions

Study conception and design: OTE, DX
Data collection: DX
Data analysis and interpretation: All authors
Drafting of the article: All authors
Critical revision of the article: OTE, SMC

References

Arshadi, N. (2011). The relationships of perceived organizational support (POS) with organizational commitment, in-role performance, and turnover intention: Mediating role of felt obligation. *Procedia-Social and Behavioral Sciences, 30*, 1103–1108. https://doi.org/10.1016/j.sbspro.2011.10.215

Asiedu, E. E. A., Annor, F., Amponsah Tawiah, K., & Dartey Baah, K. (2018). Juggling family and professional caring: Role demands, work–family conflict and burnout among registered nurses in Ghana. *Nursing Open, 5*(4), 611–620. https://doi.org/10.1002/nop2.178

Aycan, Z., & Eskin, M. (2005). Relative contributions of childcare, spousal support, and organizational support in reducing work–family conflict for men and women: The case of Turkey. *Sex Roles, 53*(7–8), 453–471. https://doi.org/s11199–005–7134-8

Bahçecik, N., & Alpar, S. E. (2009). Nursing education in Turkey: From past to present. *Nurse Education Today, 29*(7), 698–703. https://doi.org/10.1016/j.nedt.2009.05.008

Barać, I., Prlić, N., Plužarić, J., Farčić, N., & Kovačević, S. (2018). The mediating role of nurses' professional commitment in the relationship between core self-evaluation and job satisfaction. *International Journal of Occupational Medicine and Environmental Health, 31*(5), 649–658. https://doi.org/10.13075/ijomeh.1896.01256

Benligiray, S., & Sonmez, H. (2013). The analysis of demographic and work–life variables which affect the occupational commitment of nurses. *Journal of Management Development, 32*(4), 419–434. https://doi.org/10.1108/02621711311326392

Blau, P. M. (1964). *Exchange and power in social life*. John Wiley & Sons.

Casper, W. J., Martin, J. A., Buffardi, L. C., & Erdwins, C. J. (2002). Work–family conflict, perceived organizational support, and organizational commitment among employed mothers. *Journal of Occupational Health Psychology, 7*(2), 99–108. https//doi.org/10.1037/1076-8998.7.2.99

Chang, H.-Y., Chu, T.-L., Liao, Y.-N., Chang, Y.-T., & Teng, C.-I. (2019). How do career barriers and supports impact nurse professional commitment and professional turnover intention? *Journal of Nursing Management, 27*(2), 347–356. https://doi.org/10.1111/jonm.12674

Dawley, D., Houghton, J. D., & Bucklew, N. S. (2010). Perceived organizational support and turnover intention: The mediating effects of personal sacrifice and job fit. *The Journal of Social Psychology, 150*(3), 238–257. https://doi.org/10.1080/00224540903365463

Derya, S. (2008). *Crossover of work–family conflict: Antecedent and consequences of the crossover process in dual-earner couples* [Unpublished master's thesis]. Koc University, Istanbul, Turkey (Original work published in Turkish)

Durmus, S. Ç., Ekici, D., & Yildirim, A. (2018). The level of collaboration amongst nurses in Turkey. *International Nursing Review, 65*(3), 450–458. https://doi.org/10.1111/inr.12440

Durmus, V. (2011). *The relationship between perceived organizational support and organizational learning: A study about military hospitals in Ankara* [Unpublished master's thesis]. Hacettepe University, Ankara, Turkey.

Edwards, J. R., & Rothbard, N. P. (2000). Mechanisms linking work and family: Clarifying the relationship between work and family constructs. *Academy of Management Review, 25*(1), 178–199. https://doi.org/10.5465/amr.2000.2791609

Eisenberger, R., Huntington, R., Hutchison, S., & Sowa, D. (1986). Perceived organizational support. *Journal of Applied Psychology, 71*(3), 500–507. https//doi.org/10.1037/0021-9010.71.3.500

Ekici, D., Cerit, K., & Mert, T. (2017). Factors that influence nurses' work–family conflict, job satisfaction, and intention to leave in a private hospital in Turkey. *Hospital Practices and Research, 2*(4), 102–108. https//doi.org/10.15171/HPR.2017.25

Foa, E. B., & Foa, U. G. (1980). Resource theory: Interpersonal behavior as exchange. In K. J. Gergen, M. S. Greenberg, & R. H. Willis (Eds.), *Social exchange: Advances in theory and research* (1st ed., pp. 77–94). Springer.

George, J. M., Reed, T. F., Ballard, K. A., Colin, J., & Fielding, J. (1993). Contact with AIDS patients as a source of work-related distress: Effects of organizational and social support. *Academy of Management Journal, 36*(1), 157–171. https://doi.org/10.5465/256516

Ghislieri, C., Gatti, P., Molino, M., & Cortese, C. G. (2017). Work–family conflict and enrichment in nurses: Between job demands, perceived organisational support and work–family backlash. *Journal of Nursing Management, 25*(1), 65–75. https://doi.org/10.1111/jonm.12442

Grandey, A. A., & Cropanzano, R. (1999). The conservation of resources model applied to work–family conflict and strain. *Journal of Vocational Behavior, 54*(2), 350–370. https://doi.org/10.1006/jvbe.1998.1666

Greenhaus, J. H., & Beutell, N. J. (1985). Sources of conflict between work and family roles. *Academy of Management Review, 10*(1), 76–88. https://doi.org/10.5465/amr.1985.4277352

Hayes, A. F. (2018). *PROCESS: A versatile computational tool for observed variable mediation, moderation, and conditional process modeling [White paper]*. http://www.afhayes.com/public/process2012.pdf

Hobfoll, S. E., Halbesleben, J., Neveu, J. P., & Westman, M. (2018). Conservation of resources in the organizational context: The reality of resources and their consequences. *Annual Review of Organizational Psychology and Organizational Behavior, 5*, 103–128. https://doi.org/10.1146/annurev-orgpsych-032117-104640

Jacobsen, D. I., & Fjeldbraaten, E. M. (2019). Exploring the links between part-time employment and absenteeism: The mediating roles of organizational commitment and work–family conflict. *Public Organization Review, 20*, 129–143. https://doi.org/10.1007/s11115-018-00437-x

Malik, O. F., Waheed, A., & Malik, K. U. R. (2010). The mediating effects of job satisfaction on role stressors and affective commitment. *International Journal of Business and Management, 5*(11), 223–235. https://doi.org/10.5539/ijbm.v5n11p223

Mesmer-Magnus, J. R., & Viswesvaran, C. (2005). Convergence between measures of work-to-family and family-to-work conflict: A meta-analytic examination. *Journal of Vocational Behavior, 67*(2), 215–232. https://doi.org/10.1016/j.jvb.2004.05.004

Meyer, J. P., & Allen, N. J. (1991). A three-component conceptualization of organizational commitment. *Human Resource Management Review, 1*(1), 61–89. https://doi.org/10.1016/1053-4822(91)90011-Z

Meyer, J. P., Allen, N. J., & Smith, C. A. (1993). Commitment to organizations and occupations: Extension and test of a three-component conceptualization. *Journal of Applied Psychology, 78*(4), 538–551. https//doi.org/10.1037/0021-9010.78.4.538

Meyer, J. P., Stanley, D. J., Herscovitch, L., & Topolnytsky, L. (2002). Affective, continuance, and normative commitment to the organization: A meta-analysis of antecedents, correlates, and consequences. *Journal of Vocational Behavior, 61*(1), 20–52. https://doi.org/10.1006/jvbe.2001.1842

Netemeyer, R. G., Boles, J. S., & McMurrian, R. (1996). Development and validation of work–family conflict and family–work conflict scales. *Journal of Applied Psychology, 81*(4), 400–410. https://doi.org/10.1037/0021-9010.81.4.400

Nissly, J. A. (2004). *Prospective and retrospective examinations of factors related to intention to leave and turnover among public child welfare workers* [Unpublished doctoral dissertation]. The University of Southern California.

Organization for Economic Co-operation and Development. (2017). *Health at a glance*. https://data.oecd.org/healthres/nurses.htm

Peterson, M. F., Smith, P. B., Akande, A., Ayestaran, S., Bochner, S., Callan, V., Cho, N. G., Jesuino, J. C., D'Amorim, M., Francois, P. H., Hofmann, K. H., Koopman, P. L., Leung, K., Lim, T. K., Mortazavi, S., Munene, J., Radford, M., Ropo, A., Savage, G., ... Viedge, C. (1995). Role conflict, ambiguity, and overload: A 21-nation study. *Academy of Management Journal, 38*(2), 429–452. https://doi.org/10.5465/256687

Polat, S., Kutlu, L., Ay, F., Erkan, H. A., & Doğrusöz, L. A. (2018). The relationship between work–family conflict, organizational silence, and social support in nurses at a university hospital. *Journal of Psychiatric Nursing, 9*(3), 195–204. https://doi.org/10.14744/phd.2018.38278 (Original work published in Turkish)

Preacher, K. J., Rucker, D. D., & Hayes, A. F. (2007). Addressing moderated mediation hypotheses: Theory, methods, and prescriptions. *Multivariate Behavioral Research, 42*(1), 185–227. https://doi.org/10.1080/00273170701341316

Reiley, P. J., & Jacobs, R. R. (2019). Linking leader power use and performance: The mediating role of follower satisfaction and commitment. *Journal of Management & Organization*, 1–21. https://doi.org/10.1017/jmo.2019.20

Rhoades, L., & Eisenberger, R. (2002). Perceived organizational support: A review of the literature. *Journal of Applied Psychology, 87*(4), 698–714. https://doi.org/10.1037/0021-9010.87.4.698

Rousseau, D. M. (1990). New hire perceptions of their own and their employer's obligations. Study of psychological contracts. *Journal of Organizational Behavior, 11*(5), 389–400. https://doi.org/10.1002/job.4030110506

Schermelleh-Engel, K., Moosbrugger, H., & Müller, H. (2003). Evaluating the fit of structural equation models: Tests of significance and descriptive goodness-of-fit measures. *Methods of Psychological Research Online, 8*(2), 23–74.

Schulz, P., Kirschbaum, C., Prüßner, J., & Hellhammer, D. (1998). Increased free cortisol secretion after awakening in chronically stressed individuals due to work overload. *Stress Medicine, 14*(2), 91–97. https://doi.org/10.1002/(SICI)1099-1700

Sianoja, M., Kinnunen, U., Mäkikangas, A., & Tolvanen, A. (2018). Testing the direct and moderator effects of the stressor–detachment model over one year: A latent change perspective. *Work & Stress, 32*(4), 357–378. https://doi.org/10.1080/02678373.2018.1437232

Sönmez, B., Oğuz, Z., Kutlu, L., & Yıldırım, A. (2017). Determination of nurses' mental workloads using subjective methods. *Journal of Clinical Nursing, 26*(3–4), 514–523. https://doi.org/10.1111/jocn.13476

Stoeva, A. Z., Chiu, R. K., & Greenhaus, J. H. (2002). Negative affectivity, role stress, and work–family conflict. *Journal of Vocational Behavior, 60*(1), 1–16. https://doi.org/10.1006/jvbe.2001.1812

Tabachnick, B. G., & Fidell, L. S. (2013). *Using multivariate statistics.* Pearson Education.

Wasti, S. A. (1999). *Organizational commitment in a collectivist culture: The case of Turkey* [Unpublished doctoral dissertation]. The University of Illinois at Urbana-Champaign.

Yang, J., Bently, J. R., Treadway, D. C., Brouer, R. L., & Wallace, A. (2018). The role of affective commitment and political skill in the work interfering with family (WIF) conflict–voluntary turnover relationship. *The International Journal of Human Resource Management, 29*(3), 595–613. https://doi.org/10.1080/09585192.2016.1172656

Yildirim, D., & Aycan, Z. (2008). Nurses' work demands and work–family conflict: A questionnaire survey. *International Journal of Nursing Studies, 45*(9), 1366–1378. https://doi.org/10.1016/j.ijnurstu.2007.10.010

Zeytinoglu, I. U., Denton, M., Davies, S., Baumann, A., Blythe, J., & Boos, L. (2007). Deteriorated external work environment, heavy workload, and nurses' job satisfaction and turnover intention. *Canadian Public Policy, 33*(1), 31–47. https://doi.org/10.3138/0560-6GV2-G326-76PT

14

An Exploration of Factors Related to Quality of Life in Indonesian Care Workers in Home-Based Care Settings

Shu-Fen LO[1]* • Li-Jung CHANG[2] • Mark HAYTER[3] • An-Chi O YANG[4]

ABSTRACT

Background: Indonesians constituted 79% of foreign care workers for long-term care in Taiwan in 2015. Therefore, it is crucial to explore the effect of work stress and quality of life (QoL) on this population.

Purpose: This study aims to explore stress levels, social support requirements, and perceived QoL among Indonesian care workers (ICWs) who work in home care settings.

Methods: A cross-sectional design was used. Data were collected between 2014 and 2016 from a convenience sample of ICWs working in eastern Taiwan using a self-administered questionnaire that comprised the Stress Perception Scale (SPS), Social Support Scale (SSS), and World Health Organization Quality of Life-Brief scale. One hundred fifty-seven valid questionnaires were collected. The response rate was 80.51%. Data were analyzed using descriptive statistics, one-way analysis of variance, Pearson's correlation coefficient, and multiple regression analysis.

Results: The results found that the average SPS of the sample was 70.50, with low QoL scores and requirements for more social support. In addition, significant and positive correlations were found between QoL and SPS, SSS, duration of patient care, and hours of care per week. Stepwise regression analysis showed that the most predictive variables for QoL were time spent caring, preservice training, psychological stress, and emotional support, which together accounted for 60.9% of the total variance.

Conclusions/Implications for Practice: This study facilitated understanding of the stress on ICWs and the impact of social support on their QoL. The findings suggest that new immigrants in Taiwan should be introduced to foreign care workers or nursing attendants. Moreover, long-term-care-related teachers should work with home care institutions or agencies to develop a teaching model for innovative care skills to relieve the perceived stress of ICWs.

Key Words:
Indonesian care workers, quality of life, stress perception, social support.

Introduction

The world population in 2017 comprised an estimated 962 million older adults (≥ 60 years old), a population that is growing faster than all other age groups. The number of older adults worldwide is expected to more than double by 2050 and more than triple by 2100 (United Nations, 2018). This will increase workforce demands and the need for services provided by care workers. As the care burden increases, the number of foreign care workers (FCWs) increases, particularly in home care settings where FCWs are hired to alleviate the long-term-care (LTC) loading on family members (Workforce Development Agency, Ministry of Labor [MOL], Taiwan, ROC, 2017a; Wu, Lee, Lin, & Wai, 2011). FCWs are a vital and indispensable element of the workforce in current LTC systems. Since 1992, the Taiwanese government has allowed FCWs to care for people with physical or mental disorders or disabilities to meet the domestic labor shortage and the need for LTC workers (Ministry of Health and Welfare, Taiwan, ROC, 2017). However, in Taiwan, only 6.16% of FCWs work in LTC institutions (Workforce Development Agency, MOL, Taiwan, ROC, 2017b). In 2017, 76% of FCWs were Indonesians aged between 25 and 44 years (Workforce Development Agency, MOL, Taiwan, 2017b). However, many FCWs receive only short-term care training before coming to Taiwan. Thus, their care skills are not sophisticated enough to manage serious illnesses and disabilities, especially in home care settings (Chen, Liu, Li, & Kao, 2012). Most are able to speak only very limited Mandarin or Taiwanese (Huang & Yang, 2011). Inexperience, culture shock, living habits, and language problems result in conflicts between FCWs and their employers (Chen et al., 2012), which affects the quality of care provided by FCWs and their ability to adjust to their work responsibilities (Huang & Yang, 2011). This conflict of culture and language as well as the challenges of care contribute to the stress perceived by FCWs. A previous study reported that stress has

[1]*PhD, RN, Associate Professor, Department of Nursing, Tzu Chi University of Science and Technology, Nursing Technology Innovation Service Research Center, Taiwan, ROC* • [2]*MSN, RN, Assistant Professor, Department of Nursing, Tzu Chi University of Science and Technology, Taiwan, ROC* • [3]*PhD, RN, Professor, Nursing and Health Research, Faculty of Health Sciences, University of Hull, England, UK* • [4]*RN, Lecturer, Department of Nursing, Tzu Chi University, and Doctoral Program Student, School and Graduate Institute of Nursing, National Taiwan University, Taipei, Taiwan, ROC.*

a negative impact on FCWs' quality of life (QoL) and affects the quality of care they provide to patients (Chen et al., 2012; Huang & Yang, 2011). Occupational stress has harmful effects on individuals in terms of health, physical and psychological well-being, and job satisfaction, which may affect the quality of care provided to patients (Chen et al., 2012). Some studies have found that reducing occupational stress and strengthening social support and rational coping may improve QoL among FCWs (Chen et al., 2012; Wu et al., 2011). Previous studies have focused on experiences of FCWs in hospitals or LTC institutions. However, studies related to Indonesian care workers (ICWs) working in home care settings are limited. The primary purpose of this study was to examine the level of occupational stress, social support, and QoL among ICWs.

Foreign Care Workers' Stress

Lazarus (1991) defined stress as a relationship between individuals and environment. It is a function of the degree of person–environment fit (Lazarus & Folkman, 1984). Stress is a dynamic process that occurs when an individual appraises situational demands as exceeding available resources (Lazarus, 2006). Stress may be caused by either internal or external sources. The perception of stress is conceptually distinct from the amount of stress experienced by an individual and may affect health (Keller et al., 2012). Potential stressors include work stress, work overload, and limitations on resources (Admi & Moshe-Eilon, 2010). Higher levels of stress may have a negative impact on working ability. Extended periods of work stress may have psychological or physical effects, cause behavioral changes, deteriorate quality of work, increase the risk of accidents, and even endanger patient safety (Hung & Chiou, 2013).

For FCWs, stressors include workload, care abilities, and physical load. FCWs are often required to care for patients with dementia or stroke for 24 hours, particularly for patients with multiple physical or mental disorders who often need help to change position or use the toilet during the night (Huang & Lin, 2013; Yang, Wang, Wang, & Wang, 2013). FCWs average 10.2 hours/day at work (Workforce Development Agency, MOL, Taiwan, ROC, 2017b). Studies indicate that FCWs who take care of patients with functional deficits, have less than 6 months of experience working in Taiwan, or are not proficient in Chinese are more likely to have a higher level of stress perception (Wu et al., 2011). With respect to care ability, FCWs receive only 90 hours of training before coming to Taiwan (Fu, 2018). Moreover, their training addresses only basic communication skills, occupational safety, health and inspection, Taiwan work policy, and housekeeping issues (Ministry of Labor, Taiwan, ROC, 2018). Most FCWs do not receive a care training program, but FCWs' care experiences affect patient safety and quality of care. Nearly 60% of FCWs perform noninvasive techniques such as measuring blood pressure and body temperature. They also perform invasive care such as feeding medicines or milk using a nasogastric tube and sputum suction (Yang et al., 2013). These techniques are challenging for FCWs and may endanger the safety of patients if performed incorrectly (Chen, Lu, Chen, & Li, 2014).

With respect to physical load, nearly 70% of FCWs sleep less than 8 hours a day (Huang & Lin, 2013). When FCWs have insufficient time for rest, stress increases, which subsequently affects quality of care. Consequently, care accidents such as repeat hospitalizations, unexplained infections, and pressure injuries may increase (Kao, Chen, & Yang, 2013). The error rates for nasogastric tube care and trachea care are 58% and 57%, respectively (Chen et al., 2014). The stress level of FCWs affects not only perceptions of stress but also quality of care. Stress is a major factor contributing to poor quality of care and QoL in FCWs.

Social Support Needs for Foreign Care Workers

When FCWs work in an unfamiliar environment without sufficient care experience, they experience poor life adjustment and perceive greater stress. Receiving appropriate support and assistance may improve coping strategies (Koinis et al., 2015). Social support needs include emotional support in terms of self-esteem, love, compassion, listening, and comfort; instrumental support such as money, material assistance, and action intervention; and informative social support such as advice, recommendations, guidelines, and other helpful messages. A study revealed that FCWs are prone to mental health problems or substance abuse if they feel disrespected or experience poor social support (Huang & Yang, 2011). Hu, Yeh, and Wang (2009) surveyed 26 discrete social support needs of FCWs and found the demand for psychosocial support to be the most prevalent. More than 50% of FCWs required financial support, family support, stress adjustment, and emotional support. Learning caring and communication skills from their employers through support groups holds the potential to significantly increase the social support received by FCWs, resulting in enhanced quality of care.

Quality of Life of Foreign Care Workers

In 1948, the World Health Organization (WHO) defined the concept of "quality of life" as physical, psychological, social, and spiritual comfort. Thus, QoL may be defined in terms of subjective perceptions determined by culture and value systems, which includes physical function, mental status, independence, social relationships, personal beliefs, and environment. Different individuals have different interpretations of QoL (Yao, 2002). Chen et al. (2012) surveyed 300 FCWs in a medical center and nursing home in northern Taiwan. They found that younger FCWs had poor QoL and had been trained for a short period of time only, and some had not received the care training program at all. Critical predictors of QoL were available time for rest and sleep, extra bonuses or rewards, and having children. Studies indicate that job stress, social support, and self-perceived QoL dramatically affect the quality of care provided by FCWs. However, research on the stress factors affecting ICWs in home environments with respect to social support and QoL are limited. Thus, the impact of care stress and QoL in this population must be investigated.

In particular, this study was intended to answer the following research questions: (1) What are the major sources of occupational stress among ICWs? (2) What are the levels of occupational stress, social support, and QoL among ICWs? (3) What are the relationships between demographic characteristics and occupational stress, social support, and QoL in ICWs? and (4) What are the variables that best predict QoL in ICWs?

The conceptual framework was developed for this study by integrating information from the studies in the literature review (Figure 1).

Methods

Study Participants and Setting

This study employed a cross-sectional design. The ICWs were recruited from five nursing home agencies and three foreign worker agencies in eastern Taiwan between August 1, 2014, and July 31, 2016. Inclusion criteria for the ICWs were (1) aged 20 years or older; (2) able to read the Indonesian version of the questionnaire; (3) involved in the informal care of patients (e.g., helping feed and wash patients) in home care settings; and (4) willing to participate in the study. This study was approved by the Ethics Committee of the Hualien Tzu Chi Hospital (IRB No. 104–28-B); 195 participants were recruited, and 157 completed the questionnaires, a response rate of 80.5%.

Instruments

Demographic characteristics of the ICWs, including age, gender, and education level, and the marital status and demographic and disease characteristics of their patients were collected. As discussed in the following paragraphs, three instruments were used in this study.

Stress perception scale

Participant stress levels were assessed using the 29-item Stress Perception Scale (SPS; Chen et al., 2012, 2014; Wu et al., 2011), which was designed to measure stress experiences during the previous 1-month period. Total possible SPS scores range from 29 to 145, with higher scores associated with greater stress. After factor analysis, five factors were extracted: "stress of general work" (9 items), "invasive performance" (7 items), "environmental stress" (3 items), "interpersonal stress" (5 items), and "psychological stress" (5 items), which explained 77.22% of the variance. The Cronbach's α was .94.

Social support scale

The Social Support Scale (SSS) was used to measure the social support requirements of the ICWs while they provided care to patients (Lo, Hwang, Yau, & Liu, 2001; Wang, Yang, Chen, & Wang, 2013). The SSS comprises 17 items. The range of possible scores is from 17 to 68, with higher scores indicating higher levels of perceived social support. After factor analysis, three factors were extracted: "emotional support" (8 items), "substantive support" (5 items), and "informative support" (4 items), which explained 74.22% of the variance. The Cronbach's α was .91.

WHO Quality of Life-Brief Taiwan version

The WHO Quality of Life-Brief (WHOQOL-BREF) was used to measure the QoL of the ICWs. This tool comprises 28 items, including physiological, psychological, social, and environmental factors, as well as two Taiwanese localization issues (Yao, 2002). The range of possible WHOQOL-BREF scores is from 16 to 80, with higher scores indicating better QoL. After factor analysis, the five factors explained 55.89% of the variance. The Cronbach's α was .87.

Statistical Analyses

Data were analyzed using IBM SPSS Statistics Version 19.0 (IBM, Inc., Armonk, NY, USA). Descriptive statistics were

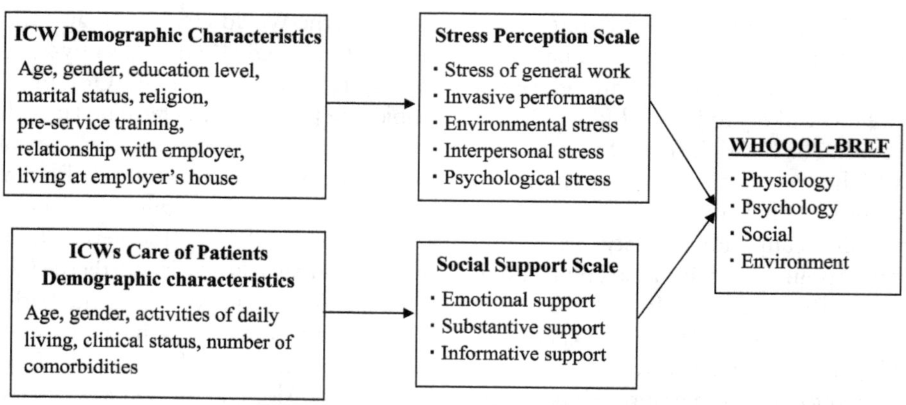

Figure 1. The conceptual framework of quality of life and its related factors among Indonesian care workers (ICWs). WHOQOL-BREF = World Health Organization Quality of Life-Brief Scale.

used to assess the participants and the general characteristics of their patients. One-way analysis of variance was used to verify the differences in QoL according to the general characteristics. Post hoc analyses were performed using Scheffe's test. The Pearson correlation coefficient was used to analyze the correlations among the SPS, SSS, and QoL of the participants. Finally, multiple regression analysis was used to identify the factors that influenced the QoL of the participants, the alpha level was set to $p < .05$.

Results

Sample Characteristics

The age of the study population ranged from 23 to 49 years (mean: 35.46 ± 6.54 years). Among the participants, 80.25% were married and Muslim. The most common educational level was junior high (55.41%), and 79.62% lived at their employers' house. The average experience with patient care was 2.74 ± 1.98 years. The average time spent on caring was 15.97 hours/day, and the average duration of sleep was 6.30 hours/day. In addition, 84.72% had not received nursing training before coming to Taiwan. Their roles varied and included caring for older adults (57.5%), cleaning the house (65.0%), and preparing meals (60%; Table 1). The average age of the patients was 78.9 years, most were male (52.22%), and 44.59% required assistance with activities of daily living (Table 2).

TABLE 1.

Demographic Characteristics of Indonesian Care Workers (N = 157)

Variable	Mean	*SD*	Range
Age	35.46	6.54	23.0–49.0
Duration of patient care (years)	2.74	1.98	0.2–9.0
Average time spent caring	15.97	5.16	6.0–24.0
Average number of sleep hours	6.30	2.81	0.5–12.0
Experience of assistant (years)	1.33	2.14	0.5–11.0
	n	%	
Gender			
Male	3	0.70	
Female	154	99.30	
Educational level			
Elementary school	16	10.19	
Junior high school	87	55.41	
Senior high school	51	32.48	
University or college	3	1.91	
Marital status			
Married	126	80.25	
Divorced or separated	20	12.74	
Widowed	11	7.00	
Religion			
None	16	10.19	
Christianity	12	7.64	
Islam	126	80.25	
Other	3	1.92	
Preservice training			
Yes	24	15.28	
No	133	84.72	
Live at their employers' house			
Yes	125	79.62	
No	32	20.38	
Relationship with employer			
Poor	3	1.92	
Okay	24	15.28	
Ordinary	75	47.77	
Good	55	35.03	

Descriptive Analysis

Table 3 presents a descriptive analysis of the SPS. The SPS scores ranged from 27 to 111, with an average stress pressure score of 70.50 (*SD* = 22.99). The stress intensity item with the highest score was psychological stress. The lowest score was for the invasive performance domain. Table 3 shows the participants' subjective perceptions of their social support needs. The SSS ranged from 17 to 68. The mean score was 50.98 (*SD* = 10.18), indicating that the degree of social support requirement was moderate, but the difference was quite large. The most important need for ICWs was emotional support, with the lowest scores in the substantive social support domain. Table 3 also presents a descriptive analysis of the WHOQOL-BREF scores, the total scores for which ranged from 41.76 to 66.70, with a mean score of 56.87 (*SD* = 5.19). The average scores for each domain were divided by 4 to calculate the scores in a range from 4 to 20. The highest score was for the environmental domain (14.67 ± 1.93), and the lowest score was for the physiological domain (12.96 ± 1.60).

Relationships Between Independent Variables and QoL

The factors influencing QoL were analyzed using one-way analysis of variance. Scheffe's post hoc test revealed that the QoL of participants who had received orientation training before coming to Taiwan was higher ($F = 6.76$, $p = .013$). The relationships between QoL and demographic variables, SPS, and SSS were analyzed, with results showing that stress perception, social support, duration of patient care, and hours of care per week were all significantly correlated with QoL. The correlation coefficients were .45, .28, .46, and .86 ($p < .05$), respectively, indicating that higher levels of pressure were associated with lower levels of social support received. In addition, longer lengths of care and more hours of care per week were both associated with poorer self-perceived QoL (Table 4).

TABLE 2.
Demographic and Disease-Related Characteristics of Indonesian Care Workers of Patients (N = 157)

Variable	n	%
Age (*M* and *SD*)	78.90	19.22
Number of comorbidities (*M* and *SD*)	1.34	0.68
Gender		
Male	82	52.22
Female	75	47.78
Activities of daily living		
Good	18	11.46
Ordinary	8	5.10
Okay	61	38.85
Poor	40	25.48
Extremely poor	30	19.11
Clinical status		
Minimal	10	6.37
Slight	35	22.29
Ordinary	85	54.14
Severity	19	12.10
Extremely serious	8	5.10

Note. Range of age of patients: 21–99 years; number of comorbidities: 1–4.

Predictors of Quality of Life

Multiple regression analyses were conducted to analyze all of the independent variables based on the significance of the results from the Pearson's correlation analyses. The

TABLE 3.
The Mean and Standard Deviation of the SPS, SSS, QoL, and Each Domain (N = 157)

Variable (Item)	Mean	SD	Rank
Stress Perception Scale (29)	70.50	22.99	
Psychological stress (5)	13.72	6.46	1
Environmental stress (3)	7.30	2.75	2
Stress of general work (9)	20.72	7.27	3
Interpersonal stress (5)	11.32	4.69	4
Invasive performance (7)	13.88	2.83	5
Social Support Scale (17)	50.98	10.18	
Emotional support (8)	24.67	5.69	1
Informative support (4)	11.45	3.60	2
Substantive support (5)	13.57	4.15	3
Quality of life (28)	56.87	5.19	
Overall domain (2)	14.10	3.00	
Environmental domain (9)	14.67	1.93	1
Psychological domain (6)	14.66	1.86	2
Social relationships domain (4)	14.56	2.06	3
Physiological domain (7)	12.96	1.60	4

Note. SPS = Stress Perception Scale; SSS = Social Support Scale; QoL = WHO Quality of Life-Brief Taiwan version.

TABLE 4.
Correlation Between QoL and Variables (N = 157)

Variable	QoL	SPS	SSS	LPC/Year	HCP/Week
QoL	1				
SPS	.45*	1			
SSS	.28*	.68**	1		
DPC/year	.46*	−.46*	−.26	1	
HCP/week	.86*	−.36*	.13	.35	1

Note. QoL = WHO Quality of Life-Brief Taiwan version; SPS = Stress Perception Scale; SSS = Social Support Scale; DPC = duration of patient care; HCP = hours of care.
$^{*}p < .05$. $^{**}p < .01$. $^{***}p < .001$ (two-tailed).

discontinuous variables were converted into dummy variables before the analysis. The results revealed that average time spent caring ($F = 5.30, p = .032$), not receiving complete training in patient care before coming to Taiwan ($F = 6.76, p = .013$), psychological stress ($F = 6.25, p = .017$), and emotional support ($F = 4.81, p = .035$) were all significant variables determining QoL, accounting for 60.9% of the total variance (Table 5). The duration spent caring each day and not receiving complete training before coming to Taiwan strongly predicted QoL in the participants.

Discussion

Previous studies have revealed low levels of stress among FCWs (Chen et al., 2012). However, this study found that the ICW participants were exposed to moderate levels of stress and that level of stress varied significantly among individual participants. Possible reasons for this variance include differences in previous working experience, the average number of hours of care provided per day, and the age of their patients. Average nursing experience was 1.33 years, and the average age of patients was 78.90 years. In addition, 44.57% of the patients had poor self-care ability. Most of the participants (84.72%) had no preservice training. According

TABLE 5.
Regression Analysis Variables Predicting QoL Total Scores (N = 157)

Independent Variable	R	SE	R^2	F	p
Constant	51.84	1.60			
Average time spent caring	.45	4.42	.21	5.30	.032
Preservice education	.39	4.83	.15	6.76	.013
Psychological stress	.38	4.85	.14	6.25	.017
Emotional support	.49	4.63	.10	4.81	.035

Note. QoL = WHO Quality of Life-Brief Taiwan version.
$^{*}p < .05$ (two-tailed).

to the policy of the Ministry of Labor, Taiwan, ROC (2018), the standard 90-hour pretraining program includes only language, occupational safety, health and inspection, Taiwan work policy, and housekeeping training. However, ICWs are otherwise required to possess nursing skills such as nasogastric tube care and trachea care, which may be sources of considerable stress. The daily duration of work was very long, with 84.4% of FCWs working in excess of 10 hours/day (Wang et al., 2013; Wu et al., 2011).

Stress Perception of ICWs

Scores were high at all levels of stress perception; however, psychological stress scores were the highest. The reasons for the latter were likely associated with autonomy of care, as the most significant psychological stress events identified in this study were "having no right to decide care job by themselves" and "facing harassment from employers." These two factors are closely linked to the fact that ICWs work and live in the same home care setting. As ICWs have little input into care-related decisions, work overload is likely to increase stress and thus affect the quality of care provided (Jetha, Kernan, Kurowski, & Pro-Care Research, 2017). The findings of this study suggest that employers should give ICWs appropriate decision-making authority to make care-related decisions based on their knowledge of care and length of stay in Taiwan. Moreover, employers should consider them as family members and address their concerns (Kang & Lee, 2010). The perception among FCWs of being harassed is also important (Hanson, Perrin, Moss, Laharnar, & Glass, 2015). FCWs should be aware of their labor rights and know how to seek help and support through channels such as the FCW 24-hour counseling and protection hotline.

Social Support Needs of ICWs

In this study, the social support needs of the participants were rated in the middle to upper range (M = 50.98), with considerable difference among individuals. The ICWs in our study seemed to be socially isolated. This feeling of isolation may be because of language barriers, which complicates seeking help from others (Kang & Lee, 2010). The results regarding social support in this study were congruent with those of previous studies (Chen et al., 2012). FCWs feel socially isolated because of the care needs of older patients, which may occur 24 hours/day without support (Chen, 2011). We found that 55.41% of the subjects reported junior high as their highest level of education and that only 40% could speak Mandarin. These individuals require considerably more support, especially emotional support, in the working environment. Furthermore, the participants required spiritual counseling and assistance.

QoL of ICWs

The QoL scores of the ICWs were moderate (mean: 56.87 ± 5.19), which is inconsistent with Chen et al. (2012), who reported a mean overall QoL score of 68 (SD = 11.34), with the highest score in the social domain and the lowest score in the environmental domain. This may be because of differences in average daily working hours. In this study, the average was 15.97 hours/day, much higher than the average reported by Chang Chien, Lee, Sun, Chou, and Yang (2012). Previous studies indicate that working hours, educational level, age, number of days off, and length of working experience each affect the QoL of FCWs (Chang Chien et al., 2012). In this study, the highest QoL subscale was the environmental domain and the lowest score was for the physiological domain. Previous studies indicate that FCWs often work for more than 12 hours/day, which requires considerable physical strength and spiritual stamina. This work pressure had an adverse impact on the time available for mental/physical rest and worsened the physical and mental health of ICWs. This poor work situation affected their QoL (Chang Chien et al., 2012; Huang & Lin, 2013).

In addition, this study found that the top three QoL items for the participants were "feeling my life was meaningful," "satisfaction with my current life," and "satisfaction with my environmental health." The lowest three items were "having frequent, negative feelings," "having little time to engage in leisure activities," and "reliance upon medical help to cope with daily life." The results of this study differed from those of Chen et al. (2012), who reported that the highest scored item for ICWs was "having frequent, negative feelings" and the lowest scored items were "having little time to engage in leisure activities" and "reliance on medical help to cope with daily life." Most ICWs worked to improve their lives, and they earned a substantial amount working overseas to help them achieve this goal. This may be the reason they felt their lives were meaningful and satisfactory. The negative feelings and low leisure activity may be because of frustrations related to their jobs and to working overtime. Previous studies have found that, when FCWs are overburdened and unable to take leave, negative feelings of inability are easily induced (Huang & Lin, 2013).

Predictors of Participant QoL

FCWs play a significant role in providing direct care to elderly patients in long-term home-based caregiving. The job stress, social support, and QoL of FCWs are factors crucial to the provision of quality patient care. This study found that the key determinants for high QoL among ICWs were social support, preservice training, and ability to cope with stress. Hours of care per week and average time spent in caregiving were also important predictors. These results were consistent with those of other studies (Chang Chien et al., 2012; Chen et al., 2012), which revealed that shorter working hours, more adequate rest, and appropriate vacation periods reduce stress and enhance physical recovery (Ha, Chong, Choo, Tam, & Yap, 2018). Working overtime and having little rest cause stress and affect the quality of care provided by FCWs (Chang Chien et al., 2012; Huang & Hsieh, 2010; Li, Ho, & Che, 2015). Chang Chien et al. (2012) noted that FCWs should have reasonable working hours and adequate rest to improve their care quality and QoL. The 2017 Foreign Nursing Workers Respite Service Program in Taiwan was intended to address these problems and help enhance the QoL of FCWs.

Appropriate training programs are essential to equip FCWs with the skills necessary to provide competent home-based patient care. Relevant training includes disease-specific caregiving skills, language training opportunities, information about available support groups, recognition of the early signs of depression, and stress management (Wu et al., 2011; Yeoh & Huang, 2010). Huang and Hsieh suggested that FCWs should undergo training courses to strengthen their caregiving skills and knowledge before beginning work. However, FCW in-service education faces several barriers, including lack of approval from Taiwanese employers, time limitations, and employer unwillingness to pay for the costs of this education (Li et al., 2015). Therefore, the use of intelligent technology (e.g., apps and QR codes) with Indonesian dubbing is proposed to help ICWs learn care skills and knowledge.

FCWs alleviate the physical, mental, and behavioral impairments of ill older adults in home care settings (Østbye, Malhotra, Malhotra, Arambepola, & Chan, 2013). However, the results of this study indicate that the psychological stress experienced by ICWs has a negative impact on their QoL. Strong evidence from several studies has shown that long work hours, multiple roles (e.g., household chores, childcare, and caregiving for the older adults), work overload, client disability care, restrictions on mobility and communication, and conflict between patients and their families affect FCWs and eventually become sources of psychological stress and burden (Ho, Chiang, Leung, & Ku, 2018; Wu et al., 2011). Taiwan's policymakers must devise standardized occupational strategies to enhance the working conditions of FCWs, such as rest days, proper accommodation, and safe working conditions.

Social support is especially crucial in mediating stress and improving QoL for FCWs (Chang Chien et al., 2012; Tam, Koh, Legido-Quigley, Ha, & Yap, 2017). Individual well-being, achieved through socioemotional support of personal capacities, may mediate stress (Østbye et al., 2013). A study in Singapore found that FCWs coped better with caring for an ailing elderly person when they received support from that person's family (Ha et al., 2018). The quality of care that FCWs provide may be expected to improve when employer–employee relationships are relatively equal (Yeoh & Huang, 2010). Ideal care worker–care receiver relationships rely on active but noninterfering participation by the families of both the care worker and the care receiver. The development of kin-like relationships with care receivers may enhance FCWs' emotional support and job satisfaction, alleviate burnout, and improve QoL (Chang Chien et al., 2012; Ho et al., 2018).

Limitations

This study has several limitations. First, data were collected in eastern Taiwan. Thus, these results may differ from those from FCWs of different cultural or religious backgrounds. Second, during this study, the Taiwan government's Long-Term Care 2.0 policy promoted FCW respite services and home-based supplementary training programs. This study could not identify the areas where this pilot project was being conducted. Future studies should be conducted to compare the provision of care in areas where the Long-Term Care 2.0 policy is and is not in effect. The cross-sectional nature of this study could not provide insight into the stressors, social support requirements, and QoL in the ongoing dynamic processes of FCWs. Therefore, longitudinal studies are required to further understand the support and assistance requirements of FCWs.

Conclusions

This study showed that the participants experienced moderate to high degrees of stress at work and perceived a low level of social support. The need for "emotional social support" was high, and participants needed to "be encouraged when frustrated," to "have someone to talk to when they encounter problems," and to have contacts with "someone who understands the situation they experienced." They often experienced negative feelings and relied on medical help to cope with daily life and did not have sufficient time to engage in leisure activities. In addition, receiving more adequate preservice training and working for reasonable amount of time per day were shown to have a positive effect on QoL. In Singapore, the Foreign Domestic Worker Association was established to help FCWs (Choon, 2017). We suggest establishing a similar association to provide skills training through affordable training programs and social support to FCWs.

At present, Chinese and Indonesian versions of care manuals are available online for healthcare workers to download. However, the care skills presented in the manuals are very complex, and FCWs who lack formal training require longer time to learn. Because most ICWs have smartphones, applications may be used to link training and care delivery resources with QR codes to make audio and video care-skill and other related resources available for download. Recent legislation has been enacted to promote the planning of respite programs for foreign nursing aides (Ministry of Health and Welfare, Taiwan, ROC, 2017). After the implementation of these programs, studies should address the effectiveness of this policy as a means of reducing work-related stress in FCWs.

Because most ICWs are Muslim, they cannot eat pork or food that has been used in worship ceremonies. However, most Taiwanese do eat meat and consume food used in traditional worship services. As the lifestyle requirements of ICWs differ from the mainstream in Taiwan, their beliefs and lifestyles should be understood and respected. Employers should consider ICWs as family members as a strategy for securing high-quality care. Furthermore, the Taiwan government should facilitate the provision of spiritual counseling and assistance to reduce the stress of FCWs through their LTC policy. In recent years, the Taiwanese government has emphasized cooperation between industry and educators. The impact on LTC-related education should be explored in the future to improve care standards, teach critical care skills, and empower FCWs. The results of this study provide information for healthcare professionals and policymakers involved in improving home-based healthcare in Taiwan as well as those involved in the welfare and training of FCWs.

Acknowledgments

The study was completed thanks to all of the participants. The authors also wish to thank Hsiu-hua Yang, the nurses of Hualien Shu Yang Nursing Home, Ms. Suhui Zhang, Hualien Hospital, and Zhuo Ruyu's Home Nursing Staff.

References

Admi, H., & Moshe-Eilon, Y. (2010). Stress among charge nurses: Tool development and stress measurement. *Nursing Economic$, 28*(3), 151–158.

Chang Chien, H. C., Lee, C. H., Sun, C. A., Chou, Y. C., & Yang, T. (2012). Factors influencing the quality of life of Vietnamese nursing aides working at medical institutions in Taiwan. *Journal of Nursing and Healthcare Research, 8*(3), 212–222. https://doi.org/10.6225/JNHR.08.3.212 (Original work published in Chinese)

Chen, C. F. (2011). Management or exploitation? The survival strategy of employer of family foreign care workers. *Taiwan: A Radical Quarterly in Social Studies, 85*, 89–155. https://doi.org/10.29816/TARQSS.201112.0004 (Original work published in Chinese)

Chen, M. J., Lu, Y. H., Chen, C. C., & Li, A. C. (2014). A project to reduce the incidence of intubation care errors among foreign health aides. *The Journal of Nursing, 61*(4), 66–73. https://doi.org/10.6224/JN.61.4.66 (Original work published in Chinese)

Chen, S. H., Liu, H. E., Li, C. L., & Kao, C. Y. (2012). An exploration of quality of life and related factors in foreign nurse aides. *The Journal of Health Sciences, 14*(1), 57–68. https://doi.org/10.6563/TJHS.2012.14 (1).5 (Original work published in Chinese)

Choon, S. S. (2017, February). *Programme to help maids adapt to working here.* Retrieved from http://www.straitstimes.com/forum/letters-in-print/programme-to-help-maids-adapt-to-working-here

Fu, H. C. (2018). *The training and management of foreign family nursing workers.* Retrieved from https://www.mohw.gov.tw/dl-2988-4717aeb4-c821-485b-8222-7066b89cda90.html (Original work published in Chinese)

Ha, N. H. L., Chong, M. S., Choo, R. W. M., Tam, W. J., & Yap, P. L. K. (2018). Caregiving burden in foreign domestic workers caring for frail older adults in Singapore. *International Psychogeriatrics, 30*(8), 1139–1147. https://doi.org/10.1017/S1041610218000200

Hanson, G. C., Perrin, N. A., Moss, H., Laharnar, N., & Glass, N. (2015). Workplace violence against homecare workers and its relationship with workers health outcomes: A cross-sectional study. *BMC Public Health, 15*, 11. https://doi.org/10.1186/s12889-014-1340-7

Ho, K. H. M., Chiang, V. C. L., Leung, D., & Ku, B. H. B. (2018). When foreign domestic helpers care for and about older people in their homes: I am a maid or a friend. *Global Qualitative Nursing Research, 5*, 1–10. https://doi.org/10.1177/2333393617753906

Hu, Y. Y., Yeh, L., & Wang, C. J. (2009). The exploratory study for home care needs: Comparison between foreign care workers and family primary caregivers. *The Journal of Long-Term Care, 13*(3), 339–350. (Original work published in Chinese)

Huang, C. H., & Lin, J. D. (2013). An exploratory study of the caring difficulties and problems of foreign care workers. *Taiwan Journal of Gerontological Health Research, 9*(1), 62–70. (Original work published in Chinese)

Huang, F. F., & Yang, H. H. (2011). The effects of nationality differences and work stressors on work adjustment for foreign nurse aides. *BMC Health Services Research, 11*, 192. https://doi.org/10.1186/1472-6963-11-192

Huang, W. Y., & Hsieh, Y. P. (2010). A study on work stress and its related factors for foreign nursing aides in nursing homes around Taichung and Changhua area. *Journal of Mei Ho Institute of Technology, 29*(1), 181–198. https://doi.org/10.7067/JMHIT.201003.0181 (Original work published in Chinese)

Hung, S. W., & Chiou, W. B. (2013). Job stress, social support and perceived health status: Evidence from general labors in healthcare institutes of southern Taiwan. *Pao-Chien Journal of Healthcare and Management, 11*(2), 20–29. (Original work published in Chinese)

Jetha, A., Kernan, L., Kurowski, A., & Pro-Care Research Team. (2017). Conceptualizing the dynamics of workplace stress: A systems-based study of nursing aides. *BMC Health Services Research, 17*(1), 12. https://doi.org/10.1186/s12913-016-1955-8

Kang, Y. L., & Lee, L. J. (2010). Indonesian family nursing laborers' work adaption and interpersonal adaptation in Taiwan. *The Journal of Regional and Social Development Research, 1*, 31–63. (Original work published in Chinese)

Kao, C. C., Chen, L. F., & Yang, M. H. (2013). The care stress, care preparation, and care skill on foreign nurse aides at home: Taking Yi-Lan and Keelung counties as examples. *The Journal of Taiwan Health Care Association, 15*, 53–74. (Original work published in Chinese)

Keller, A., Litzelman, K., Wisk, L. E., Maddox, T., Cheng, E. R., Creswell, P. D., & Witt, W. P. (2012). Does the perception that stress affects health matter? The association with health and mortality. *Health Psychology, 31*(5), 667–684. https://doi.org/10.1037/a0026743

Koinis, A., Giannou, V., Drantaki, V., Angelaina, S., Stratou, E., & Saridi, M. (2015). The impact of healthcare workers job environment on their mental–emotional health. Coping strategies: The case of a local general hospital. *Health Psychology Research, 3*(1), 12–17. https://doi.org/10.4081/hpr.2015.1984

Lazarus, R. S. (1991). *Emotion and adaptation.* New York, NY: Oxford University Press.

Lazarus, R. S. (2006). *Stress and emotion: A new synthesis.* New York, NY: Springer.

Lazarus, R. S., & Folkman, S. (1984). *Stress, appraisal, and coping.* New York, NY: Springer.

Li, H. C., Ho, H. C., & Che, H. L. (2015). A pilot study for the process of adaptation among foreign nurse aides at long-term care facility. *The Journal of Long-Term Care, 19*(1), 41–58. https://doi.org/10.6317/LTC.19.41 (Original work published in Chinese)

Lo, S. F., Hwang, S. L., Yau, K. P., & Liu, H. E. (2001). Factors associated with stress and social support for caregivers of burn patients during the stage of rehabilitation. *Formosan Journal of Medicine, 5*(1), 28–37. https://doi.org/10.6320/FJM.2001.5(1).04 (Original work published in Chinese)

Ministry of Health and Welfare, Taiwan, ROC. (2017, May). *Users of welfare institutions for disabled individuals, by age.* Retrieved from https://dep.mohw.gov.tw/DOS/lp-3550-113.html (Original work published in Chinese)

Ministry of Labor, Taiwan, ROC. (2018). *2014 survey report on the work and life of foreign workers in Taiwan.* Retrieved from http://statdb.mol.gov.tw/html/trend/103/51203.pdf (Original work published in Chinese)

Østbye, T., Malhotra, R., Malhotra, C., Arambepola, C., & Chan, A. (2013). Does support from foreign domestic workers decrease the negative impact of informal caregiving? Results from Singapore survey on informal caregiving. *The Journals of Gerontology: Series B, 68*(4), 609–621. https://doi.org/10.1093/geronb/gbt042

Tam, W. J., Koh, G. C. H., Legido-Quigley, H., Ha, N. H. L., & Yap, P. L. K. (2017). "I can't do this alone": A study on foreign domestic workers providing long-term care for frail seniors at home. *International Psychogeriatrics, 30*(9), 1269–1277. https://doi.org/10.1017/S1041610217002459

United Nations. (2018). *Ageing.* Retrieved from http://www.un.org/en/sections/issues-depth/ageing

Wang, C. J., Yang, Y. P., Chen, Y. C., & Wang, J. J. (2013). Development and validation of a questionnaire to measure self-perceived needs for care supportive among Indonesian home care aides. *Taiwan Journal of Public Health, 32*(2), 179–191. https://doi.org/10.6288/tjph2013-32-02-08 (Original work published in Chinese)

Workforce Development Agency, Ministry of labor, Taiwan, ROC. (2017a). *2017 foreign workers in productive industries and social welfare by nationality.* Retrieved from http://statdb.mol.gov.tw/html/mon/c12030.htm

Workforce Development Agency, Ministry of Labor, Taiwan, ROC. (2017b). *Foreign workers in productive industries and social welfare by industry.* Retrieved from http://statdb.mol.gov.tw/html/mon/212020.htm

Wu, C. J., Lee, W. K., Lin, W. J., & Wai, Y. W. (2011). Factors affecting the burden on foreign caregivers of long-term disabled survivors in Taiwan. *Taiwan Journal of Physical Medicine and Rehabilitation, 39*(1), 1–8. https://doi.org/10.6315/2011.39(1)01 (Original work published in Chinese)

Yang, Y. P., Wang, J. J., Wang, H. Z., & Wang, C. J. (2013). Care-support needs of Indonesian homecare workers and related factors. *Journal of Nursing and Healthcare Research, 9*(1), 65–73. https://doi.org/10.6225/JNHR.09.1.65 (Original work published in Chinese)

Yao, K. P. (2002). Introduction to the concepts and measurement of health-related quality of life. *Formosan Journal of Medicine, 6*(2), 183–192. https://doi.org/10.6320/fjm.2002.6(2).08 (Original work published in Chinese)

Yeoh, B. S., & Huang, S. (2010). Foreign domestic workers and home-based care for elders in Singapore. *Journal of Aging & Social Policy, 22*(1), 69–88. https://doi.org/10.1080/08959420903385635

15

Comparing the Effects of Simulation-Based and Traditional Teaching Methods on the Critical Thinking Abilities and Self-Confidence of Nursing Students

Mashael Hasan ALAMRANI[1]* • Kamila Ahmad ALAMMAR[2] • Sarah Saad ALQAHTANI[3]
Olfat A. SALEM[4]

ABSTRACT

Background: Critical thinking and self-confidence are imperative to success in clinical practice. Educators should use teaching strategies that will help students enhance their critical thinking and self-confidence in complex content such as electrocardiogram interpretation. Therefore, teaching electrocardiogram interpretation to students is important for nurse educators.

Purpose: This study compares the effect of simulation-based and traditional teaching methods on the critical thinking and self-confidence of students during electrocardiogram interpretation sessions.

Methods: Thirty undergraduate nursing students volunteered to participate in this study. The participants were divided into intervention and control groups, which were taught respectively using the simulation-based and traditional teaching programs. All of the participants were asked to complete the study instrument pretest and posttest to measure their critical thinking and self-confidence.

Results: Improvement was observed in the control and experimental groups with respect to critical thinking and self-confidence, as evidenced by the results of the paired samples *t* test and the Wilcoxon signed-rank test ($p < .05$). However, the independent *t* test and Mann–Whitney *U* test indicate that the difference between the two groups was not significant ($p > .05$).

Conclusions/Implications for Practice: This study evaluated an innovative simulation-based teaching method for nurses. No significant differences in outcomes were identified between the simulator-based and traditional teaching methods, indicating that well-implemented educational programs that use either teaching method effectively promote critical thinking and self-confidence in nursing students. Nurse educators are encouraged to design educational plans with clear objectives to improve the critical thinking and self-confidence of their students. Future research should compare the effects of several teaching sessions using each method in a larger sample.

KEY WORDS:
simulation, electrocardiogram, self-confidence, critical thinking.

Introduction

In the late 20th century, simulation-based clinical skill training employed optimized clinical learning activities in nursing education and promoted critical thinking to move students out of their knowledge comfort zone (Linthacum, 2011). Critical thinking and self-confidence are imperative to success in clinical practice. Simulation is intended to help nursing students learn and become more self-confident in critical thinking (Kaddoura, 2010). Moreover, simulation has been considered an important part of nursing program curricula for decades, allowing students to practice specific procedures in a controlled environment before performing these procedures on actual patients (Hicks, Coke, & Li, 2009). Simulation is used "to replace or amplify real experiences with guided experiences that evoke or replicate substantial aspects of the real world in a fully interactive manner" (Gaba, 2007).

Nurse educators are required to implement teaching strategies that promote the critical thinking skills of learners, because many important institutions (e.g., the National League for Nursing and the American Association of Colleges of Nurses) mandate these skills for baccalaureate nursing education and because critical thinking and problem-solving skills are required in professional nursing practice (Vacek, 2009). In addition, critical thinking skills help students solve problems and make sound clinical judgments in the healthcare environment (Smith-Blair & Neighbors, 2000). Critical thinking has many definitions. Halpern (1999) proposed that critical thinking refers to "the use of cognitive skills or strategies that increase the probability of a desirable outcome." Studies assessing critical thinking training have yielded inconclusive findings. One study by Sullivan-Mann,

[1]*MSN, RN, Demonstrator, Faculty of Applied Medical Science, Department of Nursing, University of Tabuk, Saudi Arabia* • [2]*MSN, RN, Nurse Educator, Nursing Education Adminstration, King Fahad Medical City, Saudi Arabia* • [3]*BSN, RN, Clinical Instructor, Nursing Education Department, AlAmal Complex for Mental Health, and Master's Student, College of Nursing, King Saud University, Saudi Arabia* • [4]*PhD, Associated Professor, Nursing Administration and Education Department, College of Nursing, King Saudi University, Saudi Arabia, and Faculty of Nursing, Nursing Administration Department, Menoufiya University, Egypt.*

Perron, and Fellner (2009) found that simulation-based teaching significantly increased critical thinking abilities, whereas another found that this mode of teaching did not significantly increase critical thinking abilities in nursing students (Shinnick & Woo, 2013). Nonetheless, simulations appear to promote self-confidence in students (Lubbers & Rossman, 2016). Confidence in nursing is a critical attribute of professional caring, which fosters mutual trust, respect, and truthful communications between nurses and their patients (Roach, 2002). High-fidelity simulation has been suggested as a new and supplemental teaching–learning strategy that improves the transfer of students' self-confidence and competence into the clinical environment (Bambini, Washburn, & Perkins, 2009); however, in one study, confidence among students who participated in simulations did not significantly differ from that among students who received traditional instruction (Brannan, White, & Bezanson, 2008). Finally, human patient simulators may increase the critical thinking abilities of students but not their self-confidence (Soucy, 2011).

Few studies have examined the effectiveness of simulation with respect to electrocardiogram (ECG) learning. ECG assists in the diagnosis, treatment, and monitoring of arrhythmias, coronary syndromes, and cardiac revascularization (Lessard et al., 2009) and is considered the gold standard in the evaluation of rhythm. Nurse educators commonly experience difficulty in teaching ECG interpretation. Moreover, only a few studies have compared ECG teaching strategies. Direct instruction, lectures, self-directed learning, and textbooks are considered traditional methods for teaching ECG interpretation. Advanced teaching methods include PC-based ECG software packages, 12-lead ECG signal generators, and advanced training mannequins (patient simulators). The data presented by Mahler, Wolcott, Swoboda, Wang, and Arnold (2011) found that using workshop and lecture-based formats is more effective than self-directed learning. Moreover, using simulation in ECG courses has been shown to improve self-confidence and critical thinking ability in students (Brown & Chronister, 2009).

In summary, although the available evidence suggests that simulation-based teaching is important, the effect of simulation on the critical thinking skills and self-confidence of students remains unclear. Additional research is necessary to compare the results of simulation technology and traditional teaching methods (Medley & Horne, 2005).

Many universities in Saudi Arabia, including King Saud University (KSU) and Princess Nourah bint Abdulrahman University, have expressed interest in simulation and have integrated simulation technology in their curriculum to overcome clinical education barriers (e.g., lack of clinical sites or preceptors). Nonetheless, few studies have evaluated simulation, which are required by nurse educators aiming to optimally promote the critical thinking ability and self-confidence of their students. Accordingly, this study compared the effect of simulation-based and traditional teaching methods on the critical thinking ability and self-confidence of students.

Methods

Design

A pretest–posttest design was used to compare the effects on critical thinking ability and self-confidence in undergraduate nursing students of an ECG interpretation course that was taught using either simulation-based or traditional teaching methods. The experimental and control groups received simulation- and lecture-based teaching, respectively.

Sample and Setting

Participants were a convenience sample of 30 eighth-level undergraduate nursing students who were recruited from the College of Nursing. Inclusion criteria were as follows: completed the fundamentals of nursing and medical–surgical nursing course, had no previous experience with ECG courses, and voluntarily provided written consent. Before implementation, the chief educator, who is certified in cardiovascular nursing, debriefed and trained the educators on the data collection procedure. The chief educator gave lecture-based training, and three educators conducted the ECG interpretation training using simulation under the supervision of the chief educator to prevent a confounding educator effect. Lectures were considered to constitute "traditional teaching." All study sessions were conducted at the Laboratory for Nursing Simulation in the College of Nursing, KSU, and simulation used a high-fidelity patient simulator.

Data Collection

After ethical approval from the College of Nursing, the researchers recruited the students on the appointed day in March 2016. Participants were assigned randomly to either the experimental or control group. The investigator explained the purpose of the study to each participant before commencing the study. All participants voluntarily provided written consent. Participants received assurance that participation was voluntary, that their results were confidential, and that their scores and participation would not affect their course grade. Participants completed an ECG pretest 30 minutes before course commencement. Both participant groups attended a 2-hour PowerPoint presentation (on the core concepts of ECG) to create a common ECG knowledge base. Control group participants continued a session of lecture lasting 60 minutes (on basic arrhythmia interpretation). During this 60-minute period, students were given an opportunity for questions and discussion with the educator. Experimental group participants subsequently completed a session of simulation training (on basic arrhythmia interpretation) lasting 60 minutes and a debriefing session of 20 minutes. The student–investigator ratio was 5:1. In the following 30 minutes, both groups completed a posttest that examined critical thinking ability and self-confidence in ECG interpretation.

Educational Activities

Lecture content

The lecture introduced the core concepts of ECG, addressing the interpretation of basic arrhythmias. A purposefully selected panel of three faculty members, who were experts in clinical and academic nursing, reviewed the lecture content.

Simulation scenario

Six scenarios were simulated. The panel of three expert faculty members had experience in the content of each scenario and had reviewed each scenario to ensure content validity and course content fidelity. The simulation session included an ECG demonstration and illustrations. A high-fidelity simulator was used (a computerized full-body manikin that simulates human functions and includes a cardiac monitor that displays hemodynamic waveforms, ECG rhythms, and vital signs).

Instruments

Critical thinking

The authors developed a 15-item multiple-choice questionnaire to measure the critical thinking ability of participants regarding ECG interpretation. A well-constructed multiple-choice questionnaire can test the cognitive skills of students (Khan & Aljarallah, 2011). Moreover, multiple-choice test items can be highly discriminating and measure the ability of a respondent to think critically when written properly (Morrison & Walsh Free, 2001). Possible scores ranged from 0 to 15, with higher scores indicating greater critical thinking ability in ECG interpretation. Each item included one correct response and three distracter responses. Participants received ECG strips for interpretation. The multiple-choice questions used in this study were drawn from a variety of sources (e.g., relevant literature, textbooks, the Internet). The test items were reviewed by a panel of experts, which included three nursing faculty members, who currently teach critical care nursing at KSU and have clinical and academic experience of more than 15 years each, and one cardiologist with experience in the critical care units at King Fahad Medical City. The panel approved the face validity of items for measuring the critical thinking ability of participants regarding ECG. The panel rated item relevance, and the item-level content validity indices ranged from 0.75 to 1.00, whereas the scale-level content validity index, using the averaging approach, was 0.95.

Self-confidence

Self-confidence was measured using the five-item C-Scale; the concurrent validity was supported by the administration of two additional instruments of confidence that had moderate to high correlations with the C-Scale (Grundy, 1993). Responses to items used a 5-point Likert scale. Grundy (1993) found that the Cronbach's α coefficient of this scale was .85, indicating good reliability.

Ethical Considerations

Ethical approval for this study was received from the College of Nursing, KSU.

The following ethical considerations were addressed by the researcher regarding this study: Participants were protected from physical and psychological harm; before commencing the study, an information sheet explaining the study purpose, process, risks, benefits, and alternative procedures, if any, were disclosed; and participants received formal assurances of anonymity and confidentiality. Participants were asked to sign a consent form attached to the questionnaire. Participants were also informed that they had the right to withdraw from the study at any time and for any reason without penalty.

Data Analysis

Data were analyzed using SPSS Version 22.0. The paired *t* test and its nonparametric equivalent, the Wilcoxon signed-rank test, were used to assess whether statistically significant differences existed between the pretest and posttest scores of critical thinking and confidence for both groups. Independent *t* tests and Mann–Whitney *U* tests were used to compare score changes between the experimental and control groups from pretest to posttest.

Results

By using paired samples *t* test and Wilcoxon signed-rank tests, the critical thinking and self-confidence scores of both groups improved significantly ($p < .05$; Table 1). Regarding self-confidence, the mean scores of the control group at pretest and posttest were 1.99 and 3.80, respectively ($p = .001$), and those of the experimental group were 2.20 and 3.89 ($p = .001$), respectively. Regarding critical thinking, the scores of the control group were 5.47 and 11.00 ($p = .001$), and those of the experimental group were 5.33 and 9.47 ($p < .05$).

In Table 2, an independent *t* test and Mann–Whitney *U* tests indicated no significant differences between the control and experimental groups with regard to gains in either self-confidence or critical thinking ($p > .05$). There were no significant differences in gains in self-confidence between the control and experimental groups ($t = 0.393$, $p = .698$; Mann–Whitney *U* test: $p = .870$, *ns*). Likewise, no significant difference in gain was found with respect to critical thinking ($t = 1.250$, $p = .222$; Mann–Whitney *U* test: $p = .512$, *ns*).

Discussion

This study compared the effects of simulation-based and traditional teaching methods on the critical thinking ability

TABLE 1.
Paired Samples t Test and Wilcoxon Signed-Rank Test Comparing Gains in CT and SC (N = 30)

	Experimental Group (n = 15)							Control Group (n = 15)						
	Pretest		Posttest				Wilcoxon Test, p Value	Pretest		Posttest				Wilcoxon Test, p Value
Variable	M	SD	M	SD	t	p		M	SD	M	SD	t	p	
CT	5.33	1.839	9.47	2.669	−4.769	.001	.002	5.47	1.506	11.00	2.591	−7.798	.001	.001
SC	2.20	0.997	3.89	0.636	−9.052	.001	.001	1.99	0.880	3.80	0.737	−7.500	.001	.001

Note. CT = critical thinking; SC = self-confidence.

and self-confidence of nursing students with regard to ECG interpretation. The results indicate that both teaching methods had beneficial effects on the examined parameters. The lack of a significant difference between the examined teaching methods may partly reflect the limited statistical power (due to the small sample) and the limited exposure. However, the present findings (drawn from a single exposure) resemble those of Ravert (2008) and Blum, Borglund, and Parcells (2010), who compared the effects of simulation and traditional education over time using a longitudinal design. This suggests that a single exposure to simulation-based education affects the critical thinking and self-confidence abilities of students similarly to multiple exposures. These findings collectively suggest that simulation-based and traditional teaching methods provide significant but approximately equal benefit to the critical thinking ability and self-confidence of undergraduate nursing students in the context of ECG interpretation.

Alternatively, the results further confirmed that well-implemented educational programs may effectively promote positive student outcomes independent of method. Student outcomes such as critical thinking ability and self-confidence are not easily influenced by teaching methods as the only valuable factor. Some studies such as that of Heston (2010), which compared the effects of simulation and traditional teaching methods on self-confidence, suggest that students' behavior and performance may be improved by applying great effort to increase their confidence, regardless of which teaching method is used by the educator. In addition, previous studies have shown that critical thinking differs significantly between learning styles and by student characteristics such as year of study, nationality, and previous experience (Andreou, Papastavrou, & Merkouris, 2014; Hunter, Pitt, Croce, & Roche, 2014). However, in the present attempt, learning style was not assessed, as participants were all in the same year of school, lacked experience, and were of the same nationality. Consequently, future empirical studies may help better define the relationship between learner characteristics and learning style and its effect on the critical thinking ability and self-confidence of students using different teaching methods.

Limitations and Future Research

This study is affected by the following limitations. The sample was small, resulting in limited statistical power. Sample size is often a concern in nursing education research because of small class size (Ravert, 2008). In our attempt, the small sample size was due to the small number of enrolled students at the targeted nursing college. In addition, the sample may not have been representative, as all participants originated from a single college and were women and of the same nationality. Accordingly, the present results should be tested in a larger sample by including students from numerous nursing colleges. Finally, future research should examine learning outcomes in a broad range of complex educational content.

TABLE 2.
Independent t Test and Mann–Whitney U Test Comparing Gains in CT and SC Between Study Groups (N = 30)

	Experimental Group (n = 15)		Control Group (n = 15)				
Variable	M	SD	M	SD	t	p	Mann–Whitney p
CT	9.47	2.669	11.00	2.591	1.250	.222	.512
SC	3.89	0.636	3.80	0.737	0.393	.698	.870

Note. CT = critical thinking; SC = self-confidence.

Conclusions

The present findings contribute to the growing body of evidence comparing critical thinking and self-confidence gains between simulation-based and traditional teaching methods, regarding complex content. Simulator-based and traditional teaching methods did not deliver significantly different outcomes after a single simulation session among undergraduate nursing students. The authors suggest that well-implemented educational programs using either teaching method will effectively promote nursing students' critical thinking ability and self-confidence. Nurse educators, based on the findings of this study, were encouraged to design educational plans with clear objectives for improving critical thinking ability and self-confidence. Ideally, future research should examine these variables in larger samples, include diverse content, address demographic variables (e.g., grade point average), and examine the influence of learning styles.

Acknowledgments

The authors are thankful to the Deanship of Scientific Research, College of Nursing Research Center at King Saud University for funding this research.

References

Andreou, C., Papastavrou, E., & Merkouris, A. (2014). Learning styles and critical thinking relationship in baccalaureate nursing education: A systematic review. *Nurse Education Today, 34*(3), 362–371. https://doi.org/10.1016/j.nedt.2013.06.004

Bambini, D., Washburn, J., & Perkins, R. (2009). Outcomes of clinical simulation for novice nursing students: Communication, confidence, clinical judgment. *Nursing Education Perspectives, 30*(2), 79–82. https://doi.org/10.1043/1536-5026-030.002.0079

Blum, C. A., Borglund, S., & Parcells, D. (2010). High-fidelity nursing simulation: Impact on student self-confidence and clinical competence. *International Journal of Nursing Education Scholarship, 7*(1), Article18. https://doi.org/10.2202/1548-923X.2035

Brannan, J. D., White, A., & Bezanson, J. L. (2008). Simulator effects on cognitive skills and confidence levels. *The Journal of Nursing Education, 47*(11), 495–500. https://doi.org/10.3928/01484834-20081101-01

Brown, D., & Chronister, C. (2009). The effect of simulation learning on critical thinking and self-confidence when incorporated into an electrocardiogram nursing course. *Clinical Simulation in Nursing, 5*(1), e45–e52. doi:10.1016/j.ecns.2008.11.001

Gaba, D. M. (2007). The future vision of simulation in health care. *Simulation in Healthcare, 2*(2), 126–135. doi:10.1097/01.SIH.0000258411.38212.32

Grundy, S. E. (1993). The confidence scale: Development and psychometric characteristics. *Nurse Educator, 18*(1), 6–9.

Halpern, D. F. (1999). Teaching for critical thinking: Helping college students develop the skills and dispositions of a critical thinker. *New Directions for Teaching and Learning, 1999*(80), 69–74. doi:10.1002/tl.8005

Heston, M. D. (2010). *The effect of human patient simulation and the role of learning styles on the self-confidence of nursing students* (ProQuest dissertations and theses). Barry University-Adrian Dominican School of Education, Ann Arbor, MI, USA. Retrieved from http://search.proquest.com/docview/853648218?accountid=142908

Hicks, F. D., Coke, L., & Li, S. (2009). The effect of high-fidelity simulation on nursing students' knowledge and performance: A pilot study. *National Council of State Boards of Nursing, 40*. Retrieved from https://www.ncsbn.org/09_SimulationStudy_Vol40_web_with_cover.pdf

Hunter, S., Pitt, V., Croce, N., & Roche, J. (2014). Critical thinking skills of undergraduate nursing students: Description and demographic predictors. *Nurse Education Today, 34*(5), 809–814. doi:10.1016/j.nedt.2013.08.005

Kaddoura, M. A. (2010). New graduate nurses' perceptions of the effects of clinical simulation on their critical thinking, learning, and confidence. *Journal of Continuing Education in Nursing, 41*(11), 506–516. doi:10.3928/00220124-20100701-02

Khan, M. U., & Aljarallah, B. M. (2011). Evaluation of modified essay questions (MEQ) and multiple choice questions (MCQ) as a tool for assessing the cognitive skills of undergraduate medical students. *International Journal of Health Sciences, 5*(1), 39–43. Retrieved from http://www.pubmedcentral.nih.gov/articlerender.fcgi?artid=3312767andtool=pmcentrezandrendertype=abstract

Lessard, Y., Sinteff, J. P., Siregar, P., Julen, N., Hannouche, F., Rio, S., & Le Beux, P. (2009). An ECG analysis interactive training system for understanding arrhythmias. *Studies in Health Technology and Informatics, 150*, 931–935. doi:10.3233/978-1-60750-044-5-931

Linthacum, M. D. (2011). *Teaching strategies that promote critical thinking in associate-degree nursing students: Perceptions of associate-degree nursing educators* (ProQuest dissertations and theses). Capella University, Ann Arbor, MI, USA. Retrieved from http://search.proquest.com/docview/897534212?accountid=142908

Lubbers, J., & Rossman, C. (2016). The effects of pediatric community simulation experience on the self-confidence and satisfaction of baccalaureate nursing students: A quasi-experimental study. *Nurse Education Today, 39*, 93–98. http://dx.doi.org/10.1016/j.nedt.2016.01.013

Mahler, S. A., Wolcott, C. J., Swoboda, T. K., Wang, H., & Arnold, T. C. (2011). Techniques for teaching electrocardiogram interpretation: Self-directed learning is less effective than a workshop or lecture. *Medical Education, 45*(4), 347–353. doi:10.1111/j.1365-2923.2010.03891.x

Medley, C. F., & Horne, C. (2005). Using simulation technology for undergraduate nursing education. *The Journal of Nursing Education, 44*(1), 31–34.

Morrison, S., & Walsh Free, K. W. (2001). Writing multiple-choice test items that promote and measure critical thinking. *The Journal of Nursing Education, 40*(1), 17–24. Retrieved from http://www.ncbi.nlm.nih.gov/pubmed/11198905

Ravert, P. (2008). Patient simulator sessions and critical thinking. *The Journal of Nursing Education, 47*(12), 557–562. doi:10.3928/01484834-20081201-06

Roach, M. (2002). *Caring, the human mode of being: A blueprint for the health* professions (2nd ed., pp. 56–58). Ottawa, Canada: Canadian Hospital Association Press.

Shinnick, M. A., & Woo, M. A. (2013). The effect of human patient simulation on critical thinking and its predictors in prelicensure nursing students. *Nurse Education Today, 33*(9), 1062–1067. doi:10.1016/j.nedt.2012.04.004

Smith-Blair, N., & Neighbors, M. (2000). Use of the critical thinking disposition inventory in critical care orientation. *Journal of Continuing Education in Nursing, 31*(6), 251–256.

Soucy, E. C. (2011). *The effects of high-fidelity simulators on nursing students' critical thinking and self-confidence* (ProQuest dissertations and theses). Northcentral University. Retrieved from http://search.proquest.com/docview/916790803?accountid=142908

Sullivan-Mann, J., Perron, C. A., & Fellner, A. N. (2009). The effects of simulation on nursing students' critical thinking scores: A quantitative study. *Newborn and Infant Nursing Reviews, 9*(2), 111–116. doi:10.1053/j.nainr.2009.03.006

Vacek, J. E. (2009). Using a conceptual approach with concept mapping to promote critical thinking. *Journal of Nursing Education, 48*(1), 45–48. doi:10.3928/01484834-20090101-11

16

Psychometric Properties of an Arabic Version of the Patient Satisfaction with Nursing Care Quality Questionnaire

Alaa ALBASHAYREH[1]* • Omar M. AL-RAWAJFAH[2] • Huda AL-AWAISI[3] • Suja KARKADA[4]
Sulaiman D. AL SABEI[5]

ABSTRACT

Background: Quality measurements are crucial to healthcare quality improvement, and patient satisfaction with nursing care is widely adopted as a key outcome indicator of the overall quality of healthcare. There is a lack of instruments to measure patient satisfaction with nursing care in an Arabic context.

Purpose: The purpose of this study was to develop and validate an Arabic version of the Patient Satisfaction with Nursing Care Quality Questionnaire and to explore patient satisfaction with nursing care across hospital units.

Methods: This was a cross-sectional, methodological research study. A forward–backward translation process and face and content validation using a panel of experts and a pilot test were used to produce an Arabic version of the Patient Satisfaction with Nursing Care Quality Questionnaire. A convenience sampling technique was employed to recruit 292 adult patients who were hospitalized for more than 48 hours. Data were collected over the first quarter of 2016 using a secure electronic survey method.

Results: The item-level content validity index ranged from .83 to 1, and the scale-level content validity index was .94. Evidence of construct validity was obtained. Exploratory factor analysis revealed a two-factor model that explained 69.3% of the total variance. Confirmatory factor analysis showed that the two-factor model fits the observed data. Internal consistency was satisfactory and similar across different hospital units. Cronbach's alpha estimates for Factors 1 and 2 were .83 and .96, respectively, with an overall Cronbach's alpha estimate of .96. Level of patient satisfaction with nursing care was quite high (mean = 4.30/5, *SD* = 0.74).

Conclusions: This study provides a 17-item, Likert-scaled, self-reporting instrument, which is psychometrically sound for its content, comprehension, readability, and practicality, to measure patient satisfaction with nursing care quality in an Arabic context.

Key Words:
nursing care, Oman, quality, patient satisfaction, Patient Satisfaction with Nursing Care Quality Questionnaire (PSNCQQ).

Introduction

Over the last two decades, increased attention has been paid on quantifying and improving quality of care. Accordingly, measuring nursing care quality has been recognized as a priority for healthcare providers and policymakers. There are two critical factors indicating the need to measure nursing care quality. First, nurses represent the largest segment of healthcare professionals, and therefore measuring nursing care quality is critical to improving practice (Freitas, Silva, Minamisava, Bezerra, & de Sousa, 2014). Second, measuring nursing care quality is a necessary step in determining the level of success that healthcare systems achieve in providing high-quality, high-value care in an equitable manner (Freitas et al., 2014). Patient satisfaction with nursing care (PSNC) is considered a principal outcome indicator of quality of care (Laschinger, Hall, Pedersen, & Almost, 2005), and it is seen as an important aspect for evaluating and improving overall healthcare (Dudkiewicz, 2014; Koy, Yunibhand, & Angsuroch, 2016). As nurses provide the key aspects of healthcare, their contribution influences significantly the level of patient satisfaction with the overall healthcare services provided (de-la-Cueva-Ariza et al., 2014; Laschinger et al., 2005).

[1]*MSN, RN, Graduate Research Assistant, College of Nursing, University of Iowa, Iowa City, Iowa, USA* • [2]*PhD, RN, Associate Professor, Acute Care Nursing, and Dean, College of Nursing, Sultan Qaboos University, Muscat, Oman, and Adjunct Associate Professor, Faculty of Nursing, Al Al-Bayt University, Mafraq, Jordan* • [3]*PhD, RN, Acting Head of Nursing Research, Directorate of Nursing, Sultan Qaboos University Hospital, Muscat, Oman* • [4]*PhD, RN, Assistant Professor and Head, Department of Fundamentals and Administration, College of Nursing, Sultan Qaboos University, Muscat, Oman* • [5]*PhD, RN, Assistant Professor, Department of Fundamentals and Administration, College of Nursing, Sultan Qaboos University, Muscat, Oman.*

The following two sections provide an overview of the literature that explores the published evidence relating to the concept of patient satisfaction and measures of PSNC.

Patient Satisfaction

As a subjective concept, patient satisfaction is difficult to measure and analyze. Moreover, inconsistencies between patient satisfaction and PSNC measures have been identified in the literature (Al-Abri & Al-Balushi, 2014; de-la-Cueva-Ariza et al., 2014; Junewicz & Youngner, 2015). Some authors attempt to provide a conceptual definition for PSNC that includes the actual outcome of the interaction between patients' expectations and previous experiences, respectively, and their perceptions of actual nursing behaviors (Abdel Maqsood, Oweis, & Hasna, 2012; Atallah, Hamdan-Mansour, Al-Sayed, & Aboshaiqah, 2013; Eriksen, 1995). Similarly, Linder-Pelz (1982) emphasizes that patient satisfaction is individual and subjective and may change based on standards of comparisons or expectations, although the quality of care may remain unchanged over time. In contrast, Pascoe (1983) describes PSNC as the emotional reaction of patients to nursing care.

The antecedents of PSNC include personal characteristics, social–economic influence, previous experience, involvement, motivation, cognition, and environment (Castro, Van Regenmortel, Vanhaecht, Sermeus, & Van Hecke, 2016; de-la-Cueva-Ariza et al., 2014; Milutinović, Simin, Brkić, & Brkić, 2012). These factors affect the ability of patients to judge quality of care. On the other hand, the consequences of PSNC include healthcare outcomes, compliance with healthcare instructions, treatment models, and intention to try the same healthcare provider or facility in the future and to recommend this provider or facility to family and friends (Castro et al., 2016; de-la-Cueva-Ariza et al., 2014; Milutinović et al., 2012).

For the purpose of this study, we define PSNC as the extent to which a patient is content with the care that is received from nurses and influenced by patient characteristics and expectations.

Measures of Patient Satisfaction

A review of the relevant literature revealed that measures of patient satisfaction vary widely and that overall patient satisfaction has often been used as a measure in place of PSNC (Al-Abri & Al-Balushi, 2014; de-la-Cueva-Ariza et al., 2014). Moreover, it has been noticed that a limited number of validated instruments are available to measure PSNC in particular. The identified scales measure dimensions such as attitude and communication, interpersonal relationships, competence, productivity, and provision of support and health information (Abdel Maqsood et al., 2012; La Monica, Oberst, Madea, & Wolf, 1986; Thomas, McColl, Priest, Bond, & Boys, 1996).

The three instruments mostly widely used to measure PSNC in the literature are (a) the 42-item La Monica–Oberst Patient Satisfaction Scale (La Monica et al., 1986), (b) the 56-item Newcastle Satisfaction with Nursing Scale (Thomas et al., 1996), and (c) the 19-item Patient Satisfaction with Nursing Care Quality Questionnaire (PSNCQQ; Laschinger et al., 2005). Evidence shows that these three instruments show sound psychometrics and that they have been used widely to assess PSNC in English-speaking patients (La Monica et al., 1986; Laschinger et al., 2005; Thomas et al., 1996). The PSNCQQ is preferred over the other instruments because it is generally believed to be the easiest to read and comprehend. Each item of the PSNCQQ has a label (e.g., "information you were given") and a question (e.g., "How clear and complete nurses' explanations were about tests, treatments, and what to expect?"). In addition, the PSNCQQ is relatively short, which helps minimize the burden on respondents and raise response rates.

The PSNCQQ measures PSNC during the hospital stay. The original English version of the instrument consists of 19 items related to PSNC (including two items related to discharge instructions and coordination of care after discharge) and two additional items related to overall quality of care and hospital recommendation. All PSNCQQ items were used in this study except the two items of discharge instructions and coordination of care after discharge because these two items are not measures of interest in this study. All items were scored using a Likert-type scale, with responses ranging from 1 (poor) to 5 (excellent). The reported Cronbach's alpha reliability estimate was .97, and the item–total correlations ranged from .61 to .89 (Laschinger et al., 2005). The PSNCQQ reliability estimates were similar across different hospital types, suggesting satisfactory readability and applicability. These results are consistent with the results from a Serbian study in which the PSNCQQ was translated into the Serbian language (Milutinović et al., 2012).

In Oman and the Middle East, the vast majority of patients are Arabic speakers. Although studies conducted in the region have translated some instruments to measure PSNC (Abdel Maqsood et al., 2012; Alasad, Abu Tabar, & AbuRuz, 2015; Atallah et al., 2013), these studies did not report evidence of a systematic transcultural adaptation and validation. Valid and reliable quality measures are integral to evaluation, planning, decision making, and research healthcare quality improvement. Therefore, there is a need for psychometrically sound instruments to measure PSNC in an Arabic context.

Study Aims

The primary aim of this study was to develop and validate an Arabic version of the PSNCQQ (PSNCQQ-Ar) to use it in an Arabic context. The secondary aim was to investigate PSNC in a tertiary hospital in Oman. This study is part of a larger project that aims to establish baseline measures of the nursing workforce and quality of patient care to gain knowledge for policy making and strategy development in Oman.

Methods

A cross-sectional, methodological design was employed to attain the study aims. Data collection was carried out in a large tertiary hospital in Oman with a total bed capacity of 500 during the first quarter of 2016. Participants were selected from different units of the hospital using a convenience sampling technique. The inclusion criteria for the current study are as follows: being an adult patient, hospitalized for more than 48 hours in the same unit, fully conscious and oriented, and able to read and understand the PSNCQQ-Ar. Selected patients were asked to respond directly using a computer-based electronic survey. Trained research assistants were available at the time of data collection to provide any technical assistance required by the participants to complete the survey.

Data were collected anonymously. Participants were asked to fill out electronic informed consent before accessing the electronic survey. After reading the study instructions, participants were asked to click "I agree to participate" to enter to the study survey. Those who clicked "I don't agree to participate" were thanked and not included in the survey. Permission to use the original instrument was obtained from the corresponding author. In addition, approval from the institutional review board at the affiliated university of the investigators and permission from the target healthcare facility were obtained.

Transcultural Adaptation

The transcultural adaptation of the PSNCQQ was guided by the work of Sousa and Rojjanasrirat (2011) and by the procedure described by Gjersing, Caplehorn, and Clausen (2010).

Translation of the tool

A forward translation from English into Arabic was done by two independent translators who are fluent in both original and target languages. The first translator has a healthcare background and is knowledgeable about the related healthcare terminologies and expressions in both languages. The second translator is not from the healthcare field but is familiar with the slang and jargon related to the relevant terminologies used in the target language by the target population. Two Arabic versions were generated.

After completing the above procedures, a third independent translator who is bilingual compared the two translated versions to generate one Arabic version. The generated version and all suggestions made by the third translator were discussed by a panel comprising the initial two translators and two investigators who are bilingual to assess the compatibility between the original and translated instruments. The panel assessed whether the generated words and items have the same meaning and confirmed that the utilized equivalent expressions did not change the cultural meaning of the words and items.

Subsequently, two independent bilingual Arabic–English translators respectively executed blind backward translations from Arabic into English. The first translator is from the healthcare field, and the other is not a health professional but is knowledgeable regarding the related terminologies and expressions. The two translators were completely blind to the original version of the PSNCQQ. Two English versions were generated.

Face and content validity

A panel of six experts looked into the overall appearance of the prefinal version of the scale to assess its accuracy in measuring PSNC. All of the potential differences in words, items, and meanings were discussed, and discrepancies were resolved through the consensus of the panel members to confirm the semantic, idiomatic, and conceptual equivalencies between the original version and the translated version. Thereafter, to support the scale's content validity index (CVI), the panel was asked to evaluate each item of the instrument using a 4-point scale (1 = *not relevant*, 2 = *somewhat relevant*, 3 = *quite relevant*, and 4 = *highly relevant*).

Pilot test

At this stage, 15 native Arabic-speaking participants were recruited from the target population. All participants expressed willingness to be included in the study. Each participant was asked to complete the PSNCQQ-Ar. The research team asked the participants to express any concerns related to the tool and its items and instructions using open-ended questions. All concerns were taken into consideration in finalizing the ready-to-use tool. The data collected in the pilot study were not included in the main study analysis.

Data Analysis

SPSS Version 23 was used for all statistical analyses with a significance level of .05. Descriptive statistics, including frequency, percentages, means, and standard deviations, were used to describe the sample. The reliability of the 17-item scale was derived using standard statistical procedures described by Cronbach, and a Cronbach's alpha higher than .80 was considered satisfactory (Cronbach, 1951).

To obtain the scale's CVI, items were dichotomized into relevant and irrelevant. The CVI for the item (I-CVI) was obtained by dividing each item score by 6, which equaled the total number of the expert raters. The CVI for the scale was obtained using the average method (S-CVI/ave; Polit & Beck, 2006). For a panel of six expert raters, the I-CVI of .78 or above and the S-CVI/ave of .90 or above were the minimum acceptable indices (Polit & Beck, 2006).

The suitability of data for factor analysis was assessed using the correlation matrix, Kaiser–Meyer–Olkin (KMO), and Bartlett's test of sphericity (Williams, Onsman, & Brown, 2010). An exploratory factor analysis (EFA) using maximum likelihood factor extraction was carried out using an oblique method of rotation (Promax, $\kappa = 4$) to clarify the data structure and to test the loading strength of the items on factors (Costello & Osborne, 2005). An item value of communality of .3 was considered as the cutoff point. Factors with eigenvalue greater than 1.0 were retained, and factor loadings greater than .4 were considered significant. For the scree plot, number of factors was determined by locating the point where the slope of the downward curve was clearly leveling off (Costello & Osborne, 2005). A confirmatory factor analysis (CFA) was performed using AMOS to assess how well the model gleaned from the EFA matches the observed data and to assess whether a one- or two-factor model fits data better. We estimated the degree of model fit with the data using normed chi-square (χ^2/df) ≤ 5, Tucker–Lewis Index (TLI) ≥ .9, Bentler's comparative fit index (CFI) ≥ .9, and root mean square error of approximation (RMSEA) ≤ .08 (Hu & Bentler, 1999; Schermelleh-Engel, Moosbrugger, & Müller, 2003; Schumacker & Lomax, 2004).

The scale's construct validity was achieved by assessing its convergent validity (Campbell & Fiske, 1959). Theoretically, perception of nursing care quality and the overall quality of care in the hospital both relate to PSNC. Convergent validity was obtained by testing the correlation between perception of nursing care quality and the overall quality of care in the hospital and then by testing patterns of intercorrelations between these two measures along with PSNC.

Patient satisfaction levels were then compared across different demographics using a *t* test and a one-way, between-subjects analysis of variance. Tukey's honestly significant difference (HSD) was used for post hoc analyses.

Results

Sample Description

Two hundred ninety-two patients completed the survey, of which 49.3% were female. The mean age of the participants was 41.5 years (*SD* = 18.6 years). Of the total sample, 54.8% were educated to the primary/secondary level. Only 3.4% of the participants worked in the healthcare field. Most of the participants (61.0%) had been hospitalized at least once. Most of the participants (55.1%) were hospitalized for 2 to less than 4 days, and the vast majority (80.1%) were accommodated in shared rooms (Table 1).

TABLE 1.
Sample Characteristics (N = 292)

Variable	*n*	%
Age (mean and *SD*; *n* = 287)	41.5	18.6
Gender		
Male	143	49.0
Female	144	49.3
Missing data	5	1.7
Educational level		
Primary/secondary	160	54.8
College/university	98	33.6
Missing data	34	11.6
Hospital ward		
Medical	137	46.9
Surgical	153	52.4
Missing data	2	0.7
Work		
Health field	10	3.4
Education field	29	9.9
Other work	240	82.2
Missing data	13	4.5
Previous hospitalization		
One to three times	178	61.0
Four to six times	38	13.0
More than six times	49	16.8
Missing data	27	9.2
Length of stay		
2 to less than 4 days	161	55.1
4–6 days	61	20.9
More than 6 days	67	23.0
Missing data	3	1.0
Hospital accommodation		
Private room	51	17.5
Shared room	234	80.1
Missing data	7	2.4

Psychometrics

In the current sample (*N* = 292), the overall Cronbach's alpha coefficient for the PSNCQQ-Ar was excellent and similar across different hospital units (.96). The split-half coefficients were .91 and .95 for Parts 1 and 2, respectively, with a Guttman split-half coefficient of .94. Analysis of responses of the six expert raters showed that the I-CVI of the 17 items ranged from .83 to 1 and that the S-CVI/ave was .94.

Before EFA, incomplete cases were treated with listwise deletion, which yielded a final sample size of 264 with over 15 subjects per item. Inspection of the correlation matrix revealed that all correlation coefficients were above .3. The KMO measure was satisfactory (.96). Bartlett's test of sphericity was significant (χ^2 = 3878.065, *df* = 136, *p* < .001). Accordingly, all assessment results fulfilled the prerequisites for conducting EFA.

Regarding the dimensionality of the PSNCQQ-Ar, EFA revealed two factors with eigenvalues greater than 1 (10.75, 1.02), suggesting a two-factor model that explained 69.3% of the variance. The scree plot showed that the downward curve leveled off after the second component, confirming the two-factor model. Table 2 shows the pattern matrix from EFA. Factor 1 was composed of Items 6–17 and explained 46.4% of the variance, whereas Factor 2 consisted of Items 1–5 and accounted for 22.9% of the variance. The Cronbach's alpha coefficients for Factors 1 and 2 were .83 and .96, respectively.

Results of the CFA showed that the one-factor model had a poor data fit, with χ^2/df = 4.56, TLI = .86, CFI = .89, and RMSEA = .11, whereas the two-factor model had relatively adequate data fit, with χ^2/df = 3.90, TLI = .90, CFI = .91, and almost acceptable RMSEA = .09.

Perception of nursing care quality and the overall quality of care in the hospital significantly and positively correlated

TABLE 2.
Pattern Matrix From Exploratory Factor Analysis[a] of the 17 Items of the PSNCQQ-Ar (N = 264)

PSNCQQ-Ar Item	Factor Loading	
	Factor 1	Factor 2
Factor 1: satisfaction with provided care		
14. How well things were done, like giving medicine and handling IVs	.933	−.096
13. How quick they were to help	.850	−.085
12. Ability of the nurses to make you comfortable and reassure you	.790	.121
11. How well they adjusted their schedules to your needs	.782	.058
16. Amount of peace and quiet	.778	.076
8. How often nurses checked on you and how well they kept track of how you were doing	.775	.097
15. The teamwork between nurses and other hospital staff who took care of you	.750	.104
10. Willingness of the nurses to be flexible in meeting your needs	.748	.150
17. Provisions for your privacy by nurses	.745	.082
9. How much nurses ask you what you think is important and give you choices	.715	.158
7. Courtesy and respect you were given; friendliness and kindness	.644	.179
6. How much they were allowed to help in your care	.445	.193
Factor 2: satisfaction with provided information		
2. How well nurses explained how to prepare for tests and operations	−.083	.878
1. How clear and complete the nurses' explanations were about tests, treatments, and what to expect	.000	.800
4. How well nurses communicated with patients, families, and doctors	.288	.562
3. Willingness of nurses to answer your questions	.392	.453
5. How well the nurses kept them informed about your condition and needs	.148	.446

Note. PSNCQQ-Ar = Arabic version of the Patient Satisfaction with Nursing Care Quality Questionnaire.
[a]Extraction method = maximum likelihood; rotation method = oblique (Promax, κ = 4).

with each other ($r = .67$, $p < .001$). PSNC scores significantly and positively correlated with perception of nursing care quality ($r = .72$, $p < .001$) and with the overall quality of care in the hospital ($r = .81$, $p < .001$), supporting the theoretical correlation between these measures and suggesting acceptable convergent validity (Campbell & Fiske, 1959).

Patient Satisfaction

The total mean score of PSNC was 4.30 of 5 ($SD = 0.74$). The average score of individual items in the PSNCQQ-Ar ranged from 3.90 to 4.51, with higher scores indicating higher PSNC (Table 3).

There was a significant difference in the scores of patients who recommended the hospital ($M = 4.39$, $SD = 0.66$) and those who did not recommend the hospital ($M = 3.25$, $SD = 0.79$; $t = 0.34$, $p < .001$). The overall patient satisfaction levels were statistically different in terms of perceived nursing care quality ($F = 164$, $p < .001$). Post hoc analysis (Tukey's HSD) revealed that patients who reported excellent nursing care were more satisfied ($M = 4.69$, $SD = 0.43$) than both those who reported good nursing care ($M = 3.83$, $SD = 0.57$) and those who reported poor nursing care ($M = 2.60$, $SD = 0.81$). In addition, the overall patient satisfaction levels were statistically different in terms of the overall quality of care ($F = 135.2$, $p < .001$). Post hoc analysis (Tukey's HSD) revealed that patients who reported excellent quality of care ($M = 4.51$, $SD = 0.49$) were more satisfied than both those who reported good quality of care ($M = 3.44$, $SD = 0.76$) and those who reported poor quality of care ($M = 2.69$, $SD = 0.65$; Table 4).

In terms of PSNC at the ward level, no significant difference was identified between medical ($M = 4.31$, $SD = 0.76$) and surgical ($M = 4.29$, $SD = 0.73$) wards ($t = 0.22$, $p < .82$).

Discussion

We sought to adapt and validate the PSNCQQ-Ar using a sample of Arabic speakers who were adult inpatients in a tertiary hospital in Oman. We employed a structured process of transcultural adaptation and used sophisticated psychometric techniques to create a scale that would be valid, reliable, and ready for use in an Arabic context.

The Cronbach's alpha for the PSNCQQ-Ar was excellent and similar to that of both the original, English scale (Laschinger et al., 2005) and the Serbian version (Milutinović et al., 2012), suggesting that each has good internal consistency (Cronbach, 1951). For content validity, six expert raters evaluated the 17 items on a 4-point scale. Analysis revealed that none of the 17 items had an I-CVI of less than .79 and that the S-CVI/ave was above .90. Accordingly, an evidence of acceptable content validity of the PSNCQQ-Ar was supported (Polit & Beck, 2006). The former two studies of the PSNCQQ did not report evidence of obtained

TABLE 3.

Means and Standard Deviations of Individual Items and Average at the Hospital Ward Level (N = 290)

PSNCQQ-Ar Item Label[a]	Medical Ward (*n* = 137)		Surgical Ward (*n* = 153)		Total	
	Mean	*SD*	Mean	*SD*	Mean	*SD*
1. Information you were given	4.41	0.78	4.39	0.79	4.40	0.79
2. Instructions	4.37	0.81	4.43	0.75	4.40	0.78
3. Ease of getting information	4.37	0.88	4. 28	0.92	4.32	0.90
4. Information given by nurses	4.36	0.82	4.38	0.83	4.37	0.83
5. Informing family or friends	3.95	1.34	3.86	1.26	3.90	1.30
6. Involving family or friends in your care	4.10	1.14	4.07	1.15	4.08	1.14
7. Concern and caring by nurses	4.47	0.79	4.54	0.79	4.51	0.80
8. Attention of nurses to your condition	4.42	0.95	4.46	0.84	4.44	0.89
9. Recognition of your opinions	4.18	1.05	4.16	1.12	4.17	1.09
10. Consideration of your needs	4.34	0.93	4.31	0.94	4.33	0.93
11. The daily routine of the nurses	4.31	0.96	4.18	1.14	4.24	1.06
12. Helpfulness	4.36	0.95	4.28	1.01	4.31	0.99
13. Nursing staff response to your calls	4.17	1.11	4.28	0.98	4.23	1.04
14. Skill and competence of nurses	4.38	0.89	4.42	0.88	4.40	0.88
15. Coordination of care	4.36	0.94	4.30	1.01	4.33	0.98
16. Restful atmosphere provided by nurses	4.24	1.03	4.20	1.12	4.22	1.08
17. Privacy	4.45	0.84	4.43	0.84	4.44	0.84
Average	4.31	0.76	4.29	0.73	4.30	0.74

Note. PSNCQQ-Ar = Arabic version of the Patient Satisfaction with Nursing Care Quality Questionnaire.
[a]Labels of items that have been used.

content validity (Laschinger et al., 2005; Milutinović et al., 2012).

Listwise deletion yielded a final sample size of 264, with over 15 subjects per item, suggesting an adequate sample size for EFA to avoid computational difficulties (Costello & Osborne, 2005; Hair, Black, Babin, & Anderson, 2010). In addition, inspection of the correlation matrix for factorability of *R* revealed that, although variables were intercorrelated, the correlations were not excessive (all variables were above 0.3 and below 0.8), indicating that the unique contribution of each of the 17 variables was maintained (Williams et al., 2010). Furthermore, the excellent KMO value (.96; Kaiser, 1974) and the significant result of Bartlett's test ($p < .001$; Hair et al., 2010) suggested sample adequacy and appropriateness for the EFA (Tabachnick & Fidell, 2013).

Maximum likelihood factor extraction is the best method when data are relatively normally distributed because "it permits statistical significance testing of factor loadings and correlations among factors" (Fabrigar, Wegener, MacCallum, & Strahan, 1999). In addition, maximum likelihood is suggested when the intention of the EFA is to obtain interpretable factors rather than to remove items (Costello & Osborne, 2005). As the data obtained in this study were relatively normally distributed and all of the 17 items of the PSNCQQ-Ar are believed to be important in measuring PSNC, maximum likelihood factor extraction is considered appropriate for this study.

Considering the fact that oblique methods allow factors to correlate but orthogonal rotations do not, Costello and Osborne (2005) argued that orthogonal methods lead to loss of valuable data if factors being studied correlate and that oblique rotations are best when factors are believed to correlate with each other. In this study, items of the PSNCQQ-Ar belong to factors that represent the study's concept of interest, PSNC. As an evolving concept, PSNC's attributes are believed to reflect the perspective of patients. Obviously, correlations among PSNC factors are inevitable in this study, and therefore the oblique rotation method is more appropriate than orthogonal rotation.

Whereas the Serbian study used principal component analysis with varimax rotation method (Milutinović et al., 2012), the extraction method that was used in the original Canadian study is not known (Laschinger et al., 2005). On the basis of the findings of previous studies (Laschinger et al., 2005; Milutinović et al., 2012), we expected either a one- or two-factor model for the PSNCQQ-Ar.

Results from this study revealed a two-factor model with eigenvalues greater than 1. CFA showed that the two-factor

TABLE 4.
Comparison of Patient Satisfaction Levels (N = 292)

Variable	Mean	*SD*	*t*/*F*	*p*
Gender			1.08	.28
Male	4.25	0.85		
Female	4.35	0.61		
Education			1.28	.20
Primary/secondary	4.31	0.79		
College/university	4.18	0.72		
Hospital ward			0.22	.82
Medical	4.31	0.76		
Surgical	4.29	0.73		
Hospital accommodation			0.30	.82
Private room	4.33	0.61		
Shared room	4.30	0.76		
Hospital recommendation			0.34	< .001
Recommended	4.39	0.66		
Not recommended	3.25	0.79		
Work			*F* = 0.03	.96
Health field	4.34	0.62		
Education field	4.30	0.71		
Other work	4.28	0.76		
Previous hospitalization (number of times)			*F* = 0.42	.66
1–3	4.32	0.71		
4–6	4.27	0.88		
> 6	4.21	0.75		
Length of stay (days)			*F* = 1.30	.28
2–3	4.32	0.73		
4–6	4.37	0.68		
> 6	4.18	0.82		
Nursing care quality			*F* = 164.00	< .001
Poor	2.60	0.81		
Good	3.83	0.57		
Excellent	4.69	0.43		
Overall quality of care			*F* = 135.20	< .001
Poor	2.69	0.65		
Good	3.44	0.76		
Excellent	4.51	0.49		

model had better fit indices than the one-factor model. In addition, CFA revealed that Factors 1 and 2 had adequate fit indices. These findings suggest that the factor structure gleaned from the EFA fits data better than the single-factor model.

Inspection of the pattern matrix indicates that Items 3, 5, and 6 are close to the cutoff of 0.4, which is considered fair (Tabachnick & Fidell, 2013). The inability of Items 3, 5, and 6 to measure well may relate to the sample size used in this study (Tabachnick & Fidell, 2013). Another potential reason may be an insufficient level of respondent awareness of the functions that are described in these three items. The functions described in the three items are theoretically related to the job of nurses, and thus respondents may not be sufficiently cognizant of these. Although these three items did not measure well, we still believe that they make important contributions to the overall PSNC. Hence, Items 3, 5 and 6 were retained in the factor structure of the PSNCQQ-Ar.

Theoretically, Items 6–17 are believed to measure patient satisfaction with actions done by nurses. Therefore, Factor 1 could be labeled "satisfaction with provided care." In addition, Factor 2 could be labeled "satisfaction with provided information" because Items 1–5 are believed to measure patient satisfaction with information provided by nurses.

Construct validity of the PSNCQQ-Ar was obtained by testing the correlations between PSNC and other constructs. Pearson's correlation coefficients revealed strong associations between PSNC quality, perceived nursing care quality, and the overall quality of care in the hospital, which is consistent with the results of the original study (Laschinger et al., 2005) and of the Serbian version (Milutinović et al., 2012).

The overall mean of patient satisfaction was quite high, suggesting that patients had a good experience with nursing care. However, comparisons across hospital wards revealed no significant differences in terms of PSNC. Patients were mostly satisfied with aspects such as "concern and caring by nurses" and "attention of nurses to your condition," suggesting that nurses pay significant attention to patient care tasks, which is the core concept of nursing. Moreover, patients were least satisfied with aspects such as "informing family or friends," "involving family or friends in your care," and "recognition of your opinions," suggesting that nurses pay less attention to involving patients and their families and friends in planning and implementing nursing care. Likewise, these findings are congruent with the findings of the Canadian and Serbian studies (Laschinger et al., 2005; Milutinović et al., 2012).

Limitations

This study was conducted in one setting. Thus, the current lack of comparability between different hospitals may limit the generalizability of the findings. In addition, because of time constraints, researchers were unable to collect data on two different occasions to obtain a test–retest estimate of reliability, which would have added value to the psychometrics of the PSNCQQ-Ar. Furthermore, the electronic survey method may have introduced confounding factors because of lack of control over the sample, stakeholder bias, unverified respondents, and nonresponse bias (Duda & Nobile, 2010). However, researchers maintained the recommended measures to ensure that only eligible participants were involved in filling out the survey, that participants filled out the survey only once, and that each participant received the required instructions.

Conclusions

In view of its sound psychometric properties for content, comprehension, readability, and practicality, the PSNCQQ-Ar is a promising instrument for measuring PSNC in an Arabic context, further equipping nurses and managers with useful information related to care strengths and weaknesses and to areas that require improvement. The information provided by the PSNCQQ-Ar has the potential to help communities of interest discriminate between different care experiences at the unit and hospital levels, which may be further used in (a) planning and resource allocation at the organizational level, (b) marketing and awareness at the community level, and (c) policy development and strategic planning at the national level. In addition, the PSNCQQ-Ar may be useful in better understanding how patients perceive what nurses actually do. Furthermore, the results of this study may serve as baseline data for future quality improvement projects and research in Oman and the Middle East.

We recommend applying the PSNCQQ-Ar in different settings and using electronic as well as traditional survey methods to collect data. In addition, we recommend using test–retest estimates of reliability. Moreover, we recommend further validation studies of the PSNCQQ-Ar to standardize this instrument for general use in Oman and across the Middle East. For Oman in particular, we recommend that healthcare stakeholders adopt the PSNCQQ-Ar to measure PSNC quality, to identify differences among hospitals, and to facilitate further improvements in quality of care.

Acknowledgments

This work was supported by a grant from Sultan Qaboos University (IG/CON/DEAN/15/01). All of the authors would like to acknowledge Sultan Qaboos University for supporting this study and facilitating its conduct. Furthermore, authors would like to thank all of the patients and research assistants for their time and efforts taken to make this study successful.

References

Abdel Maqsood, A. S., Oweis, A. I., & Hasna, F. S. (2012). Differences between patients' expectations and satisfaction with nursing care in a private hospital in Jordan. *International Journal of Nursing Practice, 18*(2), 140–146. https://doi.org/10.1111/j.1440-172X.2012.02008.x

Al-Abri, R., & Al-Balushi, A. (2014). Patient satisfaction survey as a tool towards quality improvement. *Oman Medical Journal, 29*(1), 3–7. https://doi.org/10.5001/omj.2014.02

Alasad, J., Abu Tabar, N., & AbuRuz, M. E. (2015). Patient satisfaction with nursing care: Measuring outcomes in an international setting. *The Journal of Nursing Administration, 45*(11), 563–568. https://doi.org/10.1097/NNA.0000000000000264

Atallah, M. A., Hamdan-Mansour, A. M., Al-Sayed, M. M., & Aboshaiqah, A. E. (2013). Patients' satisfaction with the quality of nursing care provided: The Saudi experience. *International Journal of Nursing Practice, 19*(6), 584–590. https://doi.org/10.1111/ijn.12102

Campbell, D. T., & Fiske, D. W. (1959). Convergent and discriminant validation by the multitrait-multimethod matrix. *Psychological Bulletin, 56*(2), 81–105. https://doi.org/10.1037/h0046016

Castro, E. M., Van Regenmortel, T., Vanhaecht, K., Sermeus, W., & Van Hecke, A. (2016). Patient empowerment, patient participation and patient-centeredness in hospital care: A concept analysis based on a literature review. *Patient Education and Counseling, 99*(12), 1923–1939. https://doi.org/10.1016/j.pec.2016.07.026

Costello, A. B., & Osborne, J. W. (2005). Best practices in exploratory factor analysis: Four recommendations for getting the most from your analysis. *Practical Assessment, Research & Evaluation, 10*(7), 1–9.

Cronbach, L. J. (1951). Coefficient alpha and the internal structure of tests. *Psychometrika, 16*(3), 297–334. https://doi.org/10.1007/BF02310555

de-la-Cueva-Ariza, L., Romero-García, M., Delgado-Hito, P., Acosta-Mejuto, B., Jover-Sancho, C., Ricart-Basagaña, M. T., ... Solà-Ribó, M. (2014). Development of an instrument to measure the degree of critical patient's satisfaction with nursing care: Research protocol. *Journal of Advanced Nursing, 70*(1), 201–210. https://doi.org/10.1111/jan.12184

Duda, M. D., & Nobile, J. L. (2010). The fallacy of online surveys: No data are better than bad data. *Human Dimensions of Wildlife, 15*(1), 55–64. https://doi.org/10.1080/10871200903244250

Dudkiewicz, P. B. (2014). Utilizing a caring-based nursing model in an interdepartmental setting to improve patient satisfaction. *International Journal for Human Caring, 18*(4), 30–33. https://doi.org/10.20467/1091-5710-18.4.30

Eriksen, L. R. (1995). Patient satisfaction with nursing care: Concept clarification. *Journal of Nursing Measurement, 3*(1), 59–76.

Fabrigar, L. R., Wegener, D. T., MacCallum, R. C., & Strahan, E. J. (1999). Evaluating the use of exploratory factor analysis in psychological research. *Psychological Methods, 4*(3), 272–299. https://doi.org/10.1037/1082-989X.4.3.272

Freitas, J. S., Silva, A. E., Minamisava, R., Bezerra, A. L., & de Sousa, M. R. (2014). Quality of nursing care and satisfaction of patients attended at a teaching hospital. *Revista Latino-Americana de Enfermagem, 22*(3), 454–460. https://doi.org/10.1590/0104-1169.3241.2437

Gjersing, L., Caplehorn, J. R., & Clausen, T. (2010). Cross-cultural adaptation of research instruments: Language, setting, time and statistical considerations. *BMC Medical Research Methodology, 10*, 13. https://doi.org/10.1186/1471-2288-10-13

Hair, J. F. Jr., Black, W. C., Babin, B. J., & Anderson, R. E. (2010). *Multivariate data analysis* (7th ed.) Retrieved from https://www.pearsonhighered.com/program/Hair-Multivariate-Data-Analysis-7th-Edition/PGM263675.html

Hu, L. t., & Bentler, P. M. (1999). Cutoff criteria for fit indexes in covariance structure analysis: Conventional criteria versus new alternatives. *Structural Equation Modeling: A Multidisciplinary Journal, 6*(1), 1–55.

Junewicz, A., & Youngner, S. J. (2015). Patient-satisfaction surveys on a scale of 0 to 10: Improving health care, or leading it astray? *The Hastings Center Report, 45*(3), 43–51. https://doi.org/10.1002/hast.453

Kaiser, H. F. (1974). An index of factorial simplicity. *Psychometrika, 39*(1), 31–36. https://doi.org/10.1007/BF02291575

Koy, V., Yunibhand, J., & Angsuroch, Y. (2016). The quantitative measurement of nursing care quality: A systematic review of available instruments. *International Nursing Review, 63*(3), 490–498. https://doi.org/10.1111/inr.12269

La Monica, E. L., Oberst, M. T., Madea, A. R., & Wolf, R. M. (1986). Development of a patient satisfaction scale. *Research in Nursing & Health, 9*(1), 43–50. https://doi.org/10.1002/nur.4770090108

Laschinger, H. S., Hall, L. M., Pedersen, C., & Almost, J. (2005). A psychometric analysis of the patient satisfaction with nursing care quality questionnaire: An actionable approach to measuring patient satisfaction. *Journal of Nursing Care Quality, 20*(3), 220–230.

Linder-Pelz, S. U. (1982). Toward a theory of patient satisfaction. *Social Science & Medicine, 16*(5), 577–582. https://doi.org/10.1016/0277-9536(82)90311-2

Milutinović, D., Simin, D., Brkić, N., & Brkić, S. (2012). The patient satisfaction with nursing care quality: The psychometric study of the Serbian version of PSNCQ questionnaire. *Scandinavian Journal of Caring Sciences, 26*(3), 598–606. https://doi.org/10.1111/j.1471-6712.2012.00969.x

Pascoe, G. C. (1983). Patient satisfaction in primary health care: A literature review and analysis. *Evaluation and Program Planning, 6*(3–4), 185–210. https://doi.org/10.1016/0149-7189(83)90002-2

Polit, D. F., & Beck, C. T. (2006). The content validity index: Are you sure you know what's being reported? Critique and recommendations. *Research in Nursing & Health, 29*(5), 489–497. https://doi.org/10.1002/nur.20147

Schermelleh-Engel, K., Moosbrugger, H., & Müller, H. (2003). Evaluating the fit of structural equation models: Tests of significance and descriptive goodness-of-fit measures. *Methods of Psychological Research Online, 8*(2), 23–74.

Schumacker, R. E., & Lomax, R. G. (2004). *A beginner's guide to structural equation modeling* (2nd ed.). Mahwah, NJ: Taylor & Francis.

Sousa, V. D., & Rojjanasrirat, W. (2011). Translation, adaptation and validation of instruments or scales for use in cross-cultural health care research: A clear and user-friendly guideline. *Journal of Evaluation in Clinical Practice, 17*(2), 268–274. https://doi.org/10.1111/j.1365-2753.2010.01434.x

Tabachnick, B. G., & Fidell, L. S. (2013). *Using multivariate statistics* (6th ed.). Boston, MA: Pearson.

Thomas, L. H., McColl, E., Priest, J., Bond, S., & Boys, R. J. (1996). Newcastle satisfaction with nursing scales: An instrument for quality assessments of nursing care. *BMJ Quality & Safety, 5*(2), 67–72.

Williams, B., Onsman, A., & Brown, T. (2010). Exploratory factor analysis: A five-step guide for novices. *Journal of Emergency Primary Health Care, 8*(3), Article 990399.

17

The Medical Futility Experience of Nurses in Caring for Critically Ill Patients

Ming-Yi Hsu[1] • Shu-Fen Su[2] • Lien-Ying Chiang[3*] • Sou-Jen Shih[4]
Yu-Chen Chen[5]

ABSTRACT

Background: Medical futility is a key bioethical concern. In Taiwan, policymakers tend to provide care standards and evaluation guidelines for critically ill and terminal patients whose treatment is medically futile. However, the current status of medical futility for critically ill patients is inadequate, and no consensus currently exists on the definition of medical futility.

Purpose: The aim of this study was to understand the medical futility experiences of intensive care nurses.

Methods: This qualitative research adopted a phenomenological perspective and was conducted in a medical center and a regional hospital in Central Taiwan. Eight nurses with at least 1 year of nursing tenure who were serving in the intensive care unit were recruited. Purposive and snowball sampling methods were used to conduct one-on-one in-depth interviews. Each of the tape-recorded interviews was transcribed before data analysis.

Results: The research results found four themes, including (a) definitions of medical futility and types of patients, (b) considerations of medical futility, (c) the occurrence of medical futility, and (d) nurses' responses to medical futility. The participants indicated that medical futility refers to the point at which the continued provision of treatment does not evidently ease the disease condition of a patient or improve his or her quality of life or when life-sustaining treatment is provided to patients to facilitate the process of death.

Conclusions: This study revealed that the major challenge in clinical cases of medical futility is for physicians, nurses, and patients to communicate effectively together during times of rapid and unanticipated change in patient condition. Thus, events of medical futility may be preventable. Past cases of medical futility involving critically ill patients may serve as references for guiding clinical care, education, and related policy formulation.

KEY WORDS:
critically ill patients, critical care nursing, medical futility.

Introduction

Although the advancement of technology has prolonged the lives of critically ill patients, there is still a limit to what medical care is able to achieve. Futile treatments are criticized as inappropriate expenditures of medical resources and as a type of medical care in which the costs exceed the benefits for the patient. Thus, medical futility has raised bioethics concerns (Downar et al., 2015; Persaud, 2006).

Previous studies of medical futility have focused primarily on life-sustaining treatment (LST) in terminally ill patients (Jox, Schaider, Marckmann, & Borasio, 2012), hospice care and palliative care, or the signing of do-not-resuscitate (DNR) forms. However, medical futility does not occur only in terminally ill patients, and the specific circumstances in which medical futility occurs remain unclear. Thus, the experiences that are associated with medical futility warrant further exploration. This study investigated the experiences of intensive care unit (ICU) nurses in cases of medical futility.

Research Objective

The aim of this study was to understand the medical futility experiences of ICU nurses.

Definitions of Medical Futility

The concept of medical futility emerged in the 1980s. The term was used to describe the point at which further medical care, as determined unilaterally by the attending physician, was adjudged as futile because of inability to achieve desired physiological results. Consultation with neither the patient nor his or her family (or surrogate) was required, often resulting in conflict and controversy (Moratti, 2009). In 1990, Schneiderman, Jecker, and Jonsen (1990) proposed quantitative and qualitative approaches for defining medical futility. Schneiderman et al. suggested that physicians should regard a treatment as futile when that treatment has been "useless" when applied in 100 consecutive cases (p. 951). He further proposed that treatments that preserve patients in a state of permanent unconsciousness or result in dependence on intensive medical care should be considered qualitatively futile. In 1995, Brody and Halevy highlighted that the existing definitions of medical futility were unclear and proposed dividing the concept into two dimensions. The first dimension further

[1]*PhD, RN, Assistant Professor, School of Nursing, Chung Shan Medical University, and Adjunct Supervisor, Department of Nursing, Chung Shan Medical University Hospital* • [2]*PhD, RN, Associate Professor, Department of Nursing, National Taichung University of Science and Technology* • [3]*MSN, RN, Department of Nursing, Taichung Veterans General Hospital* • [4]*MSN, RN, Deputy Director, Department of Nursing, Taichung Veterans General Hospital* • [5]*MSN, RN, Supervisor, Department of Nursing, Cheng-Ching General Hospital.*

divides the possible outcomes of medical treatment into the four categories of physiological futility, imminent demise futility, lethal condition futility, and qualitative futility, whereas the second dimension proposes a patient-centered definition of medical futility. In 2009, Lo further provided two clinical-condition-based definitions of medical futility, in which the strict definitions of futility remain based on objective evidence or professional medical judgment and on the unilateral identification of physicians. Unlike the widely used definitions of medical futility used before 2009, the loose definitions of futility involve value judgments and thus cannot be assessed by physicians only. Instead, patients or their surrogate must agree to the following: (a) the chance of success is extremely unlikely, (b) a desirable goal cannot be achieved, (c) the patient's quality of life (QOL) is unacceptable, and (d) the extent of resource consumption exceeds the expected benefits.

Medical futility, according to the aforementioned definitions, may be divided into four dimensions: (a) the clinical decisions and judgments made by physicians regarding the medical treatment of patients, (b) the consent of patients (or their surrogates or family members) to the decisions and judgments of physicians, (c) the value placed on patient QOL, and (d) the use of medical resources.

Studies on Medical Futility

Most related studies have investigated how medical futility influences patient physiology and QOL. Jox et al. (2012) conducted in-depth interviews with ICU and hospice care physicians and nurses at a hospital in Germany to understand how they defined medical futility when they perceived LST as futile. The results indicate that the interviewees associated futility with the failure to achieve goals of care that were intended to improve patient QOL and were proportionate to patient burden (risk, harm, and cost). Moratti (2010) researched the perceptions of medical futility among physicians in the neonatal ICU at a hospital in the Netherlands. The results indicate that these neonatologists regarded life-prolonging treatment as futile and that the following were considered in sequential order to discern whether medical treatment was futile: communication, mental condition, motor condition, dependency on medical care, self-sufficiency, pain, suffering, and multisensory impairments. Sibbald, Downar, and Hawryluck (2007) adopted the grounded theory approach to conduct in-depth interviews with physician directors, nurse managers, and respiratory therapists from 14 ICUs in Canada. The results suggest the following as a working definition of medically futile care: the use of considerable medical resources without a reasonable hope that the patient will recover to a state of relative independence or be interactive with his or her environment. Yekefallah, Ashktorab, Manoochehri, and Hamid (2015) found that participant nurses defined futile care as "useless, ineffective care giving with wastage of resources and torment of both patients and nurses having nursing and medical aspects."

The few studies that have researched medical futility in Taiwan have examined medical futility in end-of-life care for critically ill patients (Lin et al., 2010; Weng, 2012). Huang (2009) conducted in-depth interviews with physicians, nurses, and patient families and explored the boundary of medical futility and the limit of medical treatment by focusing on DNR orders. The results indicate a lack of consensus on medical futility. Huang asked interviewees "Under what conditions should first aid be administered?" and "Under what conditions is administering first aid perceived as futile?" rather than asking about their core perception of medical futility. In recent years, several hospitals have been promoting standard operating procedures for evaluating critical and terminal patients for whom treatment is medically futile. For example, the ICU at Taipei Veterans General Hospital uses Simplified Acute Physiology Score II to evaluate disease severity to screen for patients with mortality risks higher than 80%, with treatments for patients in this category deemed to be futile (Huang, 2013). However, no studies have yet elucidated the clinical situations that involve medical futility or the medical care that is offered in response to these situations.

Accordingly, this study adopted a qualitative research method to conduct an in-depth investigation of the current perspectives of medical futility in Taiwan by focusing on the experiences of ICU nurses who regularly provide clinical care to patients.

Methods

Research Design

A phenomenological perspective was adopted to assist the researchers to investigate personal experiences without precognition by the interviewees (Converse, 2012). An individual first understands a phenomenon and then interprets it; in fact, personal cultural background provides insight for interpreting the content of a phenomenon (Huang, Kellett, St. John, & Lee, 2006).

Research Sites and Participants

A medical center and a regional hospital in Central Taiwan were selected as the research sites. Purposive sampling was employed for recruiting participants, and snowball sampling was subsequently adopted for sampling personnel with a registered nurse certificate or registered professional nurse certificate who had worked for at least 1 year in the ICU and who are still working in the ICU. Nurses from pediatric ICUs were excluded because of the substantial differences in patients and treatment experiences between regular and pediatric ICUs. The interviewing stage was concluded when the content from the current interview overlapped with previously obtained interview content, indicating that data saturation had been reached. Participants were recruited from March 1, 2013, to January 22, 2014, during which time eight people were interviewed.

Data Collection

After this research project was approved by the institutional review board and confirmed to adhere to all policies and procedures of the study hospitals, the head nurses of each research unit sent emails to the nurses who met the inclusion criteria. Subsequently, these nurses contacted the researchers using the contact information that was provided in the email. After being interviewed, each participant recommended other potential participants to the researchers. The interview time and location were arranged according to the convenience of each participant. All of the participants were referred to by pseudonyms to ensure privacy. The questions that were posed during the one-on-one in-depth interviews followed the format provided by the interview guide. Examples of questions include "What do you think medical futility is?" and "Please share your experiences in providing futile care." The interviews were recorded using a recording pen and then transcribed. The longest and shortest interview times were 71.5 and 42.5 minutes, respectively. The average interview time was 56.6 minutes.

Data Analysis

The collected data were analyzed according to the seven steps for data analysis proposed by Colaizzi (1978): (a) transcribe the recorded data and read the transcripts in detail to obtain an overall understanding of the participants' experiences, (b) extract significant statements directly from the transcripts to ensure that the original meaning is obtained, (c) maintain a descriptive attitude and extract the meaning of each significant statement, (d) organize the formulated meanings into clusters of themes, (e) integrate the themes and offer an exhaustive description of the investigated phenomenon under study, (f) integrate the research results and devise a thorough portrayal of the investigated phenomenon to form its primary structure, and (g) consult the participants to confirm that the research findings reflect their experiences.

Study Rigor

The concept of trustworthiness proposed by Lincoln and Guba (1985) served as the criterion for establishing the rigor of this study. Trustworthiness is composed of four aspects: credibility, transferability, dependability, and confirmability. In terms of the credibility of the present research, the researchers had received training courses on qualitative research, and the results obtained from the analyzed data were checked and reviewed by the participants. Regarding dependability, the interviews were conducted by the researchers. Each participant was interviewed only once, and to prevent bias, participants were asked not to disclose the interview content with their referrals before the referrals' interview session. Regarding confirmability, the interviews were conducted under natural situations. The interviewers maintained neutral attitudes and refrained from expressing opinions during the interviews. Regarding transferability, the results may be generalized to ICU nurses with similar experiences and backgrounds in providing care at medical centers and regional hospitals in Central Taiwan.

Ethical Considerations

The present research project was executed after approval was obtained from the medical center (Serial number CE12306) and regional hospital (Serial number HP120027). Before the interviews, the research method and objective as well as the rights of the participants were explicitly explained to the participants. Written informed consent was obtained from each participant before his or her interview. The participants were allowed to terminate the interview or otherwise withdraw from the research at any time without providing a reason. The pseudonyms of the participants were used throughout all of the interview notes, transcripts, and audio files. Thus, the collected data contained no evidence of the participant identities. The data were encrypted and stored in a manner that is not publically accessible, were used for research purposes only, and were not disclosed or discussed with anyone outside the research team.

Results

The participants included six nurses from a medical center and two nurses from a regional hospital. Four worked in a medical ICU, three worked in a surgical ICU, and one worked in a comprehensive medical–surgical ICU. All of the participants were female. The average age of the participants was 36.6 years. In terms of education, two held a master's degree, four held a bachelor's degree, and two held a 5-year junior college degree. Regarding total nursing tenure, one had a tenure of less than 5 years, three had tenures of 6–10 years, and four had tenures of more than 10 years.

The research results showed that the medical futility experiences of the participants could be divided into four themes: definitions of medical futility and types of patients, considerations of medical futility, the occurrence of medical futility, and nurses' responses to medical futility.

Definitions of Medical Futility and Types of Patients

Almost all of the participants indicated that they considered medical care that offers no obvious benefit to a patient (e.g., absence of physiological response to the prescribed treatment) and prescribed medical treatments that do not appear to improve patient QOL as medically futile. Most also described as medically futile situations in which LST was prescribed to a patient who was expected to die in the near future.

The participants generally regarded patients whose vital signs continued to deteriorate or exhibited irreversible disease progression (e.g., terminal cancer or multiple organ failure) as having a high risk of death. If a patient was expected to die within a few days but LST was continued, then the administered treatment was deemed futile. Furthermore, more than half of the participants believed that palliative care rather than LST should be administered to these patients. For example:

> *In the emergency department...we confirmed a patient as having terminal cancer.... The patient's family had previously signed a DNR form...[the patient is] not on endo [intubation]. After the VS [Visiting staff] checked on the patient, the patient was transferred to the ICU.... The patient's family should have accompanied him on his last journey, instead of transferring him to the ICU for active treatment...as the treatment couldn't bring him (patient) back.* (Nurse G)

Considerations of Medical Futility

The participants reported that, after receiving medical treatment, the physiological signs and QOL of patients were observed to determine whether the specific treatment and the overall medical treatment were futile. In addition, the participants were often unable to ascertain the thoughts of patients because of their being in a coma or under sedation. Therefore, on the basis of their personal opinions, the participants were required to make judgments regarding the types of QOL patients would not accept. If, after treatment, patient QOL deteriorated below a participant-determined level, the participant deemed treatment to be futile. According to the participants, when LST could not stop the progression of patient organ failure and when a patient was considered moribund, LST was regarded as medically futile. For example, as Nurse C described the condition of a patient with triple organ failure:

> *...according to experience [and] theory, is it generally not true that more than three failing organs is associated with a mortality rate of 90% or more?* (Nurse C)

The Occurrence of Medical Futility

Despite realizing that a medical treatment is possibly or definitely futile, the participants were required to continue administering that treatment. Provision of futile treatment occurs for the following reasons: unpredictable changes in disease condition, different individual perceptions of medical futility, lack of timely or skilled communication, families unwilling to let go, and cultural customs.

Most of the participants believed that medical futility is a conclusion drawn from the result of the implemented treatment procedure. Whether patients face a high risk of deterioration or death, because changes in disease conditions cannot be predicted, whether medical treatment will be futile cannot be judged accurately. The participants mentioned that insufficient time for communication was a problem in the ICU. When faced with urgent situations, family members often feel overwhelmed and find it difficult to accept the changes in patient condition, rendering them incapable of making appropriate decisions immediately. This was illustrated by one participant's example of a patient whose condition deteriorated from facing a high risk of deterioration to facing a high risk of death:

> *By judging from the progress of the patient's disease...the physician indicated that the disease could no longer be controlled by medical treatment.... At the surgical ward, they [the visiting physician] performed surgery and were free only on [nurses'] evening shifts. However, the patient's family visited him [the patient] during the morning or afternoon and did not have time to visit at night...so there was no time [for both the patient's family and physician] to communicate.... If they [the patient's family] had received insight [into the patient's condition],... they would have been willing to let him go [die] because what the patient's families wanted for him was for him to [get out of the bed and] walk again.... Many patient families had such [unrealistic] expectations.* (Nurse B)

Furthermore, family members would sometimes ask the participants or other health professionals to conceal the truth about the patient's condition from their other family members for fear that these members could not bear to learn the true situation. Some family members adhered to the Confucian custom of deferring to the most senior family members. Thus, when a patient deteriorated to a high risk of death, the opinions of senior family members were given the most weight. Patients' children also believed this deference to seniority to be an expression of care and filial piety when all treatment options had been exhausted. In addition, some patient families selected specific times for patient death because of spiritual beliefs that the selected dates were auspicious and would benefit the patients and families. For example:

> *The patient had already informed that he did not want CPR, but his family still wanted CPR to be performed.... The purpose was not to let the patient die in the seventh lunar month; they would rather let him [the patient] suffer, even though he had already stated his wish to not receive CPR. I think it's difficult. We still perform CPR because people would think that if you [the family] don't save the patient, you're unfilial.... It's something that you [the family] can't bear.* (Nurse C)

Nurses' Responses to Medical Futility

Participants shared that nurses are prone to being sued by patient families when they care for critical patients whose treatment is deemed as either possibly futile or definitely futile. Thus, nurses are under pressure and constrained by legal consequences. Some participants expressed that, because they feel obligated to assist with the medical treatment of physicians, they must follow physician orders and administer the prescribed medical treatments even if they believe the treatment to be futile to avoid conflict with physicians. Participants endeavor to ensure patient comfort such as by helping patients remove their sputum or maintain a comfortable supine position.

> *We [nurses] do not have enough authority.... When encountering conflicts (with physicians' decisions), we can only comply.... I can only do my best to inform the families about what's best for the patient.... If the physician orders a vasopressor, even though we [the nurse] know that this treatment is futile, are we allowed to disobey that physician's order?...* (Nurse H)

Moreover, the participants were worried that the negative emotional status of patient families could engender medical disputes. Participants thus work to avoid being involved in disputes in which the wishes of family members come into conflict with the stated wishes of the patient. Thus, even if the patient had signed a DNR form, medical team members are often afraid of the legal action that family members might take against them after the patient dies and thus choose to ignore the patient's wishes and follow the family's demands for futile treatment.

> *...The patient signed the DNR, and then both of them [the wife and a witness] had also signed it.... The patient started breathing harder, and his wife then said yes [to intubate]...the patient was back on endo.... I think nowadays everyone is afraid of being sued.... If you refuse [to perform intubation] you may be sued.* (Nurse F)

Most of the participants considered communication as the most critical factor for easing medical-futility-related problems. They stated the importance of fostering a consensus among medical teams, patients, and patients' families to reduce the gap in their perceptions of a patient-related event.

> *...When a discrepancy in opinions occurs between us [nurses] and the physicians on duty, we, in principle, would ask our supervisor or leader for assistance...to understand the physicians' perceptions on the patient condition. The conflicts between physicians and nurses nowadays are caused by the perception gap.* (Nurse H)

Discussion

The key findings of this study are discussed in depth in this section based on the following categories of issues: uncertainty of disease conditions, futile medical treatment and communication, and factors affecting nurse reactions to medical futility.

Uncertainty of Disease Conditions

This study found that the participants regarded treatment that did not evidently benefit patient condition or QOL as medically futile. This finding is similar to the three themes of medical futility found in a concept analysis by Bahramnezhad et al. (2014), which included "low quality of life," "lack physiologic return to life," and "performing nonprofessional duties." The results were also similar to those reported by Schneiderman et al. (1990), Brody and Halevy (1995), and Lo (2009), all of which identified the physiology and QOL of the patient as key factors in assessing medical futility. Jox et al. (2012) reported that medical futility was related to the inability of a treatment to improve the QOL of a patient. However, unless the disease condition had deteriorated to end-of-life conditions, determining whether medical treatment had achieved its limit is difficult. In a review of studies examining the health-related QOL of patients with cancer, Lo and Hu (2008) found that health-related QOL refers to how a person in a specific situational and cultural context subjectively perceives his or her activities of daily living and the environment while under the influence of his or her disease condition and treatment. The results of this study indicate that, although many of the participants shared that they had experienced medical futility in their jobs, they were not able to terminate the related medical treatments because disease conditions may change unexpectedly. Chao (2007) reported that, because life is full of uncertainties, physicians tend to overtreat moribund patients. Gabbay et al. (2010) employed quantitative data to define medical futility and indicated that a powerful and consistent statistical approach for making such prognoses was lacking.

The findings of this study show that most of the participants observed the physiological signs of their high-death-risk and high-deterioration-risk patients to determine whether treatment was medically futile. Existing systems for evaluating the degree of disease severity have been widely applied in ICUs for medical resource evaluation and prognosis prediction (Breslow & Badawi, 2012). Different evaluation systems have been employed for different purposes. For example, more accurate data may be obtained when multiple evaluation systems are integrated and when data are measured repeatedly (e.g., at hospital admission and at 24 hours postadmission; Vincent & Moreno, 2010). However, although evaluation systems are able to predict mortality rates and identify those patients at a high risk of death, these systems are not able to predict deterioration risk. Lin et al. (2010) regarded medical futility as related to personal feelings and, as such, unable to be assessed using the physiological responses of patients alone. Weng (2012) proposed using the four quadrant approaches to clinical ethics proposed by Jonsen, Siegler, and Winslade (2010) and discussing medical futility from the four aspects of medical indications, patient preferences, QOL, and contextual features to more accurately determine medical futility in borderline or difficult-to-determine cases.

Futile Medical Treatment and Communication

The findings of this study revealed that different individuals (e.g., members of the medical team, physicians, and patients) hold different perspectives on the meaning of the term "futile." Inconsistencies in medical care influence follow-up treatments, resulting in medical futility. The participants in this study reported having experienced ethical dilemmas when judging whether a treatment was medically futile. On the basis of the principle of autonomy, patients are granted the right to make their own decisions. However, critical patients are generally unconscious. Thus, health professionals are often unable to determine the current wishes of their patients. Conflicts arise when patients, their families, and medical teams hold different opinions regarding medical treatment (Thompson, 2011). Bahramnezhad et al. (2014) reported that lack of coordination between a doctor's diagnosis and nurse and doctors' opting for trial and error sometimes lead to administering futile care. Moreover, Downar et al. (2015) found substitute decision-makers who do not understand the limitations of treatment or who cannot accept a poor prognosis to be responsible for nonbeneficial treatments (90% agreement for each cause). They stated that the most promising strategies to reduce nonbeneficial treatment were improved advance care planning and communication training for healthcare professionals. Zier et al. (2009) researched the reactions to physician judgments of medical futility of patient surrogates in the United States, finding that physicians and patients defined medical futility differently and that 64% of the surrogates doubted physicians' characterization of medical treatment as futile. On the basis of the principles of benefit and no harm, Day (2009) stated that the difficulty with defining medical futility was that people, in accordance with their roles and positions, held differing approaches to judging the discomfort of treatment, which is administered to extend the lives of patients who are expected to die in the near future.

This study found that clinical medical teams lacked sufficient time to guide the unprepared families of patients to overcome their reluctance to accept patient death and to assist them to understand and accept the patient's terminal condition. Consequently, the patient families are likely to request medically futile LST. Huang (2009) and Kadooka, Asai, Fukuyama, and Bito (2014) indicated that medical futility is caused by medical teams lacking communication time and relevant skills. Williams et al. (2010) reported that most ICU patients died within 10 days of being transferred to an ICU. In their study on ICU patients who suddenly deteriorated and lost consciousness and on those who received emergency first aid, Sibbald et al. (2007) revealed that physicians had no time or information to discuss patient prognosis or palliative treatment with patient families and thus had to perform LST on patients. In other words, a major challenge in clinical practice is discerning medical futility rapidly and then communicating related information to patients or patient families in a timely manner.

Factors Affecting Nurse Reactions to Medical Futility

The results of this study show that the participants regarded providing futile medical care as a legally required provision of medical care as well as that Chinese cultural customs (e.g., filial piety, first considering the opinions of senior family members, concealing actual disease conditions, and the selection of a specific day on which to withdraw a patient's life-sustaining device) critically influenced the attitudes of patient families toward medical treatment. Despite social changes, traditional definitions of filial piety remain deeply rooted in modern Chinese societies (Chen, 2010). Confucianism requires that children exercise filial piety while their parents are alive. Thus, many patient families request that medical treatment be performed to extend the lives of parents (Singer, 2009). Studies (Chao, 2007; Huang, 2009; Sibbald et al., 2007) have revealed that, even when patients have signed DNR forms, physicians are often concerned that patient families may file legal proceedings against them. Thus, to avoid potential trouble, physicians tend to comply with family demands for patient resuscitation. Whereas the Nursing Personnel Act and Medical Care Act stipulates that healthcare professionals should administer adequate first aid to critically ill patients, the Hospice Palliative Care Act states that, if a patient has signed a DNR form and related documents, then healthcare professionals may decline to administer futile treatments. However, as Huang (2009) reported, some nurses perceive themselves as duty-bound to perform CPR even when resuscitation is known to be ineffectual. Although medical futility does not merely occur in terminally ill patients, our research findings reveal the need for further research to elicit the process that nurses use to determine when and how to provide futile medical care to high-deterioration-risk patients and to terminally ill patients who, while protected under the Hospice Palliative Care Act, are facing deteriorating health conditions.

Conclusions

This study identified several crucial dimensions that medical teams should consider in judging medical futility. These dimensions include changes and declines in patient physiological signs and the influence of these on the QOL of patients and their significant others. These dimensions may provide a productive framework for medical teams to discuss issues that relate to medical futility. Most of the patients who receive futile treatment are those at a high risk of deterioration or death. Thus, the timing of communication and the related skills and content are key factors that lead to medical futility. When treatment options are exhausted, the only option that is available to patients is to sign the DNR form under informed consent of the third rule of the Hospice Palliative Care Act. Nevertheless, as shown in this study, determining the optimal time for communication, comforting patient families, and communicating changes in the disease condition of critical patients are critical elements in preventing or reducing the need to administer futile medical care.

Acknowledgments

We express our gratitude to the Taiwan Nurses Association for their research project grant (Number 1022007) and to Chung Shan Medical University for a further research project grant (Number CSMU-INT-102-19) that made this study possible. We further express our gratitude to the participants for sharing their experiences and to the participating organizations for their assistance.

References

Bahramnezhad, F., Cheraghi, M. A., Salsali, M., Asgari, P., Khoshnava Fomani, F., Sanjari, M., & Farokhnezhad Afshar, P. (2014). Futile care; concept analysis based on a hybrid model. *Global Journal of Health Science, 6*(5), 301–307. doi:10.5539/gjhs.v6n5p301

Breslow, M. J., & Badawi, O. (2012). Severity scoring in the critically ill: Part 1—Interpretation and accuracy of outcome prediction scoring systems. *Chest, 141*(1), 245–252. doi:10.1378/chest.11-0330

Brody, B. A., & Halevy, A. (1995). Is futility a futile concept? *The Journal of Medicine and Philosophy, 20*(2), 123–144. doi:10.1093/jmp/20.2.123

Chao, C. S. (2007). *The life and death in doctor.* Taipei City, Taiwan, ROC: Aquarius. (Original work published in Chinese)

Chen, C. Y. (2010). *The experience of adult children in singing parent's DNR (do not resuscitate) consent* (Unpublished master's thesis). China Medical University, Taichung City, Taiwan, ROC. (Original work published in Chinese)

Colaizzi, P. F. (1978). *Psychological research as a phenomenologist views it.* New York, NY: Oxford University Press.

Converse, M. (2012). Philosophy of phenomenology: How understanding aids research. *Nurse Researcher, 20*(1), 28–32. doi:10.7748/nr2012.09.20.1.28.c9305

Day, L. (2009). Medical futility, personal goods, and social responsibility. *American Journal of Critical Care, 18*(3), 279–282. doi:10.4037/ajcc2009490

Downar, J., You, J. J., Bagshaw, S. M., Golan, E., Lamontagne, F., Burns, K., ... Canadian Critical Care Trials Group. (2015). Nonbeneficial treatment Canada: Definitions, causes, and potential solutions from the perspective of healthcare practitioners. *Critical Care Medicine, 43*(2), 270–281. doi:10.1097/ccm.0000000000000704

Gabbay, E., Calvo-Broce, J., Meyer, K. B., Trikalinos, T. A., Cohen, J., & Kent, D. M. (2010). The empirical basis for determinations of medical futility. *Journal of General Internal Medicine, 25*(10), 1083–1089. doi:10.1007/s11606-010-1445-3

Huang, H. S. (2013). *Health checkup report on the National Health Insurance.* Taipei City, Taiwan, ROC: The Control Yuan, Taiwan, ROC. (Original work published in Chinese)

Huang, L. H. (2009). *The boundary of the medical futility and the extreme limit of the medicine—An aspect of DNR analysis* (Unpublished master's thesis). Nanhua University, Chiayi County, Taiwan, ROC. (Original work published in Chinese)

Huang, Y. P., Kellett, U. M., St. John, W., & Lee, S. (2006). Analysis phenomenology and application to nursing research. *The Journal of Nursing, 53*(2), 49–58. doi:10.6224/JN.53.2.49 (Original work published in Chinese)

Jonsen, A. R., Siegler, M., & Winslade, W. J. (2010). *Clinical ethics: A practical approach to ethical decisions in clinical medicine* (7th ed.). New York, NY: McGraw-Hill.

Jox, R. J., Schaider, A., Marckmann, G., & Borasio, G. D. (2012). Medical futility at the end of life: The perspectives of intensive care and palliative care clinicians. *Journal of Medical Ethics, 38*(9), 540–545. doi:10.1136/medethics-2011-100479

Kadooka, Y., Asai, A., Fukuyama, M., & Bito, S. (2014). A comparative survey on potentially futile treatments between Japanese nurses and laypeople. *Nursing Ethics, 21*(1), 64–75. doi:10.1177/0969733013484490

Lin, F. R., Huang, S. J., Wu, C. K., Huang, M. L., Lin, Y. L., Su, L. H., ... Lin, H. M. (2010). Medical futility in critical end-of life care. *Journal of Emergency and Critical Care Medicine, 21*(4, Suppl.), 1–8. (Original work published in Chinese)

Lincoln, Y. S., & Guba, E. G. (1985). *Naturalistic inquiry.* London, England: Sage.

Lo, B. (2009). *Resolving ethical dilemmas: A guide for clinicians* (4th ed.). Philadelphia, PA: Lippincott Williams & Wilkins.

Lo, S. F., & Hu, W. Y. (2008). The critical review of health-related quality of life (HRQL) concept and measure instrument for cancer patients. *Taiwan Journal of Hospice Palliative Care, 13*(1), 42–57. doi:10.6537/TJHPC.2008.13(1).4 (Original work published in Chinese)

Moratti, S. (2009). The development of "medical futility": Towards a procedural approach based on the role of the medical profession. *Journal of Medical Ethics, 35*(6), 369–372. doi:10.1136/jme.2008.027755

Moratti, S. (2010). Non-treatment decisions on grounds of "medical futility" and "quality of life": Interviews with fourteen Dutch neonatologists. *Issues in Law & Medicine, 26*(1), 3–11.

Persaud, R. (2006). "Futile" care in the intensive care unit. *Mayo Clinic Proceedings, 81*(11), 1506–1507. doi:10.4065/81.11.1506-a

Schneiderman, L. J., Jecker, N. S., & Jonsen, A. R. (1990). Medical futility: Its meaning and ethical implications. *Annals of Internal Medicine, 112*(12), 949–954. doi:10.7326/0003-4819-112-12-949

Sibbald, R., Downar, J., & Hawryluck, L. (2007). Perceptions of futile "care" among caregivers in intensive care units.

Canadian Medical Association Journal, 177(10), 1201–1208. doi:10.1503/cmaj.070144

Singer, P. A. (2009). *Bedside bioethics: A clinician's guide* (F. C. Tsai, Trans.). Taipei City, Taiwan, ROC: Taiwan Joint Commission on Hospital Accreditation. (Original work published in Chinese)

Thompson, R. J. (2011). Medical futility: A commonly used and potentially abused idea in medical ethics. *British Journal of Hospital Medicine, 72*(2), 96–99. doi:10.12968/hmed.2011.72.2.96

Vincent, J. L., & Moreno, R. (2010). Clinical review: Scoring systems in the critically ill. *Critical Care, 14*(2), 207. doi:10.1186/cc8204

Weng, Y. C. (2012). End-of-life care in intensive care unit. *VGH Nursing, 29*(3), 220–224. doi:10.6142/VGHN.29.3.220 (Original work published in Chinese)

Williams, T. A., Ho, K. M., Dobb, G. J., Finn, J. C., Knuiman, M., Webb, S. A., & Royal Perth Hospital ICU Data Linkage Group. (2010). Effect of length of stay in intensive care unit on hospital and long-term mortality of critically ill adult patients. *The British Journal of Anaesthesia, 104*(4), 459–464. doi:10.1093/bja/aeq025

Yekefallah, L., Ashktorab, T., Manoochehri, H., & Hamid, A. M. (2015). Nurses' experiences of futile care at intensive care units: A phenomenological study. *Global Journal of Health Science, 7*(4), 235–242. doi:10.5539/gjhs.v7n4p235

Zier, L. S., Burack, J. H., Micco, G., Chipman, A. K., Frank, J. A., & White, D. B. (2009). Surrogate decision makers' responses to physicians' predictions of medical futility. *Chest, 136*(1), 110–117. doi:10.1378/chest.08-2753

18

The Experiences of Couples Affected by Stroke and Nurses Managing Patient Rehabilitation: A Descriptive Study in Singapore

Sheena RAMAZANU[1] • Doris LEUNG[2] • Vico Chung Lim CHIANG[3*]

ABSTRACT

Background: Stroke in a family affects both patients and their spousal caregivers. Despite advances in the medical management of stroke, less is known about the social and cultural factors that impact couples regarding stroke recovery.

Purpose: The purpose of this study was to explore the experiences of stroke from the perspectives of couples affected by stroke and the nurses managing patient rehabilitation.

Methods: An interpretive descriptive study was conducted. Purposive sampling was used to enroll 17 participants, comprising eight nurses, five spousal caregivers, and four stroke survivors. Individual, in-depth interviews were performed at a rehabilitation hospital in Singapore in June 2018.

Results: The primary theme was the diverse meanings of stroke recovery attributed to limited conversations about the care decisions made by couples and rehabilitation nurses. The second theme was the challenges in nursing responsibilities that hindered the recovery of patients with stroke.

Conclusions/Implications for Practice: The meaning of recovery differs between patients and their informal and formal care providers. This issue should be explored in patient–provider conversations, as these conversations highlight the values and preferences that affect the stroke recovery trajectory. Enhancing shared decision making by patients, spousal caregivers, and healthcare providers during the stroke trajectory may promote the alignment of values that are critical to the stroke recovery experience. Further research into whether and how to incorporate shared decision making in rehabilitation hospital settings as an interventional component is warranted to better support stroke survivors before discharge.

Key Words:
stroke, couples, rehabilitation, nurses, recovery, experiences.

Introduction

Stroke is an acute condition in which the blood supply to the brain is disrupted because of either a burst blood vessel (hemorrhagic stroke) or blockage by a clot (ischemic stroke). Both scenarios reduce the supply of oxygen and nutrients to the brain (World Health Organization, 2019). Stroke is a chronic disability affecting 15 million people globally (National Institute of Neurological Disorders and Stroke, 2018). Of these, five million patients with stroke die, whereas another five million experience permanent disabilities, such as hemiplegia, incoordination, loss of sensation, swallowing difficulties, bladder and bowel incontinence, aphasia, cognitive deficits, and diminished mobility and self-care skills (Palmer & Palmer, 2011). In Asian countries such as Taiwan, Korea, Japan, and urbanized parts of China, the burden of stroke is serious, with reports of higher mortality rates compared with North America and Europe. This may be attributed in part to a more rapidly aging population in this region than other parts of the world (Kim, 2014).

In Singapore, stroke is the fourth leading cause of death, contributing to 10%–12% of all deaths. The burden of stroke in Singapore is expected to rise, causing challenges to the healthcare system (SingHealth Group, 2019). In 2016, Singapore's public hospital system admitted 7,413 patients with stroke (National Registry of Diseases Office, Health Promotion Board, 2018).

Stroke is a more significant health problem in Asia than in Europe or the Americas (Feigin et al., 2014). In Asia, stroke occurrence is highly related to vascular risk factors like hypertension, diabetes, and hypercholesterolemia (Kim et al., 2016) as well as tobacco consumption (Venketasubramanian et al., 2017). According to the 2016 Singapore Stroke Registry Annual Report, the number of stroke episodes in the Singaporean Chinese, Malay, and Indian populations has increased since 2007 (National Registry of Diseases Office, Health Promotion Board, 2018). Although the medical conceptualization of stroke is well established, little is known about the social and cultural factors that affect couples' recovery after a stroke. Knowing the social factors of stroke

[1]MClin Res, RN, Doctoral Candidate, The Hong Kong Polytechnic University, Hong Kong; and Staff Nurse, Yishun Community Hospital, Singapore • [2]PhD, Adjunct Assistant Professor, School of Nursing, The Hong Kong Polytechnic University, Hong Kong • [3]PhD, RN, Associate Professor, School of Nursing, The Hong Kong Polytechnic University, Hong Kong.

recovery helps healthcare professionals understand how stroke couples perceive and respond to stroke illness (Goffman, 2009). On the other hand, cultural factors affecting stroke recovery target the recovery-related cultural beliefs of couples (Conrad & Barker, 2010).

"Stroke recovery" refers to the gradual improvement of physical and cognitive functions after an episode of stroke (Palmer & Palmer, 2011, p. 15). Stroke recovery varies from one individual to another, with some fully recovering and others suffering long-term disabilities such as paralysis (Centers for Disease Control and Prevention, 2018).

Couples affected by stroke report that stroke is a significant life-changing event for patients that affects the marital relationship (Coombs, 2007). In particular, spouses often express "feeling lost" upon their partner's discharge home from the hospital. Spouses often engage in a trial-and-error process to support their partner with little guidance or support provided by healthcare professionals (Satink et al., 2018). In another qualitative study, family caregivers expressed their feeling overwhelmed by the enormity of the tasks before them when patients with stroke were discharged home (Lutz et al., 2011). This was reported by caregivers who felt responsible for providing care 24 hours a day. The Stroke Foundation of Australia (2019) reiterated that both patients with stroke and their caregivers, often spouses, grieve after a stroke. This may be attributed to the poststroke losses of normal life routines, independence, and mobility.

Nurses, as the primary healthcare providers working in close proximity to patients and their families (Petera & Liaschenko, 2004), are vulnerable to moral ambiguity regarding their responsibility to support these couples (i.e., stroke dyads) reach their goals and fulfill their expectations of recovery from stroke. Together with other healthcare professionals, rehabilitation nurses work together with patients with stroke and their spousal caregivers at the front lines of managing stroke recovery. Thus, the authors of this study assert that the experiences of patients with stroke, spousal caregivers, and rehabilitation nurses should be illuminated before developing supportive interventions for stroke recovery. Singapore was the focus in this article.

Community hospitals in Singapore are designed to provide rehabilitative services for patients and family members after acute care, to facilitate patient recovery to an optimal level of functional abilities, and to resume activities of daily living before returning home (Ministry of Health, Singapore, 2017). Stroke-related healthcare in Singapore is predominantly focused on providing care to individual patients with stroke. Support for patients with stroke and their spousal caregivers, as couples in recovery from stroke, is lacking. In choosing this target group, the authors hope that the findings enable rehabilitation healthcare professionals to systematically plan and develop suitable interventions for stroke couples in the Singaporean context.

Aim and Objectives

The overall aims of this study were to enhance the theoretical understanding of the meaning of stroke recovery to stroke couples and to nurses involved in their predischarge hospital care. The specific objectives of this study were to (a) gain an in-depth understanding of how couples cope with stroke recovery; (b) explore the social and cultural factors affecting couples' recovery after a stroke; (c) identify how nurses perceive what supports and hinders couples' recovery in the community; and (d) explore the meaning of stroke recovery for patients with stroke, spousal caregivers, and rehabilitation nurses.

Methods

Study Design

Interpretive description was selected to address the understanding of clinical practice in terms of health, illness, and experiences within a healthcare context (Hunt, 2009; Sandelowski, 1986; Thorne et al., 1997). This approach has been used successfully to uncover knowledge regarding what drives nursing practice (Forbes et al., 2012; Stevenson et al., 2015) and is anticipated to guide the future development of a support intervention for couples after a stroke in a Singaporean context.

Sampling Strategies and Setting

Purposive sampling was adopted by the research team to recruit participants based on their rich, firsthand knowledge of the subject matter (Polit & Beck, 2010). With reference to Thorne (2008, p. 94), "An interpretive description can be conducted on samples of any size, in that the vast majority of studies have sample sizes between five to 30 participants." Participants were recruited from one urban stroke rehabilitation hospital in Singapore.

Inclusion and Exclusion Criteria

Couples who fulfilled the following inclusion criteria were invited to participate in the study: (a) at least 21 years old and able to provide written consent, (b) patient experienced either an ischemic or hemorrhagic stroke episode, (c) spouses who self-identify as both a spouse and the primary family caregiver to the patient with stroke, and (d) able to communicate comfortably in English. Nurses were recruited who met the following inclusion criteria: (a) at least 21 years old and (b) have working experience in the stroke rehabilitation ward of the target hospital.

Exclusion criteria included patients with stroke with cognitive impairment, as assessed using the Abbreviated Mental Test score (total score for the Abbreviated Mental Test is 10). In this regard, patients with stroke who scored less than 7 were excluded because of cognitive impairment. In addition, patients with stroke with severe dysarthria as determined by a speech therapist assessment report were excluded to prevent the risk of becoming emotionally distressed during interviews (Savage, 2006).

Data Collection

Data collection using individual interviews with patients with stroke, spousal caregivers, and rehabilitation nurses took place from June 1, 2018, to June 30, 2018. The duration of each interview ranged from 20 to 60 minutes. A semistructured interview guide with open-ended questions was used to conduct the interviews (Table 1). The interview guide for this study was systematically developed using a framework for the development of a qualitative semistructured interview guide. The steps in this framework were as follows: (a) identify the need for semistructured interviews; (b) retrieve and synthesize knowledge and gaps related to the research topic; (c) develop a preliminary, semistructured interview guide; (d) conduct a pilot test of the guide; and (e) complete the semistructured interview guide (Kallio et al., 2016).

Data Analysis

Data analysis began with independent coding of the transcripts by three members in the research team. On the basis of Thorne's (2008) interpretive description, the transcribed data were "chunked" into meaning units or codes. Patterns were then organized by relationships and associations. Attention was focused on identifying participants' emotions that signaled important concerns. After coding and consensus of the first three transcripts for an initial coding structure, the remainder of the transcripts were coded and modified, building on this structure every three to five transcripts. Theorization occurred by inductively building a coherent whole using an iterative reasoning process that focused on how patterns operated and how the preliminary findings were shaped. Reconceptualization occurred when the themes provided a coherent structure of constructs, informing patterns of ideas on care management for stroke couples and the meaning of stroke recovery in the rehabilitation hospital (Thorne, 2008). The codes and coding structure were managed by the first author using NVivo 11 software (QSR International, Melbourne, Australia).

Rigor and Reflexivity

Rigor or trustworthiness was determined using the criteria proposed by Tobin and Begley (2004), which were credibility, dependability, reflexivity, and transferability. Credibility was determined by scrutinizing the findings for coherence in conveying participants' experiences. A particular challenge for the first author as a researcher was reflexivity, to keep her assumptions in abeyance, as she was a nurse with 6 years of experience in caring for patients with stroke and their families. As such, she was conscious of the dynamics of the interviewer–interviewee relationship and reflected on how her role shaped the creation of different knowledge in a reflexive diary. Credibility was also established using peer debriefing with the second and third research team members, who had expertise in qualitative methodology (Spillett, 2003) and had over 18 years of combined experience in qualitative research. To improve dependability, two of the researchers engaged in the process of coding and recoding for data analysis. Any discrepancies were verified with the third team member to achieve consensus. Finally, transferability was ensured by considering the applicability of findings (Marshall & Rossman, 1999) to the context of rehabilitation hospitals in Singapore. Although this study may not have attained data saturation, the participants provided rich descriptive data, and the research design employed a unique context that ensured the significance and relevance of the findings (Jeanfreau & Jack, 2010).

Ethical Considerations

Ethical approval was obtained from the Human Subjects Ethics Applications Review System of the Hong Kong Polytechnic University (Reference Number HSEARS20180205008) and the National Healthcare Group Domain Specific Review Board in Singapore (Reference Number 2018/00117). In light

Table 1

Semistructured Interview Guide for Research Participants

Semistructured interview guide for couples with stroke
• I would like to hear more about your experiences on how you manage yourself after the stroke situation.
(a) Perhaps, would you like to tell your story of how you (the patient) and partner first experienced the stroke event?
(b) Then, what experience stood out for you as challenging?
(c) What experience stands out for you as important in the recovery when they were going to be discharged home?
(d) What might you tell someone else wanting advice as to how to cope?
Prompts to get at social or cultural forces that shaped their experiences: Can you tell me more about how you decided to…? Can you tell me more about what made you want to…?
Semistructured interview guide for nurses
• I would like to hear more about your experiences on how you provide care for stroke patients and their spouses in the ward.
(a) What is a typical day for you caring for patients with stroke and their spouses?
(b) What makes your work with them challenging?
(c) What facilitates your work with them?
(d) What advice would you give a new nurse who is working with patients with stroke and their spouses in the community?

of the ethical importance of maintaining participant anonymity and confidentiality in human research (Clarke, 1991) and of the relative ease of recognizing participant identities because of the in-depth interactions and rapport between interviewers and interviewees in qualitative inquiries (Fouka & Mantzorou, 2011), in this study, participants' names were replaced with pseudonyms for transcription and analysis to ensure anonymity and confidentiality. Furthermore, these pseudonyms will be used in any future dissemination of research findings.

Nonmaleficence refers to the avoidance of causing unnecessary harm to participants of a study (Gillon, 1985, p. 130). Unnecessary harm to participants was avoided by identifying and mitigating potential risks to participants beforehand. If distress in a participant was encountered during the interview process, referrals for counseling services would be made with the consent of that participant. The risk of harm to participants in qualitative studies is generally considered to be low. No participant in this study required a referral for counseling services.

Table 2
Subject Demographic Characteristics

Item	*n*	%	Mean	*SD*
Patients with stroke (*n* = 5)				
Gender				
Female	1	20		
Male	4	80		
Age (years)			51.4	4.7
Ethnicity				
Chinese	0	0		
Malay	4	80		
Indian	1	20		
Incidence of strokes				
First time	4	80		
Second time	1	20		
Days after stroke			135.0	158.7
Barthel Index score			18.4	2.2
Spousal caregivers (*n* = 4)				
Gender				
Female	3	75		
Male	1	25		
Age (years)			50.8	4.6
Years of marriage			19.5	10.9
Ethnicity				
Chinese	0	0		
Malay	2	50		
Indian	2	50		
Employment status				
Working	4	100		
Not working	0	0		
Nurses (*n* = 8)				
Gender				
Female	5	62.5		
Male	3	37.5		
Age (years)			27.3	3.5
Ethnicity				
Chinese	2	25.0		
Malay	2	25.0		
Indian	1	12.5		
Filipino	3	37.5		
Years of experience in nursing			4.9	2.9

Results

Participant Demographics

Five patients with stroke, four spousal caregivers, and eight registered nurses were interviewed. The mean age of patients was 51.4 years (*SD* = 4.7), the mean age of spousal caregivers was 50.8 years (*SD* = 4.6), and the mean duration for the marital relationship of the spouses was 19.5 years. All four of the spousal caregivers were employed. Eight full-time registered nurses were interviewed individually. The mean duration of clinical working experience for the nurses was 4.9 years (range from 1 to 8; Table 2).

Perceptions of Stroke Recovery

Primary theme: Diverse meanings of stroke recovery

The primary theme identified was diverse meanings for patients, their spousal caregivers, and nurses, as these three groups held different perceptions of stroke recovery. As indicated in Figure 1, the different perspectives were rooted in differing values of stroke recovery. Moreover, these different perceptions hindered the effective coordination of care by nurses for both patients with stroke and their spousal caregivers. This was attributed to the limited conversations held between rehabilitation nurses, patients with stroke, and their spousal caregivers regarding how care decisions would be made. In particular, rehabilitation nurses perceived that spousal caregivers were skeptical and lacked trust about their nursing care because they did not perceive nurses as willing or competent to care for patients. In this regard, stroke recovery was not optimized for patients.

> *There are some family caregivers who refuse to take part in caregiver training. They feel that while the patient is in hospital, the nurses have to care for the patient's every need, and that they are paying for us, so they refuse to learn. We keep trying to teach them and tell them that we are trying to help them care for the patient at home. Sometimes they are still not receptive to learning. That is the challenge.* (Registered Nurse 3)

> *When a wife, for example, is the main caregiver but she does not want to learn anything because she is paying...we need to explain, explain, and explain until she accepts the need to learn. That is the most challenging part.* (Registered Nurse 2)

> *Despite providing health education, I think sometimes they (spousal caregivers) are going against us, I think this is mainly because trust in the nurses is*

Figure 1

The Perceptions of Stroke Recovery

Primary theme: Diverse meanings of stroke recovery

- limited conversations about care decisions
- nurses perceive spousal caregivers as unwilling to participate in care and lacking trust in healthcare providers
- spousal caregivers want to resume work to contribute to their family financially
- stoke patients believe that they will fully recover while in rehabilitation hospitalization and resume their normal life after discharge
- Muslim couples believe that the stroke and recovery have been predicted and planned by God

Second theme: Challenges in nursing responsibilities that hinder the recovery of patients with stroke

- language barriers between rehabilitation nurses and stroke couples
- nurses perceive that nursing staffing shortages and heavy workload impact the recovery of patients
- nurses are uncertain about how to develop a strategic care plan to meet the needs of spousal caregivers who are working

Perceptions of stroke recovery

> *not there. The health awareness is not there and they feel that the consequences will be very mild.* (Registered Nurse 1)

The spousal caregivers in this study primarily expressed financial-related concerns. They were uncertain about the degree to which patients would recover and considered resuming work to support the family, in conflict with their desire to care for the patient at home:

> *But even if it is taught to me, I would not be fully prepared to learn—aahhh—I mean with him because I am also working. I go, I leave my house at eight, I mean I leave my house at six a.m. and I come back in the evening at about eight p.m., and then I do not have much time to spend with him.* (Spousal Caregiver 1)

> *I think it is very difficult, as I am the only one working and my children are all studying. It is so hard for me to manage alone. I need to pay all the bills.* (Spousal Caregiver 3)

As a result of spouses working, patients with stroke relied on their peers, rather than on their spouse, for emotional support both in the clinical setting and after discharge:

> *So, you need somebody to talk to, you need somebody to give you moral support. During my hospitalization, I made friends with a group of patients there. Even after discharge, we get together and talk. I think that as human beings, if we have any problems, we need to communicate.... My wife is working and does not help me much.* (Patient With Stroke 3)

In contrast, patients with stroke expressed optimism about the chances for a full recovery by the end of their stay in the rehabilitation hospital. Furthermore, patients stated that they expected to resume work and volunteer in initiatives to support the rehabilitation of other patients after their stroke:

> *I am confident that my legs and hands will support me, and I hope there will not be any issues with work. So, when I go back to work from nine a.m. to 10:30 p.m., I need to stand and wait for the IT personnel as a form of respect, lah, and I hope I can do that.* (Patient With Stroke 4)

> *I want to volunteer to support other patients with stroke.... I will never forget the good things that people did for me. One day I will come back as a volunteer to help others.* (Patient With Stroke 4)

Patients with stroke expressed a strong desire that their lives would return to normal after discharge, as they feared being a burden on their families:

I do not like to put a burden on my children to take care of me, to support me financially, even to take time off work to take me to the hospital. For me, if you can be independent, you might as well do it yourself. So, no choice, my children still depend on me and need to come to me for support. (Patient With Stroke 3)

I do not have to give up and I cannot give up. Oh God, if I had given up, what would have happened to me by now? I must be strong for my wife and children. (Patient With Stroke 4)

Alternatively, Muslim patients with stroke believed that their stroke was a consequence of God's plans for them. They engaged in spiritual coping and self-rationalization to come to terms with why God had chosen them to have a stroke and to accept this in the context of their recovery:

The first thing that I asked myself, I will be honest with you, is why me? I asked God, why did you choose me? When God chooses you, you are the only selected one. God tests you for no formal reason. Whatever a patient with stroke has to go through, the hassles of life after a stroke, just take it as a gift from God. (Patient With Stroke 4)

This one God gives. Because God has decided everything, whether you can walk, or cannot walk, all is by God.... Everything you suffering from now, is God's way of punishing you. He makes you remember your past sins. Really you know, every sickness that happens is God punishing you. When God gives you a stroke, you must know how to take care of yourself. You know what it is being a Muslim. (Patient With Stroke 1)

Spousal caregivers of Muslim patients also believed strongly that God had reasons for what had happened to them. Similar to patients, the caregivers in this study perceived that a stroke was a way of "cleansing past sins" and, thus, they should accept their experiences and make sense of it in their lives:

Malay call this God knowing whatever is going to happen to us. It means that God has already predicted what will happen to us now and in the future. So, we have to accept it, lah. Sometimes in Islam the way is that, you know why you get a sickness? It is because God loves you. It is God's way of cleaning up all of your sins. (Spousal Caregiver 2)

Second theme: Challenges in nursing responsibilities that hinder the recovery of patients with stroke

The lack of care decisions in aligning diverse meanings of stroke recovery for patients with stroke, spousal caregivers, and nurses was intensified within three clinical contexts. First, language barriers were evident between rehabilitation nurses and stroke couples. Rehabilitation nurses were unable to adequately educate patients with stroke and their spousal caregivers before discharge, as they were not always able to speak and comprehend the others' language:

I think we have problems with a language barrier, since most older patients with stroke and caregivers use the old language. For this kind of situation, right, the main spoken language for us is English, because we are not from this country and we mostly speak English, so we are not used to speaking their languages, such as Hokkien and Mandarin. If they cannot understand, we need an interpreter, and we use another staff member to interpret for us. (Registered Nurse 2)

Yes! Very much, because some can speak Malay, some can speak Chinese, and only a few can speak English, so it is difficult to speak with patients and spouses. (Registered Nurse 5)

Second, rehabilitation nurses perceived that nursing staffing shortages and their own heavy workloads impacted the recovery of their patients. Staffing shortages made it difficult for nurses to juggle routine care and to provide sufficient support to stroke couples in the clinical setting:

I think that human resources are lacking because we take charge of 16 to 18 patients and there are only two nurses to take charge. Let us say that one patient calls for the toilet, and another patient also calls for the toilet. Then there is really a lack of staffing. It is very difficult to address all patient concerns at the same time. (Registered Nurse 7)

One staff nurse is in charge of 17 patients, making the workload even heavier. (Registered Nurse 8)

Third, the rehabilitation nurses in this study were uncertain regarding how to develop a strategic care plan to meet the needs of spousal caregivers, many of whom were working. Nurses reported plans to engage stroke dyads in rehabilitation activities together. However, education to explore the coping of these dyads, including rebuilding their marriage after a stroke, was lacking:

So, some of them are working, some spousal caregivers are available in the morning, while others are available in the evening. So, when we conduct bedside education in the morning, we will miss those who can only come at night. If we come at night, we will miss those who can only come in the morning. (Registered Nurse 2)

If they want a regular time, we will arrange it on Fridays and Saturdays, which are not so busy. Because on Saturdays and Sundays, patients are so free, just lying down as there are no therapy sessions with physiotherapists and occupational therapists. They will also do nothing. So maybe we can provide some entertainment and activities for them. (Registered Nurse 4)

Discussion

The primary theme identified in this study was the diverse meanings of stroke recovery that prevailed because of limited conversations and failure of discussions between couples and rehabilitation nurses about care decisions. A secondary theme was the challenges in nursing responsibilities that hindered the recovery of patients with stroke. In particular, this study highlights the need for further exploration of how the diverse meanings of stroke recovery for patients with stroke, spousal caregivers, and nurses may be better explored and aligned to improve care coordination.

The experiences of rehabilitation nurses revealed that spousal caregivers were not interested in the care of patients with stroke at home in the community. To support the family financially, spousal caregivers prioritized the resumption of work over care for their spouse. King et al. (2010) recognized that most caregivers struggled to provide for their family while caring for patients who experienced disabilities after a stroke. Informal caregivers depend on nurses for assistance with issues with their daily lives such as how to balance caregiving schedules with other commitments, including work. Therefore, the utmost priority for rehabilitation nurses may be to discuss decisions about caregiver training, meaning, and planning stroke recovery for couples and the types of support required so that appropriate assistance may be rendered in a timely manner (Camak, 2015).

One way of ensuring coordinated care among patients with stroke, spousal caregivers, and rehabilitation nurses is to practice shared decision making in a clinical context. Shared decision making refers to collaboration among patients with stroke, spousal caregivers, and nurses that considers the preferences and values of each during the stroke recovery process as well as evidence to inform the best possible decisions (Armstrong et al., 2016). Shared decision making allows patients and their family members to choose the best option available based on their respective values and goals for care (Armstrong, 2017). In a recent systematic review, shared decision making was reported to improve patients' knowledge and understanding of their clinical condition and their satisfaction and trust in healthcare professionals, thereby leading to better health outcomes (Shay & Lafata, 2015). In another systematic review, results highlighted that "knowledge alone is not power," recognizing the need for shared decision making in clinical settings (Joseph-Williams et al., 2014).

A study by Charles et al. (2006) argued that shared decision making should only be practiced when the cultural context of patients and their family members is taken into consideration. Indeed, in this study, ethnic norms affected the meaning of recovery less than the cultural and societal norms and the spiritual beliefs of stroke dyads. Similarly, in a study conducted in an Indian Muslim community in Africa, 59% of stroke caregivers held shared beliefs that stroke etiology was God's will and that they were not in a position to question what God had planned for them (Bham & Ross, 2005). The study highlighted important findings regarding the effect of stroke-related cultural and religious beliefs on patient expectations during stroke recovery. In particular, the findings of this study in terms of the primary theme "diverse meanings of stroke recovery" support that the attitudes, values, and beliefs of the three key stakeholders (i.e., patients, their spouses, and nurses) affect poststroke recovery. Hence, the assertion that shared decision making is necessary for families in Asia is justified, as it facilitates overall understanding in terms of health awareness between patients and their caregivers (Deber, 1996; Saint-Germaine & Longman, 1993).

Shared decision making in stroke care is an evolving approach in which recent research has predominantly focused on treatment decisions involving the use of oral anticoagulants for stroke prevention (Eckman et al., 2015; Ferguson & Hendriks, 2017; Kaiser et al., 2015; Visvanathan et al., 2017). Less research has been conducted in psychosocial areas involving decisions such as the engagement of couples in social support and in strategies for rebuilding a marriage after a stroke. In a recent systematic review (Anderson et al., 2017), chaos in marriage was found to be a prominent factor affecting poststroke recovery. It was recommended that support be provided to couples affected by stroke and that marital relationships be reestablished by managing the expectations of ideal and current poststroke marital contexts (Anderson et al., 2017).

The rehabilitation nurses in this study expressed a need for more time for training on how to involve patients with stroke and their spousal caregivers in postdischarge care, including training in (a) setting the stage for life after stroke; (b) how stroke affects patients and their marriage; (c) shared decision making on social support after a stroke; (d) balancing the roles of spousal caregiver and marriage partner; (e) strategies for rebuilding a marriage after stroke; and (f) safe lifting, transferring, feeding, and blood pressure monitoring (Palmer & Palmer, 2011). Overall, training should enable nurses to better support spousal caregivers as well as patients before patient discharge from the hospital.

Study Limitations

Although the participants may have been underrepresented in each group, the themes that emerged out of the patients–caregivers–staff mix of data were sufficient, as the rigor of this study ensured discovery of experience on the recovery of couples after stroke in Singapore. Insights on the theorization of a suitable intervention for stroke couples in a Singaporean context were introduced. Even with the small number of participants in this study, data saturation does not depend on a large sample size but rather on the incidents or events identified from the collected data (Corbin & Strauss, 2014). Another limitation of this study is that relatively more independent patients with stroke (mean Barthel Index score of 18.4 points) were interviewed. A future study that includes more patients with stroke with disabilities such as dysphagia or dysarthria is recommended because of inadequate representation in this study.

Conclusions

The meaning of recovery differs between patients and their informal and formal care providers. This issue should be explored in patient–provider conversations, as conversations shape values and preferences in the stroke recovery trajectory. Enhancing shared decision making by patients, spousal caregivers, and healthcare providers during the stroke trajectory may allow the alignment of values critical to the stroke recovery experience. Further research is warranted as to whether and how to incorporate shared decision making as an interventional component to better support couples at the rehabilitation hospital before patient discharge.

Author Contributions

Study conception and design: All authors
Data collection: SR
Data analysis and interpretation: All authors
Drafting of the article: SR
Critical revision of the article: DL, VCLC

References

Anderson, S., Keating, N., & Wilson, D. (2017). Reconciling marriage and care after stroke. *Canadian Journal on Aging, 36*(3), 386–401. https://doi.org/10.1017/S0714980817000241

Armstrong, M. J. (2017). Shared decision-making in stroke: An evolving approach to improved patient care. *Stroke and Vascular Neurology, 2*(2), 84–87. https://doi.org/10.1136/svn-2017-000081

Armstrong, M. J., Shulman, L. M., Vandigo, J., & Mullins, C. D. (2016). Patient engagement and shared decision-making: What do they look like in neurology practice? *Neurology Clinical Practice, 6*(2), 190–197. https://doi.org/10.1212/CPJ.0000000000000240

Bham, Z., & Ross, E. (2005). Traditional and western medicine: Cultural beliefs and practices of south African Indian Muslims with regard to stroke. *Ethnicity & Disease, 15*(4), 548–554.

Camak, D. J. (2015). Addressing the burden of stroke caregivers: A literature review. *Journal of Clinical Nursing, 24*(17–18), 2376–2382. https://doi.org/10.1111/jocn.12884

Centers for Disease Control and Prevention. (2018). *Recovering from stroke.* https://www.cdc.gov/stroke/recovery.htm

Charles, C., Gafni, A., Whelan, T., & O'Brien, M. A. (2006). Cultural influences on the physician-patient encounter: The case of shared treatment decision-making. *Patient Education and Counselling, 63*(3), 262–267. https://doi.org/10.1016/j.pec.2006.06.018

Clarke, J. (1991). Moral dilemmas in nursing research. *Nursing Standard, 5*(50), 22–25. https://doi.org/10.7748/ns.5.50.22.s64

Conrad, P., & Barker, K. K. (2010). The social construction of illness: Key insights and policy implications. *Journal of Health and Social Behavior, 51*(Suppl.), S67–S79. https://doi.org/10.1177/0022146510383495

Coombs, U. E. (2007). Spousal caregiving for stroke survivors. *Journal of Neuroscience Nursing, 39*(2), 112–119. https://doi.org/10.1097/01376517-200704000-00008

Corbin, J., & Strauss, A. (2014). *Basics of qualitative research: Techniques and procedures for developing grounded theory* (4th ed.). SAGE.

Deber, R. B. (1996). Shared decision making in the real world. *Journal of General Internal Medicine, 11*(6), 377–378. https://doi.org/10.1007/BF02600052

Eckman, M. H., Wise, R. E., Naylor, K., Arduser, L., Lip, G. Y., Kissela, B., Flaherty, M., Kleindorfer, D., Khan, F., Schauer, D. P., Kues, J., & Costea, A. (2015). Developing an atrial fibrillation guideline support tool (AFGuST) for shared decision making. *Current Medical Research and Opinion, 31*(4), 603–614. https://doi.org/10.1185/03007995.2015.1019608

Feigin, V. L., Forouzanfar, M. H., Krishnamurthi, R., Mensah, G. A., Connor, M., Bennett, D. A., Moran, A. E., Sacco, R. L., Anderson, L., Truelsen, T., O'Donnell, M., Venketasubramanian, N., Barker-Collo, S., Lawes, C. M. M., Wang, W., Shinohara, Y., Witt, E., Ezzati, M., Naghavi, M., ... Global Burden of Diseases, Injuries, and Risk Factors Study 2010 (GBD 2010) and the GBD Stroke Experts Group. (2014). Global and regional burden of stroke during 1990–2010: Findings from the Global Burden of Disease Study 2010. *The Lancet, 383*(9913), 245–254. https://doi.org/10.1016/S0140-6736(13)61953-4

Ferguson, C., & Hendriks, J. (2017). Partnering with patients in shared decision-making for stroke prevention in atrial fibrillation. *European Journal of Cardiovascular Nursing, 16*(3), 178–180. https://doi.org/10.1177/1474515116685193

Forbes, D. A., Finkelstein, S., Blake, C. M., Gibson, M., Morgan, D. G., Markle-Reid, M., Culum, I., & Thiessen, E. (2012). Knowledge exchange throughout the dementia care journey by Canadian rural community-based health care practitioners, persons with dementia, and their care partners: An interpretive descriptive study. *Rural and Remote Health, 12*(4), 2201.

Fouka, G., & Mantzorou, M. (2011). *What are the major ethical issues in conducting research? Is there a conflict between the research ethics and the nature of nursing? Health Science Journal [Online], 5*(1), 3–14. http://www.hsj.gr/medicine/what-are-the-major-ethical-issues-in-conducting-research-is-there-a-conflict-between-the-research-ethics-and-the-nature-of-nursing.php?aid=3485

Gillon, R. (1985). "Primum non nocere" and the principle of non-maleficence. *British Medical Journal, 291*(6488), 130–131. https://doi.org/10.1136/bmj.291.6488.130

Goffman, E. (2009). *Stigma: Notes on the management of spoiled identity*. Simon and Schuster.

Hunt, M. R. (2009). Strengths and challenges in the use of interpretive description: Reflections arising from a study of the moral experience of health professionals in humanitarian work. *Qualitative Health Research, 19*(9), 1284–1292. https://doi.org/10.1177/1049732309344612

Jeanfreau, S. G., & Jack, L. Jr. (2010). Appraising qualitative research in health education: Guidelines for public health educators. *Health Promotion Practice, 11*(5), 612–617. https://doi.org/10.1177/1524839910363537

Joseph-Williams, N., Elwyn, G., & Edwards, A. (2014). Knowledge is *not* power for patients: A systematic review and thematic synthesis of patient-reported barriers and facilitators to shared decision making. *Patient Education and Counselling, 94*(3), 291–309. https://doi.org/10.1016/j.pec.2013.10.031

Kaiser, K., Cheng, W. Y., Jensen, S., Clayman, M. L., Thappa, A., Schwiep, F., Chawla, A., Goldberger, J. J., Col, N., & Schein, J. (2015). Development of a shared decision-making tool to assist patients and clinicians with decisions on oral anticoagulant treatment for atrial fibrillation. *Current Medical Research & Opinion, 31*(12), 2261–2272. https://doi.org/10.1185/03007995.2015.1096767

Kallio, H., Pietila, A. M., Johnson, M., & Kangasniemi, M. (2016). Systematic methodological review: Developing a framework for a qualitative semi-structured interview guide. *Journal of Advanced Nursing, 72*(12), 2954–2965. https://doi.org/10.1111/jan.13031

Kim, J. S. (2014). Stroke in Asia: A global disaster. *International Journal of Stroke, 9*(7), 856–857. https://doi.org/10.1111/ijs.12317

Kim, Y. D., Jung, Y. H., & Saposnik, G. (2016). Traditional risk factors for stroke in East Asia. *Journal of Stroke, 18*(3), 273–285. https://doi.org/10.5853/jos.2016.00885

King, R. B., Ainsworth, C. R., Ronen, M., & Hartke, R. J. (2010). Stroke caregivers: Pressing problems reported during the first months of caregiving. *Journal of Neuroscience Nursing, 42*(6), 302–311. https://doi.org/10.1097/JNN.0b013e3181f8a575

Lutz, B. J., Young, M. E., Cox, K. J., Martz, C., & Creasy, K. R. (2011). The crisis of stroke: Experiences of patients and their family caregivers. *Topics in Stroke Rehabilitation, 18*(6), 786–797. https://doi.org/10.1310/tsr1806-786

Marshall, C., & Rossman, G. B. (1999). *Designing qualitative research* (3rd ed.). Sage.

Ministry of Health, Singapore. (2017). *Community hospital care—Handbook for patients*. https://www.moh.gov.sg/docs/librariesprovider5/resources-statistics/educational-resources/handbook-on-ch-care-for-patients_210617.pdf

National Institute of Neurological Disorders and Stroke. (2018). *Stroke statistics*. http://www.strokecenter.org/patients/about-stroke/stroke-statistics/

National Registry of Diseases Office, Health Promotion Board. (2018). *Singapore stroke registry annual report* 2016. https://www.nrdo.gov.sg/docs/librariesprovider3/Publications—Stroke/singapore-stroke-registry-annual-reprot-2016_upload_nrdo_website.pdf?sfvrsn=0

Palmer, S., & Palmer, J. B. (2011). *When your spouse has a stroke: Caring for your partner, yourself, and your relationship*. Johns Hopkins University Press.

Petera, E., & Liaschenko, J. (2004). Perils of proximity: A spatiotemporal analysis of moral distress and moral ambiguity. *Nursing Inquiry, 11*(4), 218–225. https://doi.org/10.1111/j.1440- 1800.2004.00236.x

Polit, D. F., & Beck, C. T. (2010). *Essentials of nursing research: Appraising evidence for nursing practice* (7th ed.). Lippincott Williams & Wilkins.

Saint-Germaine, M. A., & Longman, A. J. (1993). Breast cancer screening among older Hispanic women: Knowledge, attitudes, and practices. *Health Education Quarterly, 20*(4), 539–553. https://doi.org/10.1177/109019819302000412

Sandelowski, M. (1986). The problem of rigor in qualitative research. *Advances in Nursing Science, 8*(3), 27–37. https://doi.org/10.1097/00012272-198604000-00005

Satink, T., Cup, E. H. C., de Swart, B. J. M., & Sanden, M. W. G. N. (2018). The perspectives of spouses of stroke survivors on self-management—A focus group study. *Disability & Rehabilitation, 40*(2), 176–184. https://doi.org/10.1080/09638288.2016.1247920

Savage, T. A. (2006). Ethical issues in research with patients who have experienced stroke. *Topics in Stroke Rehabilitation, 13*(4), 1–10. https://doi.org/10.1310/tsr1304-1

Shay, L. A., & Lafata, J. E. (2015). Where is the evidence? A systematic review of shared decision making and patient outcomes. *Medical Decision Making, 35*(1), 114–131. https://doi.org/10.1177/0272989X14551638

SingHealth Group. (2019). *Stroke*. https://www.singhealth.com.sg/patient-care/patient-education/stroke

Spillett, M. A. (2003). *Peer debriefing: Who, what, when, why, how*. https://www.thefreelibrary.com/Peer+debriefing%3a+who%2c+what%2c+when%2c+why%2c+how.-a0111848817

Stevenson, K. N., Jack, S. M., O'Mara, L., & LeGris, J. (2015). Registered nurses' experiences of patient violence on acute care psychiatric inpatient units: An interpretive descriptive study. *BMC Nursing, 14*, 35. https://doi.org/10.1186/s12912-015-0079-5

Stroke Foundation of Australia. (2019). *Grief after stroke*. https://strokefoundation.org.au/Blog/2015/05/19/Grief-after-stroke

Thorne, S. (2008). *Interpretive description*. Left Coast Press.

Thorne, S., Kirkham, S. R., & MacDonald-Emes, J. (1997). Interpretive description: A noncategorical qualitative alternative for developing nursing knowledge. *Research in Nursing* and *Health, 20*(2), 169–177. https://doi.org/10.1002/(SICI)1098-240X(199704)20:2<169::AID-NUR9>3.0.CO;2-I

Tobin, G. A., & Begley, C. M. (2004). Methodological rigour within a qualitative framework. *Journal of Advanced Nursing, 48*(4), 388–396. https://doi.org/10.1111/j.1365-2648.2004.03207.x

Venketasubramanian, N., Yoon, B. W., Pandian, J., & Navarro, J. C. (2017). Stroke epidemiology in South, East, and South-East Asia: A review. *Journal of Stroke, 19*(3), 286–294. https://doi.org/10.5853/jos.2017.00234

Visvanathan, A., Dennis, M., Mead, G., Whiteley, W. N., Lawton, J., & Doubal, F. N. (2017). Shared decision making after severe stroke—How can we improve patient and family involvement in treatment decisions? *International Journal of Stroke, 12*(9), 920–922. https://doi.org/10.1177/1747493017730746

World Health Organization. (2019). *Stroke, cerebrovascular accident*. http://www.emro.who.int/health-topics/stroke-cerebrovascular-accident/index.html

Identifying and Ranking the Factors Affecting the Choice of Nursing Discipline Among Nursing Students in Iran: A Fuzzy Hierarchical Analysis

Zohreh HOSSEINI MARZNAKI[1] • Khatere KHANJANKHANI[2] • Waliu Jawula SALISU[3] • Fatemeh HAJIHOSSEINI[4] • Saeed BARZEGARI[5]*

ABSTRACT

Background: Choosing a career in nursing is frequently a complicated decision that is influenced by multiple factors.

Purpose: This study was designed to identify and rank the main factors that influence individuals to choose to pursue a career in nursing.

Methods: This cross-sectional study was conducted at Mazandaran University of Medical Sciences, Iran. A comprehensive review of the literature was conducted to identify the factors that people consider when making a choice to pursue a career in nursing. The face and content validities of these factors were evaluated. A sample of 250 participants was invited to assess the factors using exploratory factor analysis. Finally, the analytical hierarchy process, in combination with fuzzy logic, was used to rank the criteria and related factors.

Results: Twenty factors were identified and extracted from 50 published studies. After confirming the face and content validity of each, these 20 factors were distinguished into four criteria, including (a) external motivation, (b) social dignity, (c) internal motivation, and (d) usefulness of discipline. Each criterion had an eigenvalue greater than 1. External motivation and usefulness of discipline were respectively identified as the most and least important criteria (38.60% vs. 16.11%) in terms of influencing individuals to pursue a nursing career.

Conclusions/Implications for Practice: The results of this study show that exposure to positive recommendations from family and friends, receiving positive information about studying nursing, positive perceptions regarding the general usefulness of nursing knowledge, and migration opportunities to other countries are the primary factors that influence individuals in Iran to pursue a career in nursing.

KEY WORDS:
fuzzy logic, nursing students, discipline, analytic hierarchical process.

Introduction

Nurses are at the forefront of healthcare in most health systems, and their contribution is vital to achieving societal health goals and providing safe and effective healthcare (Lim & Muhtar, 2016). Understanding why individuals choose to pursue a career in nursing is critical to the survival and success of this profession and especially important for related leaders and academics. Understanding the factors affecting choice of discipline may be used to help drive the curriculum to better meet student needs and expectations (Cho et al., 2010).

In Iran, withdrawal from nursing education is a common problem. Students experience steady lowering of educational standards, which imposes great economic costs on the educational system and psychologically impacts other students. One of the most important reasons for student withdrawal is the lack of awareness when choosing the nursing discipline (Farahani et al., 2017). Many factors, including career image, future personal plans, and prospects for success in life, are known to influence discipline-selection decision making (Elibol & Seren, 2017). A conscientious search for information about a particular academic field before choosing that field can influence an individual's satisfaction and commitment (Wilkes et al., 2015). A review of the literature found choosing nursing as a career to be influenced by factors such as willingness to help and care for others, job opportunities,

[1]*MSc, RN, Instructor, Amol Faculty of Nursing and Midwifery Sciences, Department of Nursing, Mazandaran University of Medical Sciences, Sari, Iran* • [2]*Doctoral Candidate, Researcher, Department of Health Policy, School of Public Health, Tehran University of Medical Sciences, Tehran, Iran* • [3]*PhD, RN, Cambridge Liver Unit, Cambridge University Hospitals NHS Foundation Trust, Addenbrookes Hospital, Cambridge, United Kingdom* • [4]*PhD, RN, Assistant Professor, Amol Faculty of Nursing and Midwifery Sciences, Department of Nursing, Mazandaran University of Medical Sciences, Sari, Iran* • [5]*PhD, Assistant Professor, Amol Faculty of Paramedical Sciences, Department of Health Information Technology, Mazandaran University of Medical Sciences, Sari, Iran.*

social status, income, personal environmental factors, experience caring for a loved one, having a close relative who is a nurse, and experiencing the hospitalization of relatives or friends (Ergün & Güzel, 2016; Liaw et al., 2016; Önder et al., 2014).

When the criteria affecting a particular goal are numerous, the analytic hierarchy process (AHP), which is one of the methods of multiple-criteria decision making, may be used in combination with Fuzzy Analytical Hierarchy Process (FAHP) to determine the weight and ranking of each criterion (Önder et al., 2014). Fuzzy logic allows decisions and judgments to be made that are closer to rigid numbers than human logic (Ahmed & Kilic, 2019). Because no study has been conducted in Iran to determine and rank the specific factors that affect choosing to pursue a career in nursing, this study was performed using the FAHP method.

Methods

This cross-sectional and analytic study was conducted in 2019 in four phases. The research population consisted of two groups: academic faculty and nursing students. The ethics committee of Mazandaran University of Medical Sciences approved the study (approval no.: IR.MAZUMS.REC.1398.064).

In Phase 1, the literature was reviewed to identify and extract the factors affecting the decision to pursue a career in nursing. To accomplish this, a search was conducted in international databases such as PubMed, Scopus, Science Direct, Google Scholar, Cochrane Library, CINAHL, and a local database (Scientific Information Database) for articles published between 2008 and 2018. The following keywords were used: "nursing profession," "student choice," "career decision," "careers," "career choice," "chosen profession," "career selection," "discipline choice," "nursing," "nursing student," and "criteria" and "factors." Only articles published in Persian or English were selected. To search the Persian electronic databases, the Farsi equivalents of the English keywords were used. Finally, 20 factors that affect choosing a career in nursing were extracted from the 50 studies identified. Details on the identified studies are in Figure 1.

In the second phase, an expert panel consisting of 10 nursing professors was formed. Their role was to evaluate the qualitative and quantitative face and content validities of the factors identified in Phase 1. The inclusion criterion for panelists was having at least 5 years of work experience as a nurse faculty member.

In the qualitative face validity phase, the grammatical and semantic problems of the factors were corrected. Both content validity index (CVI) and content validity ratio (CVR) were used to confirm quantitative content validity. CVI was used to assess the simplicity, relevance, and transparency of the factors. The experts categorized the factors into four significant criteria and scored each on a scale of 1 (*strongly disagree*) to 4 (*strongly agree*; Lin et al., 2014). To obtain the CVI for each factor, the number of panelists who scored 3 and 4 was divided by the total number of panelist respondents, and factors earning a CVI greater than .79 were retained (Maasoumi et al., 2013). CVR was used to assess

Figure 1

Flowchart of the Analytic Hierarchy Process: Questionnaire Design Process

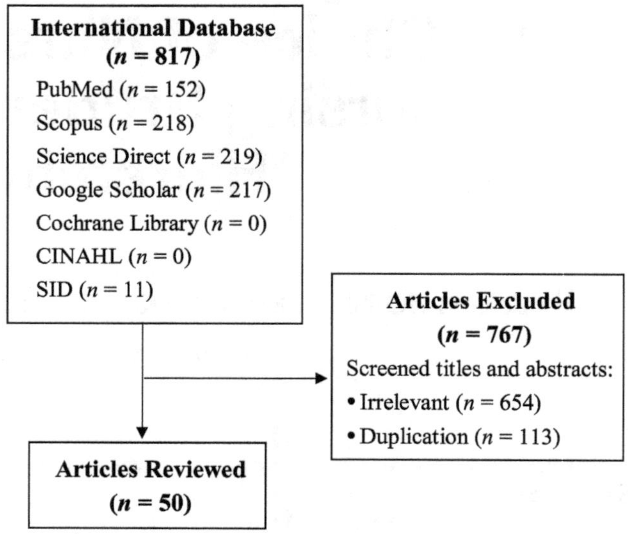

Note. SID = Scientific Information Database.

the necessity of each factor. The CVR for the 10-member panel of experts was at least .62, as determined using the Lawshe table (Lawshe, 1975).

In Phase 3, a sample of students was invited to use the exploratory factor analysis (EFA) approach to assess the factors that were extracted and validated in Phases 1 and 2.

We presented the factors to a study sample of 250 nursing students in a questionnaire scored using a 5-point Likert scale with 5 = *very high importance*, 4 = *high importance*, 3 = *medium importance*, 2 = *low importance*, and 1 = *very low importance*. Because the minimum sample size required for EFA is 10 per criterion, 250 students were invited to participate in this study (MacCallum et al., 1999). Principal component analysis and promax rotation were used to extract the factors. The cutoff level for the eigenvalue was ≥ 1.

The final phase was set to label and rank the factors. The experts reviewed the results obtained using the EFA and assigned each factor to an associated criterion. A hierarchical structure was then created that included the criteria and factors. Chang's triangular FAHP method was used to rank the criteria and factors affecting the choice of a nursing career. The AHP is one of the approaches in multivariate decision support systems that was introduced by Thomas Saati in 1983. The purpose of the AHP is to rank the criteria and related factors by pairwise comparison and then weigh each (Shafii et al., 2016). The formation scheme of the AHP questionnaire in this study is presented in Figure 2. The purpose of multicriteria decision-making techniques is not to prove a hypothesis or statistical study but rather to rank the related criteria. In this phase of the study, 20 nursing students were selected randomly from the primary study sample of 250 to complete the paired comparisons matrix. In the first phase of this study, participants were asked to compare the importance of each criterion in terms of its effect on choosing to pursue a career in nursing and to compare the relevance of each criterion to the other using linguistic variables. The researchers then converted the linguistic variables to their corresponding triangular fuzzy numbers. The linguistic variables and their corresponding triangular fuzzy numbers included absolute importance (7, 9, 9), very strong importance (5, 7, 9), strong importance (3, 5, 7), weak importance (1, 3, 5), and equal importance (1, 1, 3). Participants were then asked to determine the significance of the factors in each criterion separately and comparatively. Finally, the weight of the criteria and factors were determined using the Chang's FAHP and were ranked accordingly.

The consistency ratio was calculated to check the validity of each pairwise comparison matrix (Wedley, 1993).

$$Consistency\ ratio = Consistency\ Index\ /\ Random\ Consistency\ Index$$

The Random Consistency Index is a constant value that varies according to the dimensions of the pairwise comparison matrices and is equal to 0.9, 1.12, and 1.24 for the 4 × 4, 5 × 5, and 6 × 6 matrices, respectively. The following formula was used in this study to calculate the Consistency Index (CI):

$$CI = \frac{\lambda_{max} - n}{n-1}$$

In this formula, λ_{max} or principal eigenvalue is calculated by averaging the matrix eigenvector, and n also indicates the number of dimensions of the pairwise comparison matrix (Sun, 2010). If a matrix is consistent, the principal eigenvalue (λ_{max}) is equal to the matrix dimension (Alonso & Lamata, 2006). Descriptive factor analysis/EFA and FAHP analyses were performed using IBM SPSS Version 19 (IBM, Corp., Armonk, NY, USA) and MATLAB Version 9.7 (MathWorks, Natick, MA, USA) software, respectively.

Results

After reviewing the literature, 20 factors were identified that affect the choice of individuals to pursue a career in nursing. In the second phase of this study, experts edited the factors grammatically and semantically. All 20 factors were included in the subsequent assessment and analysis phase because of their appropriateness in terms of qualitative and quantitative face and content validities. In the third phase of this study, 250 nursing students with a mean age of 21.18 ± 1.99 years were invited to participate. All of the participants submitted complete and valid questionnaires. Most (148, 59.2%) were female and single (97.2%). The demographic characteristics of the participants are presented in Table 1.

In terms of demographic data, a significant and positive relationship was found with the educational level of parents (mothers and fathers; $p < .001$, $r = .245$), whereas significant and negative relationships were found between grade average and age ($p = .011$, $r_s = -.160$) and between grade average and semester ($p < .001$, $r_s = -.233$).

On the basis of the results of the EFA, all four criteria had an eigenvalue ≥ 1 and a variance of 64.16. The factor loading and commonalities of each criterion were ≥ .5, and the Kaiser-Meyer-Olkin index was .84, which is considered desirable (Table 2). In addition, the internal consistencies of

Figure 2

Flowchart of the Analytic Hierarchy Process—Questionnaire Design Process

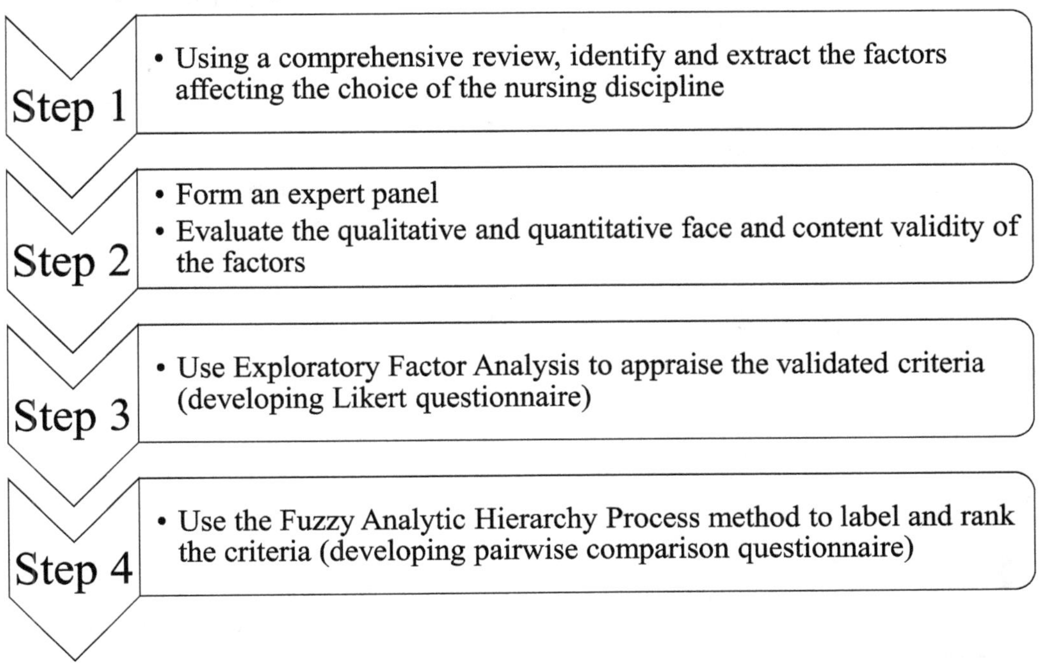

all items (.76) and each criterion (.83–.88) were acceptable. The results are presented in Table 2.

The experts reviewed and approved the criteria appraised using the EFA. The results were categorized and placed in a hierarchical structure (Figure 3).

The main criteria identified were as follows: (a) external motivation, (b) social dignity, (c) internal motivation, and (d) usefulness of discipline. The factors included in each criterion are also specified in the corresponding structure.

In the fourth phase of this study, some of the selected participants completed the pairwise comparisons matrix, which was used to conduct a pairwise comparison of each criterion and factor. Participants presented their preferences in the form of linguistic variables. The linguistic variables were converted to corresponding triangular fuzzy numbers, and the weights of the criteria and factors were calculated using the FAHP method (Table 3).

The "external motivation" and "usefulness of discipline" criteria were ranked, respectively, as the most (38.6%) and least (16.11%) important in terms of affecting the decision to pursue a career in nursing. The effect of the external motivation criterion in determining the discipline of nursing was found to be 1.56, 1.87, and 2.40 times stronger, respectively, than the social dignity, internal motivation, and usefulness of discipline criteria.

In terms of factors, the normalized weight of the "recommendations from others" factor (55.69) was 3.48–4.26 times higher than the other factors included under the external motivation criterion, "getting positive information about studying in the field" (30.19) weighed 1.23–2.86 times more than the other factors under the social dignity criterion, "the usefulness of nursing knowledge in personal life" (24.14) weighed 1.06–8.97 times higher than the other factors under the same criterion, and "immigration opportunities to other countries" (44.30) weighed 1.85–8.26 times more than other factors under the same criterion of usefulness of discipline.

The principal eigenvalues for the matrices were very close to the magnitude of each matrix dimension, which indicates that the results exhibited appropriate consistency (Table 3). On the other hand, the CI for each of the five matrices was lower than the Random Consistency Index, and the consistency ratio was lower than 0.1 for all of the matrices, indicating that all pairwise comparisons obtain reasonably good results and that the findings in this study were consistent.

Table 1

Demographic Characteristics of Participants (N = 250)

Characteristic	n	%
Gender		
Male	102	40.8
Female	148	59.2
Father's education		
Illiterate	15	6.0
Diploma	129	51.6
Academic education	106	42.4
Mother's education		
Illiterate	14	5.6
Diploma	150	60.0
Academic education	86	34.4
Marital status		
Single	243	97.2
Married	57	2.8
Residence		
A native of the province	193	77.2
Nonnative	57	22.8
Semester		
1	31	12.4
2	97	38.8
3	69	27.6
4	53	21.1
University entrance examination		
1	163	65.2
2	53	21.2
3	30	12.0
4	4	1.6

Discussion

In this study, a four-phase approach was used to identify and prioritize factors that influence students to choose a career in nursing.

The findings highlighted the primary importance of external motivation in selecting nursing as a career. This is in contrast to the results of a study by Manzour et al., which found that most participants considered personal interest as having the most significant impact on career choice (Manzoor et al., 2010). In this study, the two factors "recommendations from others (family, friends, and teachers)" and "media (television, Internet, and social networks)" earned the highest and lowest coefficients for importance, respectively, under the external motivation criterion. Similar external factors such as parental recommendations (Lim & Muhtar, 2016; Wu et al., 2015), employment of a family member in the profession (Manzoor et al., 2010), and the influence of others' suggestions and encouragement (Crawford & Turvey, 2019; Mooney et al., 2008) have been identified in other related studies as considerations in choosing a career in nursing. Given that family, friends, and teachers are important influencers in a person's life, their role in a future job search may be expected to be crucial and significant (Mphahlele, 2011).

A survey of the significant coefficients of each factor found the most significant coefficient under the social dignity criterion to be "getting positive information about studying in this field." Mooney et al. (2008) also found "having professional knowledge" as an essential factor in choosing a nursing career. The high importance of this factor reflects the high impact of extrinsic motivation dimensions that can be received in various ways such as through family, friends, and the media. Further evaluation showed "having a positive impression of nursing in the society" to be of minimal

Table 2
Exploratory Factor Analysis

Factor (Criteria)	Communality	Factor Loading	Explained Variance	Cronbach's Alpha
External motivation			15.07	.88
Recommendations from others (family, friends, and teachers)	.725	.85		
Having patterns in this field among friends and relatives	.740	.86		
Religious issues	.737	.86		
Media (television, Internet, and press)	.796	.88		
Social dignity			15.19	.83
Getting positive information about studying in this field	.669	.81		
Suitable social position of the profession	.580	.75		
Ability to communicate with medical team members	.580	.75		
Existence of excellent human relations in the field	.636	.79		
Having a positive impression of nursing in society	.556	.73		
Internal motivation			17.92	.86
Usefulness of nursing knowledge for personal life	.716	.84		
Being interested in the nursing profession	.510	.70		
Distance to the faculty	.543	.73		
Having a caring experience (e.g., taking care of a patient at home)	.537	.73		
Field proximity to medicine	.630	.79		
Willingness to help others	.676	.82		
Usefulness of discipline			15.98	.86
Immigration opportunity (to other countries)	.686	.81		
Having postgraduate job opportunities	.743	.86		
Opportunity for further education and academic progress	.660	.79		
Having a good income while studying	.591	.76		
Opportunity to access welfare facilities while studying	.521	.72		

Figure 3
Flowchart of the Article Selection Process

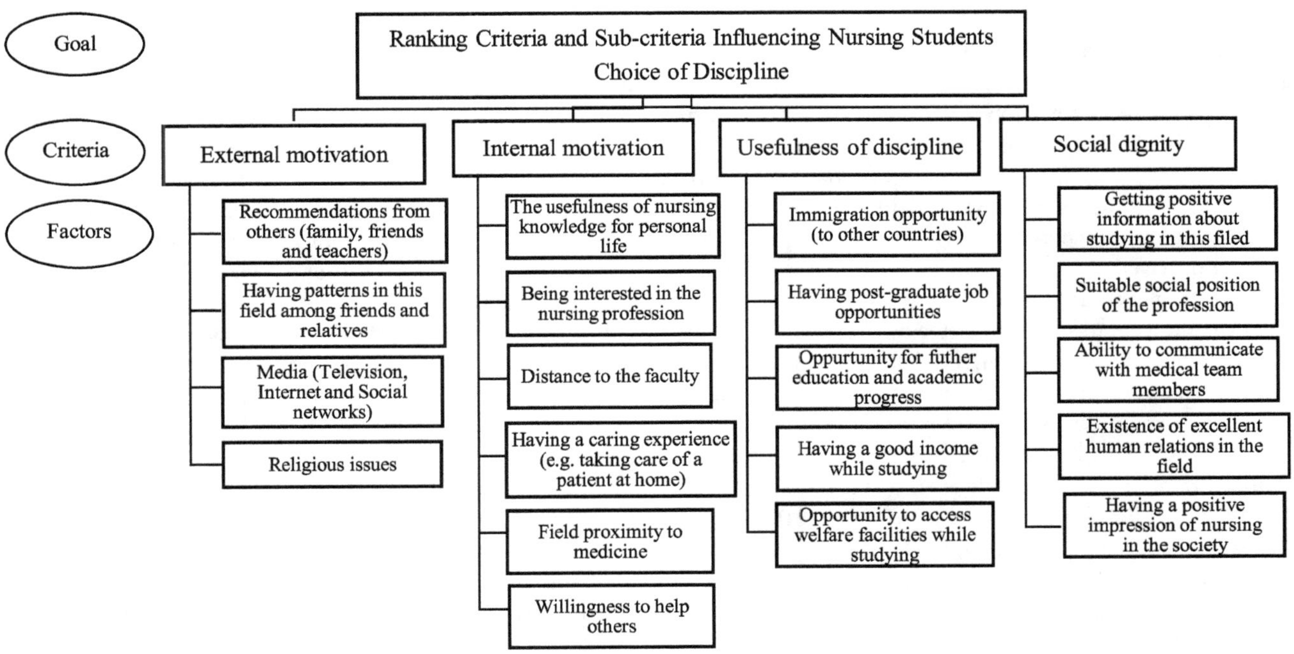

Table 3

Weight of Criteria and Factors for Choosing a Nursing Career

Criteria and Factor	Weight (w)	Matrix Dimension	RI (a)	λ (b)	CI (c)	CR (d)
Criteria		4	0.9	4.14	.050	.054
External motivation	38.60					
Social dignity	24.71					
Internal motivation	20.59					
Usefulness of discipline	16.11					
Factors (external motivation)		4	0.9	4.11	.059	.066
Recommendations from others (family, friends, and teachers)	55.69					
Having patterns in this field among friends and relatives	16.00					
Religious issues	15.22					
Media (TV, Internet, and press)	13.08					
Factors (social dignity)		5	1.12	5.41	.096	.086
Getting positive information about studying in this field	30.19					
Suitable social position of the profession	24.60					
Ability to communicate with medical team members	21.93					
Existence of excellent human relations in the field	12.72					
Having a positive impression of nursing in society	10.56					
Factors (internal motivation)		6	1.24	6.18	.054	.043
Usefulness of nursing knowledge for personal life	24.14					
Being interested in the nursing profession	22.77					
Distance to the faculty	22.56					
Having a caring experience (e.g., taking care of a patient at home)	15.51					
Field proximity to medicine	12.32					
Willingness to help others	2.69					
Factors (usefulness of discipline)		5	1.12	5.36	.089	.079
Immigration opportunity (to other countries)	44.30					
Having postgraduate job opportunities	23.99					
Opportunity for further education and academic progress	14.10					
Having a good income while studying	12.25					
Opportunity to access welfare facilities while studying	5.36					

Note. RI = Random Consistency Index; CI = consistency index; CR = consistency ratio.

significance. Contrary to the results of this study, the results of a qualitative study in the United Kingdom showed that nurses expressed pride in their profession and in being nurses (McCabe & Sambrook, 2013). The results of a previous study conducted in Iran indicate that nursing students believe that the nursing profession in Iran lacks necessary value (Joolaee et al., 2016). Although public perception of the nursing profession in Iran has improved in recent years, it seems that this profession in Iran has yet to achieve sufficient value and dignity.

Under the internal motivation criterion, "the usefulness of nursing knowledge for personal life" and "willingness to help others" were respectively scored as the most and least important factors. However, contrary to this finding, internal factors presented in other studies such as "tendency to care and help others" (Lindberg et al., 2020; McCabe & Sambrook, 2013; Patidar et al., 2011; Wu et al., 2015), "being able to communicate with people," and "having the opportunity to work with people" (Eley et al., 2010) were identified as crucial factors in choosing the nursing profession. It is evident that, different from other studies, the participants in this study did not place high priorities on willingness to help others and working with people. However, the usefulness for personal life was identified as important to the participants in the present research. Although this difference may be rooted in the gaps between cultures and research population, it may be inferred that, in this study, the participants were focused primarily on their personal improvement and growth. Under the usefulness of discipline criterion, "existence of migration opportunities (to other countries)" and "opportunity to access welfare facilities during study" were respectively ranked as the most and least important factors. In Lim and Muhtar (2016), "providing accommodations during education," "simultaneity of education and work," "travel opportunities," and "rapid support in entering the field" were identified as the main factors that motivated respondents to choose a career in nursing.

Because many countries face a shortage of nursing graduates and offer attractive salaries for practitioners, studying nursing provides an opportunity for graduates to experience better working conditions in other countries.

Because many countries face a shortage of nursing graduates and offer attractive salaries for practitioners, studying nursing provides an opportunity for graduates to experience better working conditions in other countries.

Limitations

Decision making is a systematic approach. Thus, the components of each problem could not be considered separately in this study. In other words, the different elements of decision making are correlated in real-world situations. Moreover, because human ideas are subject to dynamic change, the results of this study may be different from other samples of participants. Finally, the findings are not representative of all nursing students in Iran and are intended only to capture the situation among a subgroup of students in one particular school in Iran.

Conclusions

Recommendations from others (family, friends, and teachers), receiving positive information about studying in the field, the usefulness of nursing knowledge for personal life, and the existence of migration opportunities (to other countries) were the most significant factors found to affect choosing to pursue a career in nursing. The first two factors refer more to the external and social aspects of the discipline, whereas the other factors emphasize the internal elements and usefulness of the discipline. Therefore, the results support strengthening these aspects of the nursing profession and giving these aspects sufficient attention from stakeholders.

Acknowledgments

This study was supported financially by Mazandaran University. The authors would like to thank the Deputy of Research at Mazandaran University of Medical Sciences.

Author Contributions

Study conception and design: ZHM, SB
Data collection: ZHM
Data analysis and interpretation: SB
Drafting of the article: ZHM, KK, WJS
Critical revision of the article: ZHM, FH, WJS

References

Ahmed, F., & Kilic, K. (2019). Fuzzy analytic hierarchy process: A performance analysis of various algorithms. *Fuzzy Sets and Systems, 362*, 110–128. https://doi.org/10.1016/j.fss.2018.08.009

Alonso, J. A., & Lamata, M. T. (2006). Consistency in the analytic hierarchy process: A new approach. *International Journal of Uncertainty, Fuzziness and Knowledge-Based Systems, 14*(4), 445–459. https://doi.org/10.1142/S0218488506004114

Cho, S. H., Jung, S. Y., & Jang, S. (2010). Who enters nursing schools, and why do they choose to nurse? A comparison with female non-nursing students using longitudinal data. *Nurse Education Today, 30*(2), 180–186. https://doi.org/10.1016/j.nedt.2009

Crawford, R., & Turvey, J. (2019). Influences on indigenous and pacific students' health career choices: A longitudinal cohort study. *Contemporary Nurse, 55*(2–3), 250–260. https://doi.org/10.1080/10376178.2019.1647109

Eley, R., Eley, D., & Rogers-Clark, C. (2010). Reasons for entering and leaving nursing: An Australian regional study. *Australian Journal of Advanced Nursing, 28*(1), 6–13.

Elibol, E., & Seren, A. K. H. (2017). Reasons nursing students choose the nursing profession and their nursing image perceptions: A survey study. *Nursing Practice Today, 4*(2), 67–78.

Ergün, G., & Güzel, A. (2016). Analysis of the factors affecting the choice of profession of the first and last students at nursing department in the school of health. *Journal of Human Sciences, 13*(1), 1271–1284. https://doi.org/10.14687/ijhs.v13i1.3664

Farahani, M. A., Ghaffari, F., Oskouie, F., & Tafreshi, M. Z. (2017). Attrition among Iranian nursing students: A qualitative study. *Nurse Education in Practice, 22*, 98–104. https://doi.org/10.1016/j.nepr.2017.01.002

Joolaee, S., Farahani, M. A., Amiri, S. R. J., & Varaei, S. (2016). Support in clinical settings as perceived by nursing students in Iran: A qualitative study. *Nursing and Midwifery Studies, 5*(1), Article e31292.

Lawshe, C. H. (1975). A quantitative approach to content validity. *Personnel Psychology, 28*(4), 563–575. https://doi.org/10.1111/j.1744-6570.1975.tb01393.x

Liaw, S. Y., Wu, L. T., Holroyd, E., Wang, W., Lopez, V., Lim, S., & Chow, Y. L. (2016). Why not nursing? Factors influencing healthcare career choice among Singaporean students. *International Nursing Review, 63*(4), 530–538. https://doi.org/10.1111/inr.12312

Lim, S. G., & Muhtar, M. A. B. (2016). Factors influencing nursing students' decision to choose nursing. *International e-Journal of Science, Medicine & Education, 10*(2), 3–10.

Lin, Y.-H., Chang, L.-R., Lee, Y.-H., Tseng, H. W., Kuo, T. B. J., & Chen, S. H. (2014). Development and validation of the Smartphone Addiction Inventory (SPAI). *PLOS ONE, 9*(6), Article e98312. https://doi.org/10.1371/journal.pone.0098312

Lindberg, M., Carlsson, M., Engström, M., Kristofferzon, M. L., & Skytt, B. (2020). Nursing student's expectations for their future profession and motivating factors—A longitudinal descriptive study from Sweden. *Nurse Education Today, 84*, Article 104218. https://doi.org/10.1016/j.nedt.2019.104218

Maasoumi, R., Lamyian, M., Montazeri, A., Azin, S. A., Aguilar-Vafaie, M. E., & Hajizadeh, E. (2013). The Sexual Quality of Life-Female (SQOL-F) questionnaire: Translation and psychometric properties of the Iranian version. *Reproductive Health, 10*, Article No. 25. https://doi.org/10.1186/1742-4755-10-25

MacCallum, R. C., Widaman, K. F., Zhang, S., & Hong, S. (1999). Sample size in factor analysis. *Psychological Methods, 4*(1), 84–99. https://doi.org/10.1037/1082-989X.4.1.84

Manzoor, I., Daud, S., Hashmi, N. R., Zafar, M., Khan, M., Zafar, J., & Babar, S. (2010). Reasons for the selection of nursing profession in Pakistan. *The Professional Medical Journal, 17*(4), 728–734.

McCabe, T., & Sambrook, S. (2013). Psychological contracts and commitment amongst nurses and nurse managers: A discourse analysis. *International Journal of Nursing Studies, 50* (7), 954–967. https://doi.org/10.1016/j.ijnurstu.2012.11.012

Mooney, M., Glacken, M., & O'Brien, F. (2008). Choosing nursing as a career: A qualitative study. *Nurse Education Today, 28*(3), 385–392. https://doi.org/10.1016/j.nedt.2007.07.006

Mphahlele, N. E. (2011). *School leavers' perceptions of nursing as a career of choice.* [Master's thesis, Nursing Science, University of Witwatersrand]. https://core.ac.uk/reader/39669703

Önder, E., Önder, G., Kuvat, Ö., & Taş, N. (2014). Identifying the importance level of factors influencing the selection of nursing as a career choice using AHP: Survey to compare the precedence of private vocational high school nursing students and their parents. *Procedia-Social and Behavioral Sciences, 122,* 398–404. https://doi.org/10.1016/j.sbspro.2014.01.1361

Patidar, A. B., Kaur, J., Sharma, S. K., & Sharma, N. (2011). Future nurses' perception towards the profession and career plans: A cross-sectional survey in state Punjab. *Nursing and Midwifery Research Journal, 7*(4), 175–185. https://doi.org/10.33698/NRF0131

Shafii, M., Rafiei, S., Abooee, F., Bahrami, M. A., Nouhi, M., Lotfi, F., & Khanjankhani, K. (2016). Assessment of service quality in teaching hospitals of Yazd University of Medical Sciences: Using multi-criteria decision-making techniques. *Osong Public Health and Research Perspectives, 7*(4), 239–247. https://doi.org/10.1016/j.phrp.2016.05.001

Sun, C. C. (2010). A performance evaluation model by integrating fuzzy AHP and fuzzy TOPSIS methods. *Expert Systems with Applications, 37*(12), 7745–7754. https://doi.org/10.1016/j.eswa.2010.04.066

Wedley, W. C. (1993). Consistency prediction for incomplete AHP matrices. *Mathematical and Computer Modelling, 17*(4–5), 151–161. https://doi.org/10.1016/0895-7177(93)90183-Y.

Wilkes, L., Cowin, L., & Johnson, M. (2015). The reasons students choose to undertake a nursing degree. *Collegian, 22*(3), 259–265. https://doi.org/10.1016/j.colegn.2014.01.003

Wu, L. T., Low, M. M., Tan, K. K., López, V., & Liaw, S. Y. (2015). Why not nursing? A systematic review of factors influencing career choice among healthcare students. *International Nursing Review, 62*(4), 547–562. https://doi.org/10.1111/inr.12220

20

The Impact of Organizational Support on Practice Outcomes in Nurse Practitioners in Taiwan

Li-Hui HO[1] • Shu-Chen CHANG[2] • Kevin KAU[3] • Shu-Ying SHIU[4] • Sheng-Shiung HUANG[5] • Ya-Jung WANG[6] • Shiow-Luan TSAY[7]*

ABSTRACT

Background: Nurse practitioners (NPs) in Taiwan have practiced mainly in acute care hospitals since 2006. Although organizational support and level of support have been associated with the successful integration of NP roles and effective practice outcomes, organizational support in the context of NPs in inpatient settings is an area that has been rarely explored in the literature.

Purpose: The purpose of this study was to investigate the relationship between organizational support and the practice outcomes of job satisfaction, care effectiveness, and intention to leave in NPs.

Methods: A national survey of 512 NPs was conducted that included a demographic characteristics datasheet, the Nurse Practitioner Primary Care Organizational Climate Questionnaire, the Misener Nurse Practitioner Job Satisfaction Scale, and the Nurse Practitioner Care Effectiveness Scale. Multiple regression analysis was applied to explore the specific factors associated with job satisfaction. The statistical significance level was set at .05 with a two-tailed test. All statistical analyses were conducted using SPSS Statistics Version 22.0 software.

Results: More than half of the participants were found to be dissatisfied with their hospital managers (54.8%) and with each dimension of organizational support. Overall, 82.1% of the participants were satisfied with their current practice. A multiple regression analysis showed that the participants who perceived higher levels of organizational support in the workplace ($\beta = .53$, $p < .001$), expressed satisfaction with working with their managers ($\beta = .25$, $p < .001$), or perceived better care outcomes ($\beta = .10$, $p < .001$) reported higher job satisfaction. In addition, the participants who expressed intention to leave within 1 year ($\beta = -.09$, $p < .001$) and those with higher patient loads ($\beta = -.09$, $p < .001$) reported lower job satisfaction. Organizational support was found to explain 50% of the variance in job satisfaction.

Conclusions/Implications for Practice: The results of this study highlight organizational support as the most important factor affecting job satisfaction in NPs. Therefore, administrators work to promote organizational support and improve the work environment to enhance the job satisfaction, increase the clinical practice retention, and improve the care outcomes of NPs.

Key Words:
organizational support, job satisfaction, care outcomes, intent to leave, nurse practitioners.

Introduction

The vast majority (99.8%) of the population in Taiwan is covered under the public National Health Insurance program (Ministry of Health and Welfare, Taiwan, ROC, 2019), which makes access to healthcare easy and affordable for covered individuals. Various factors in recent years, including healthcare system reform, a rapidly aging population, increasing acuity in hospitalized patients, restrictions on working hours for residents and physicians, and a consistently high public demand for quality care, have led to a rising demand for healthcare services. Thus, the burden on the healthcare system and the quality of care in acute care hospitals have become important concerns. To address growing healthcare demands and the shortfall in healthcare provider capabilities, the government of Taiwan introduced a formal nurse practitioner (NP) program that has been delivering healthcare using physician-nurse practitioner team-based care models for inpatients since 2006 (Chiu et al., 2016; Tsay et al., 2019). Most of Taiwan's 8,849 licensed NPs (as of May 2020) work in acute care hospitals (Ministry of Health and Welfare, Taiwan, ROC, 2020).

Although the government has mandated regulations for the education, licensing, and practice of NPs (Tsay et al., 2019), the healthcare organizations that employ NPs significantly influence the actual role played by NPs in patient care. Specific

[1]MS, RN, NP, Department of Neurosurgery, China Medical Hospital, Taiwan, Republic of China • [2]PhD, RN, Director, Department of Nursing, Chunghwa Christian Hospital, and Adjunct Assistant Professor, College of Nursing and Health Sciences, Da-Yeh University, Taiwan, Republic of China • [3]MA, Lecturer, Academic Writing Education Center, National Taiwan University, Taiwan, Republic of China • [4]MS, RN, NP, Emergency Room, Department of Nursing, Chunghwa Christian Hospital, Taiwan, Republic of China • [5]PhD, Assistant Professor, College of Nursing and Health Sciences, Da-Yeh University, Taiwan, Republic of China • [6]PhD, RN, Assistant Professor, Department of Nursing, Da-Yeh University, Taiwan, Republic of China • [7]PhD, RN, NP, Professor, College of Nursing and Health Sciences, Da-Yeh University, Taiwan, Republic of China.

roles for NPs are often defined by the employing organization. Moreover, organizational support has been related to factors including the successful integration of the NP role, NP job satisfaction, intention to continue working as an NP, and care outcomes (Poghosyan et al., 2020; Poghosyan, Nannini, & Clarke, 2013). Although NPs are increasingly relied upon in hospitals to provide healthcare, systematic review studies have shown that NPs are capable of delivering high-quality, cost-effective care to patients in primary-care office, inpatient, outpatient surgical, and other practice settings as well (Stanik-Hutt et al., 2013). However, studies have shown that the practice of NPs is often not supported within their organizations (Poghosyan et al., 2020; Poghosyan, Nannini, & Clarke, 2013). In addition, each acute care hospital in Taiwan has its own administrative system. Thus, NPs are evaluated by managers who may be physicians, non-NPs, or NP supervisors who are unfamiliar with NP roles and functions and, therefore, may not provide to NPs adequate organizational support, resources, and rewards. The impact of organizational support on the practice outcomes of NPs in acute care settings is an issue that has received little research attention.

Organizational climate/support is one of the important factors associated with outcomes for healthcare professionals (Aiken et al., 2011). The findings of Albashayreh et al. (2019) indicate that a good work environment is positively correlated with job satisfaction. In a cross-national study, better work environments were shown to reduce the likelihood of job dissatisfaction (Aiken et al., 2011). Poghosyan et al. (2017) reported similar results, with NPs with higher scores for organizational climate showing higher levels of satisfaction with their jobs ($OR = 1.24$, 95% CI [1.12, 1.39]). In addition, a descriptive, correlational study showed that the relationship between NPs and staff was also correlated with job satisfaction (LaMarche & Tullai-McGuinness, 2009). Another large, cross-sectional online survey conducted by Halcomb and Ashley (2017) found collegiality to be the most satisfying professional aspect of work (Halcomb & Ashley, 2017).

Practice outcomes often include job satisfaction, intent to leave, and care quality (Poghosyan et al., 2020). Job satisfaction is defined as the perceived satisfaction of NPs with their clinical practice in several dimensions, including intrapractice partnership/collegiality; challenge/autonomy; professional, social, and community interaction; professional growth; time; and benefits (Misener & Cox, 2001). Moreover, job satisfaction is integral to retention efforts (Albashayreh et al., 2019), and several studies have found a correlation between job satisfaction and intention to change jobs (Applebaum et al., 2010; Masum et al., 2016; Poghosyan et al., 2017). For instance, Applebaum et al. showed that job satisfaction is inversely linked with intention to quit (Applebaum et al., 2010). The results of a study by Masum et al. (2016) also confirmed an association between higher job satisfaction and lower turnover ($r = -.57$, $p < .01$; Masum et al., 2016). Furthermore, Poghosyan et al. (2017) found that the odds of job satisfaction factors increased by approximately 20%, whereas the odds of turnover intention decreased by approximately 20%. Apart from this, the practice of NPs has been found to encompass a variety of dimensions, including providing direct patient care services, patient counseling, and health promotion education and performing administrative responsibilities, which, added together, generate heavy workloads. The results of Miller et al.'s (2005) study indicate that maintaining reasonable working hours enhances job satisfaction in NPs. One study conducted using both quantitative and qualitative methods indicates that both working hours and the duration of time worked in one's current job are statistically and significantly related to job satisfaction in NPs (Steinke et al., 2018). Patient workload is positively associated with work stress in NPs and thus negatively associated with job satisfaction (Ramoo et al., 2013). Furthermore, increased satisfaction with one's work as an NP has been shown to improve not only retention but also patient outcomes (Horner, 2017). Watts (2019) noted that work satisfaction affects patient safety and care. One review study also found that NPs experience dissatisfaction when a patient outcome is not in line with the expected outcome (Jaeger et al., 2016).

In summary, NP job satisfaction is affected by specific factors, such as organizational support, the relationship between NPs and staff, turnover intention, workload, and care outcomes. However, the studies on this issue in the literature are limited by their use of small sample sizes, specific geographic areas, and convenience sampling methodology (J.-Y. Hu et al., 2018). Little is known about which factors affect job satisfaction. Furthermore, the association between these factors and job satisfaction among NPs requires further examination using more representative samples, for example, NPs in Taiwan. Therefore, this study was designed to investigate the relationship between organizational support and the practice outcomes of job satisfaction, care effectiveness, and intention to leave using a national sample of nursing practitioners.

Organizational support theory was adopted as the framework for this study. According to this theory, the beliefs of employees relate to the extent to which the employer values their contributions and cares about their well-being. Organizational support is also valued as assurance that resources will be available when they are needed to carry out one's job effectively (Eisenberger et al., 1986). Thus, organizational support is expected to have different effects on different employee outcomes such as job satisfaction (Rhoades & Eisenberger, 2002), healthcare outcomes (Aiken et al., 2011), and turnover intention (Arshadi, 2011; Poghosyan et al., 2020). For NPs, organizational support is essential to promoting NP performance and outcomes, including improving job satisfaction and quality of care as well as reducing turnover (Poghosyan et al., 2020). In light of these concerns, the organizational support theory offers a good framework for pursuing the aims of this study.

Methods

Design and Participants

The researchers conducted a nationwide survey of NPs using a cross-sectional design. The participants were recruited from the membership of the Taiwan Association of Nurse Practitioners, which includes approximately 90% of all licensed NPs in Taiwan. The data were collected between October 2016 and November 2016. The inclusion criteria included holding active membership in the Taiwan Association of Nurse Practitioners, holding national NP certification, and being employed in a hospital or practice as an NP for at least 1 year. The eligible NPs were invited to participate via email. Those NPs who agreed to participate and provided informed consent were then asked to complete an anonymous survey online. The survey consisted of a demographic characteristics questionnaire, a work-related information datasheet, the Nurse Practitioner Primary Care Organizational Climate Questionnaire (NP-PCOCQ), the Misener Nurse Practitioner Job Satisfaction Scale (MNPJSS), and the Nurse Practitioner Practice Outcome Scale. Three thousand NPs were invited to participate in this study, and 512 NPs completed the survey, yielding a response rate of 17.1%. Approval for this study was granted by the institutional review board of China Medical University and Hospital Research Ethics Committee (approval number: 13MMHIS231).

Measures

Organizational support

In this study, practice environment was assessed using the NP-PCOCQ, which is an NP-specific tool that was designed to measure organizational support in primary and acute care settings. The NP-PCOCQ has been shown to have satisfactory internal consistency (Cronbach's alpha = .87–.95) and construct validity (Poghosyan, Nannini, Finkelstein et al., 2013).

The NP-PCOCQ consists of 29 items in the four dimensions of (a) NP–physician relations (measuring the relationship between NPs and physicians), (b) NP–administration relations (measuring the collaboration between NPs and managers), (c) independent practice and support (measuring the support or resources for NPs in practice), and (d) professional visibility (measuring the visibility of NPs in practice; Poghosyan et al., 2019). Each item is rated on a 5-point scale ranging from *strongly disagree* (0) to *strongly agree* (4). Individual dimension scores were calculated as the sum of the items within the dimension. The total score was calculated by summing all 29 items. Higher scores indicated higher levels of the associated characteristic in the practice and, thus, a better practice environment in terms of the associated dimension. The Chinese version of the NP-PCOCQ has also shown good reliability (Cronbach's alpha = .87–.95) and construct validity, with a Cronbach's alpha value of .90 in this study.

Practice outcomes examined in this study included job satisfaction, care effectiveness, and intention to leave one's current job.

Job satisfaction

NP job satisfaction was measured in this study using the MNPJSS, which encompasses 44 self-administered items measured on a 6-point scale ranging from (1) *very dissatisfied* to (6) *very satisfied*. This scale includes the six dimensions of intrapractice partnership/collegiality; challenge/autonomy; professional, social, and community interaction; professional growth; time; and benefits. Dimension scores are calculated by summing all the items within a dimension. The MNPJSS total score is calculated by summing all of the items, with higher scores associated with greater job satisfaction. The Cronbach's alpha value for the entire scale was .96, with subscale alphas ranging from .79 to .94 (Misener & Cox, 2001). The Chinese version of the MNPJSS also has good reliability (entire scale: .97; subscales: .80–.93) and construct validity (C.-Y. Hu et al., 2014). The Cronbach's alpha for this study was .92.

Care effectiveness

NP care effectiveness was evaluated in this study using the Nurse Practitioner Care Effectiveness Scale (NPCES), which was developed by coauthor Dr. S. L. Tsay using a literature review and qualitative interviews with a large number of NPs. This scale consists of 18 items scored on a 5-point scale ranging from (1) *strongly disagree* to (5) *strongly agree* and includes the two dimensions of efficacy of care (measuring the efficacy of care in practice) and cost of care (measuring the cost of care in practice). Dimension scores represent the sum of all items in the associated dimension. The NPCES total score is calculated by summing all 18 items, with higher scores associated with better care effectiveness in NP practice. The results of the exploratory factor analysis in this study indicate that the two dimension factors explained 74.14% of the total variance and that each item had a factor loading of over .45. Thus, the NPCES is a reliable and valid scale that may be used to evaluate care outcomes in NPs. The Cronbach's value for this scale was .94 in this study.

Intent to leave

Intent to leave one's current job was measured using a dichotomous item asking the NPs whether they intended to leave their positions within 1 year (yes/no). This measure has been used with NPs in previous research (Poghosyan et al., 2020).

Data Analysis

Demographic characteristics and NP practice-related information are presented in this study as percentages, means, and standard deviations (*SDs*). The correlations between the variables were examined using multiple methods. Dichotomous variables and continuous variables were examined using point-biserial correlation. The correlations between continuous variables were examined using Pearson product–moment correlation. The correlations between ordinal variables were examined using Spearman's rank correlation. The correlations between categorical variables and continuous variables were examined using the contingency coefficient.

Stepwise linear regression analysis was used to explore the factors affecting job satisfaction. Only the significant variables in the correlation analysis were entered into the stepwise linear regression model. The standardized regression coefficients (β) and adjusted R^2 were also estimated by the regression models. All of the analyses were conducted using SPSS Statistics Version 22.0 (IBM, Armonk, NY, USA). Statistical significance was determined using an alpha level of .05, presented as a p value of < .05 and two-sided tests.

Results

Two thirds (66.1%) of the NPs were in the 36- to 46-year age group, most (80.3%) had over 12 years of registered nurse (RN) practice, and 53.4% reported having less than 4 years of experience as an NP (1–2 years: 26.3%, 3–4 years: 27.1%). Most worked in either medical centers (50.9%) or regional hospitals (36%). Generally, the participants reported that their practice was trusted by doctors (94.7%), RNs (92.6%), and patients (94.9%). The NP job description primarily involved direct patient care and included providing physical assessments (94.6%); discussing patient care with physicians (94.1%); taking patient histories (92.3%); prescribing medications, laboratory tests, or treatments (90.2%); performing medical procedures (87.2%); making differential diagnoses (86.6%); analyzing patient data (84.7%); providing patient education (85.8%); arranging patient transfers (79.3%); and arranging patient discharges (71.1%). The average daily care load was 11–21 patients (67.2%), and 21.4% of the NPs reported an intention to leave within 1 year (Table 1).

Organizational support subscale scores (range: 0–4) were as follows: NP–physician relations (mean = 2.99, SD = 0.35), independent practice and support (mean = 2.77, SD = 0.32), professional visibility (mean = 2.63, SD = 0.50), and NP–administration relations (mean = 2.37, SD = 0.51). Job satisfaction subscale scores (range: 1–6) were as follows: professional, social, and community interaction (mean = 4.33, SD = 0.80); intrapractice partnership/collegiality (mean = 4.16, SD = 0.86); challenge/autonomy (mean = 4.13, SD = 0.79); time (mean = 3.87, SD = 0.88); professional growth (mean = 3.55, SD = 0.99); and benefits (mean = 3.12, SD = 0.96). Overall, 82.1% of the NPs were satisfied with their practice. The mean item scores for care effectiveness were as follows: cost of care (mean = 4.42, SD = 0.93) and efficacy of care (mean = 2.71, SD = 0.67; Table 2).

The correlations among organizational support, job satisfaction, and care effectiveness are summarized in Table 2. Organizational support was positively correlated with job satisfaction (r = .32, p < .01) and care outcomes (r = .35, p < .01) as well as with the following variables: age, years of RN practice, doctors' trust, RNs' trust, patients' trust, cooperation with doctors, and cooperation with managers (r = .21–.46, p < .01). Care outcomes showed significant relationships with the following variables: years of NP practice, doctors' trust, RNs' trust, patients' trust, cooperation with doctors, and cooperation with managers (r = .01–.19, p < .05). In addition, job satisfaction was positively correlated with the following variables: doctors' trust, RNs' trust, patients' trust, cooperation with doctors, and cooperation with managers (r = .17–.53, p < .01). Furthermore, intention to leave within 1 year was found to be negatively correlated with organizational support (r = –.25, p < .01) and job

Table 1

NP Demographic and Practice-Related Variables (N = 513)

Variable	n	%
Age (years)		
25–35	93	18.1
36–46	339	66.1
≥ 47	81	15.8
Years of RN practice		
3–5	19	3.7
6–8	37	7.2
9–11	45	8.8
≥ 12	412	80.3
Years of NP practice		
1–2	135	26.3
3–4	139	27.1
5–6	118	23.0
7–8	121	23.6
Average number of daily patients cared for		
5–10	20	3.9
11–16	148	28.8
17–21	197	38.4
22–26	63	12.3
27–31	36	7.0
> 31	49	9.6
Hospital type		
Medical center	261	50.9
Regional hospital	188	36.6
District hospital	64	12.5
Direct patient care [a]		
Physical assessment	494	94.6
Discussing patient care with MD	491	94.1
History taking	482	92.3
Prescribing meds, laboratory tests, treatments	471	90.2
Medical procedures	455	87.2
Making differential diagnoses	452	86.6
Analyzing patients' data	442	84.7
Patient education	448	85.8
Arranging patient transfers	414	79.3
Arranging patient discharges	371	71.1
Indirect patient care [a]		
Medical charting	467	89.5
Attending meetings	468	89.7
Coordination patient care	448	85.8
Filling out medical forms	439	84.1
Administration duty	387	74.1
Educating others (residents, nurses, etc.)	363	70.3
Intention to leave within 1 year		
Yes	110	21.4
No	403	78.6

Note. RN = registered nurse; NP = nurse practitioner; MD = medical doctor.
[a] This item was multiple choice.

Table 2

Distributions of Main Research Variables (N = 513)

Item	Mean	*SD*
Organizational support (range: 0–4)		
NP–physician relations	2.99	0.35
NP–administration relations	2.37	0.51
Independent practice and support	2.77	0.32
Professional visibility	2.63	0.50
Subtotal	77.68	9.01
Job satisfaction (range: 1–6)		
Intrapractice partnership/collegiality	4.16	0.86
Challenge/autonomy	4.13	0.79
Professional, social, and community interaction	4.33	0.80
Professional growth	3.55	0.99
Time	3.87	0.88
Benefits	3.12	0.96
Subtotal	164.77	34.27
Care outcome (range: 1–5)		
Efficacy of care	2.71	0.67
Cost of care	4.42	0.93
Subtotal	64.11	13.63

Note. NP = nurse practitioner.

satisfaction ($r = -.31, p < .01$). The average number of daily patients cared for also showed a negative correlation with job satisfaction ($r = -.14, p < .01$; Table 3).

The results of stepwise multiple linear regression show that the participants with higher levels of organizational support ($\beta = .53, p < .001$), satisfactory levels of cooperation with their managers ($\beta = .25, p < .001$), and better care effectiveness ($\beta = .10, p < .001$) reported higher levels of job satisfaction. In addition, those who expressed the intention to leave within 1 year ($\beta = -.09, p < .001$) and those who had a higher-than-average patient load ($\beta = -.09, p < .001$) reported significantly lower levels of job satisfaction. Fifty-eight percent of the variance in job satisfaction was explained by this model ($F = 90.9, p < .01, R^2 = .58$, adjusted $R^2 = .57$). Organizational support was shown to be the most important predictor of higher job satisfaction, explaining 50% of the total variance in job satisfaction (Table 4).

Discussion

The results of this study support the precepts of organizational support theory, which posits a positive, reciprocal, and dynamic relationship between organizational support and practice outcomes related to job satisfaction. Good organizational support, better cooperation with managers, and favorable care effectiveness were each shown to strengthen NP practice. NPs who perceive higher levels of organizational support show higher levels of job satisfaction. In contrast, organizational support, intention to leave, and a high daily patient load were each shown to reduce job satisfaction. Thus, improving perceived organizational support is key to improving NP job satisfaction.

Table 3

The Correlations Among Organizational Support, Care Outcome, Job Satisfaction, and Intent to Leave (N = 513)

Variable	1	2	3	4	5	6	7	8	9	10	11	12	13
1. Organizational support	1.00												
2. Care outcome	.35**	1.00											
3. Job satisfaction	.32**	.32**	1.00										
4. Age	.11*	.05	.09	1.00									
5. Years of RN practice	.12**	.08	.08	.29**	1.00								
6. Years of NP practice	.07	.10*	.02	.42**	.15**	1.00							
7. Doctors' trust	.32**	.15**	.25**	.04	.16**	−.01	1.00						
8. Registered nurses' trust	.32**	.15**	.29**	.08	.19**	.07	.29***	1.00					
9. Patients' trust	.23**	.13**	.17**	.07	.15**	.02	.37***	.23***	1.00				
10. Cooperation with doctors	.21**	.19**	.21**	.18**	.10*	.02	.31***	.26***	.11*	1.00			
11. Cooperation with managers	.46**	.09**	.53**	.50**	.13**	.05	.09*	.15***	.07	.11*	1.00		
12. Patient load	−.06	−.04	−.14**	−.06	−.06	−.03	.09	.11	.13	.10	.09	1.00	
13. Apply for another job within 1 year	−.25**	−.07	−.31**	−.26**	−.12**	−.01	.21***	.18***	.05	.20***	.29***	.11	1.00

Note. The correlations between dichotomous variables and continuous variables were examined using point-biserial correlations. The correlations between continuous variables were examined using Pearson product–moment correlations. The correlations between ordinal variables were examined using Spearman's rank correlations. The correlations between categorical variables and continuous variables were examined using contingency coefficients. NP = nurse practitioner; RN = registered nurse.

* $p < .05$. ** $p < .01$. *** $p < .001$.

Table 4

Stepwise Multiple Linear Regression Predicting Job Satisfaction

Step	β	*t*	R^2	Adjusted R^2	*F*
Organizational support	.53	15.09***	.50		
Cooperation with managers	.25	7.55***	.05		
Care outcome	.10	3.19***	.01		
Intention to leave within 1 year	−.09	−3.06***	.01		
Daily patient load	−.09	−3.01***	.01		
Model fit			.58	.57	90.9**

$^{**}p < .01$. $^{***}p < .001$.

The findings of this study identified organizational support as the most important factor affecting job satisfaction in NPs. This result is consistent with the results of prior studies (Aiken et al., 2011; Albashayreh et al., 2019; Poghosyan et al., 2017), which also found a positive relationship between organizational environment quality and job satisfaction. This finding may be attributed to good organizational support fostering positive interactions among managers, NPs, and other colleagues. This positive interaction may be viewed as the organization's contribution to a positive reciprocal dynamic with NPs (Baran et al., 2012). Generally, NPs who perceive higher levels of organizational support tend to perform better when reciprocating received feedback and to report better job satisfaction. Furthermore, the participants in this study who reported being satisfied with the working relationship with their managers ($\beta = .25, p < .001$) reported higher job satisfaction. Other studies have reported similar findings with regard to the associations and relationships among managers, colleagues, and NPs. For example, Poghosyan, Nannini, and Clarke (2013) noted that the relationships among NPs, doctors, and managers are significant aspects of the work environment. NPs with favorable practice environments, which include better working relations with physicians and administrators, are more likely to be satisfied with their jobs (Poghosyan et al., 2017). In evidence, doctors have reported that NPs improve the quality of patient care, patient compliance levels, and productivity. Thus, the motivation of NPs improves their cooperation, which improves the effectiveness of provided healthcare and improves job satisfaction (Holleman et al., 2010; Running et al., 2008). Our results also support the inference that the vast majority of NPs (98.4%) are satisfied with their current level of collaboration with doctors. In addition, we also found a correlation between satisfaction with one's managers and job satisfaction, which is in line with the findings of a previous study (Poghosyan et al., 2017). Hospital administrators provide sufficient resources and support to promote the autonomy of NPs in practice, especially in acute care settings. NPs who perceive adequate support channel their reciprocation efforts toward better levels of job satisfaction. Thus, it is important to support the practice environment and to decrease the perception of NPs that their practice is restricted by managers.

However, the findings of this study indicate that fewer than half (45.2%) of the participants were satisfied with the support provided by managers, and the scores for organizational support also show an inadequately supportive working environment for NPs (scores ranged from 2.37 to 2.99), which is consistent with the results of a cross-national study (Aiken et al., 2011). These results may be explained by the fact that, although national NP practice policies have been implemented for over 10 years, hospitals and NPs continue to struggle to set an appropriate practice model for acute care settings. Although the regulation allowing "nurse practitioners to perform medical care with the supervision of physicians" was issued in 2016 to protect the rights of the NP practice, some hospitals currently require NPs to perform medical care on an unlimited number of patients, which significantly increases workload stress and reduces job satisfaction in NPs. Organizational support helps NPs cope more effectively with occupational stress, whereas managers affect the work environment both positively and negatively, directly impacting job satisfaction (Ribelin, 2003). Furthermore, favorable relations with healthcare administrators have been shown to improve NP job satisfaction (Poghosyan et al., 2017). The results of this study may provide a reference for hospital management. Managers should provide adequate NP staffing and organizational support to facilitate advanced levels of practice and NP job satisfaction.

Moreover, daily patient load was highlighted in this study as a risk factor affecting job satisfaction in NPs, echoing the findings of prior studies (Miller et al., 2005; Ramoo et al., 2013; Steinke et al., 2018). The NP–patient ratios in regional hospitals and medical centers in Taiwan are much higher than those in other countries (4.7–11.7 vs. 1–8.6, respectively; Aiken et al., 2012; Kleinpell et al., 2015; Morioka et al., 2017; National Health Insurance Administration, Ministry of Health and Welfare, Taiwan, ROC, 2020). In the context of organizational support theory, higher patient load represents poor job conditions that may decrease the organizational support perceived by NPs. Although the government of Taiwan defined in 2019 the range of nurse–patient ratios allowed for different levels of hospitals as fewer than nine in medical centers, fewer than 12 in regional hospitals, fewer than 15 in district hospitals, and fewer than 15 in psychiatric hospitals, no regulations currently address the NP–patient ratio. Therefore, regulation of the NP–patient ratio is needed in the near future to establish an appropriate NP–patient ratio. In the meantime, medical institutions should recruit more NPs to decrease the overall workload. Creating a more appropriate nurse–patient ratio should improve job satisfaction in NPs and allow additional time for NPs to enhance their skills and knowledge to provide better quality of care.

The results of this study are consistent with those of prior studies showing that better care outcomes increase job satisfaction (Horner, 2017; Jaeger et al., 2016; Watts, 2019). Job satisfaction is derived not only from income but also from the feelings engendered from work performed. A good practice outcome may be viewed as a work achievement. On the basis of the organizational support theory, NPs who perceive adequate organizational support should be better prepared to engage in teamwork and perceive more job satisfaction and achieve better quality of care in their practice (Poghosyan et al., 2020). If patient care outcomes do not align with expected outcomes, NPs will experience dissatisfaction (Jaeger et al., 2016). In addition to these factors, we found significant negative correlations between NP job satisfaction and intent to leave within 1 year, which is consistent with the findings of previous studies (Applebaum et al., 2010; Masum et al., 2016; Poghosyan et al., 2017). Rambur et al. (2003) reported a stronger association between intention to leave and job dissatisfaction than with career advancement (Rambur et al., 2003). Hence, administrators view fostering good work environments as a strategy for retaining NPs and increasing their job satisfaction (Poghosyan et al., 2017). In addition, our data showed that only 45.2% of the NPs in this study were satisfied with their managers. In other words, the relationship between managers and NPs is a major barrier in the NP practice. Thus, it is necessary to promote effective communication to decrease conflicts between NPs and managers.

This study was affected by several limitations. First, this study was performed in Taiwan. Thus, the findings of this study may not be generalizable to broader populations of NPs. Second, the results may be affected by response bias, as the data were collected using a self-report questionnaire. However, a combination of anonymous questionnaire design and computer technology was used in this study to mitigate potential response error. Third, the findings were limited with regard to causal inferences because of the cross-sectional design. Future research using a longitudinal design would clarify causal inferences. The dynamic interaction of these factors may affect NP job satisfaction continuously in long-term observations. Finally, low response rates are an inevitable issue in population-based questionnaire surveys. Unfortunately, the authors had no way of accessing the demographic data of nonresponse NPs without their consent. Hence, the results should be interpreted and inferred with caution. As one recent national survey on the practice of NPs also reported a low response rate (9.9%; Kleinpell et al., 2018), our response rate (17.1%) may be considered within an acceptable range. Larger sample sizes and strategies to improve the response rate are needed in future studies. Nonetheless, the results of this study provide national-based information from Taiwan. We hope that these findings will prove helpful in addressing factors affecting NP job satisfaction and will be used as a reference for management, policymaking, and efforts to improve the work environment for NPs in medical organizations.

Conclusions

In conclusion, this study highlighted the potential factors affecting job satisfaction and practice outcomes in NPs. Organizational support was identified as the most important of these factors. Organization administrators play an important role in developing strategies and policies for improving organizational support in support of NP practice. Favorable organizational support positively affects NP job satisfaction and decreases intention to change jobs, which improves NP retention rates and stabilizes NP manpower, providing positive outcomes for administrators, NPs, and patients.

Acknowledgments

The authors express their gratitude to all of the nurse practitioners who responded to the online survey questionnaire used in this study.

Author Contribution

Study conception and design: LHH, SLT
Data collection: SCC, KK, SYS
Data analysis and interpretation: SYS, SSH, YJW
Drafting of the article: LHH, KK, SLT
Critical revision of the article: LHH, SLT

References

Aiken, L. H., Sermeus, W., Van den Heede, K., Sloane, D. M., Busse, R., McKee, M., Bruyneel, L., Rafferty, A. M., Griffiths, P., Moreno-Casbas, M. T., Tishelman, C., Scott, A., Brzostek, T., Kinnunen, J., Schwendimann, R., Heinen, M., Zikos, D., Sjetne, I. S., Smith, H. L., & Kutney-Lee, A. (2012). Patient safety, satisfaction, and quality of hospital care: Cross sectional surveys of nurses and patients in 12 countries in Europe and the United States. *BMJ, 344,* Article e1717. https://doi.org/10.1136/bmj.e1717

Aiken, L. H., Sloane, D. M., Clarke, S., Poghosyan, L., Cho, E., You, L., Finlayson, M., Kanai-Pak, M., & Aungsuroch, Y. (2011). Importance of work environments on hospital outcomes in nine countries. *International Journal for Quality in Health Care, 23*(4), 357–364. https://doi.org/10.1093/intqhc/mzr022

Albashayreh, A., Al Sabei, S. D., Al-Rawajfah, O. M., & Al-Awaisi, H. (2019). Healthy work environments are critical for nurse job satisfaction: Implications for Oman. *International Nursing Review, 66*(3), 389–395. https://doi.org/10.1111/inr.12529

Applebaum, D., Fowler, S., Fiedler, N., Osinubi, O., & Robson, M. (2010). The impact of environmental factors on nursing stress, job satisfaction, and turnover intention. *The Journal of Nursing Administration, 40*(7–8), 323–328. https://doi.org/10.1097/NNA.0b013e3181e9393b

Arshadi, N. (2011). The relationships of perceived organizational support (POS) with organizational commitment, in-role performance, and turnover intention: Mediating role of felt obligation. *Procedia - Social and Behavioral Sciences, 30*, 1103–1108. https://doi.org/10.1016/j.sbspro.2011.10.215

Baran, B. E., Shanock, L. R., & Miller, L. R. (2012). Advancing organizational support theory into the twenty-first century world of work. *Journal of Business and Psychology, 27*(2), 123–147. https://doi.org/10.1007/s10869-011-9236-3

Chiu, H.-J., Tsay, S.-L., & Tung, H.-H. (2016). A giant leap in the development of nurse practitioners in Taiwan: From statute to regulation. *Journal of the American Association of Nurse Practitioners, 28*(11), 622–627. https://doi.org/10.1002/2327-6924.12405

Eisenberger, R., Huntington, R., Hutchinson, S., & Sow, A. D. (1986). Perceived organizational support. *Journal of Applied Psychology, 71*(3), 500–507. https://doi.org/10.1037/0021-9010.71.3.500

Halcomb, E., & Ashley, C. (2017). Australian primary health care nurses most and least satisfying aspects of work. *Journal of Clinical Nursing, 26*(3–4), 535–545. https://doi.org/10.1111/jocn.13479

Holleman, J., Johnson, A., & Frim, D. M. (2010). The impact of a 'resident replacement' nurse practitioner on an academic pediatric neurosurgical service. *Pediatric Neurosurgery, 46*(3), 177–181. https://doi.org/10.1159/000321922

Horner, D. K. (2017). Mentoring: Positively influencing job satisfaction and retention of new hire nurse practitioners. *Plastic Surgical Nursing, 37*(1), 7–22. https://doi.org/10.1097/PSN.0000000000000169

Hu, C.-Y., Chen, M.-H., & Lin, S.-Y. (2014). Psychometric testing of the Chinese version of the nurse practitioner's job satisfaction scale. *Journal of Nursing and Healthcare Research, 10*(3), 240–250. https://doi.org/10.6225/JNHR.10.3.240 (Original work published in Chinese)

Hu, J.-Y., Tung, H.-H., Tsay, S.-L., & Lin, W.-C. (2018). An outcome analysis of nurse practitioner care in a community hospital in Taiwan. *Journal of the American Association of Nurse Practitioners, 30*(8), 464–471. https://doi.org/10.1097/JXX.0000000000000066

Jaeger, C. B., Acree-Hamann, C., Zurmehly, J., Buck, J., & Patrick, T. (2016). Assessment of neonatal nurse practitioner workload in a level IV neonatal intensive care unit: Satisfaction. *Newborn and Infant Nursing Reviews, 16*(3), 138–148. https://doi.org/10.1053/j.nainr.2016.07.007

Kleinpell, R., Cook, M. L., & Padden, D. L. (2018). American Association of Nurse Practitioners National Nurse Practitioner sample survey: Update on acute care nurse practitioner practice. *Journal of the American Association of Nurse Practitioners, 30*(3), 140–149. https://doi.org/10.1097/JXX.0000000000000030

Kleinpell, R., Ward, N. S., Kelso, L. A., Mollenkopf, F. P. Jr., & Houghton, D. (2015). Provider to patient ratios for nurse practitioners and physician assistants in critical care units. *American Journal of Critical Care, 24*(3), e16–e21. https://doi.org/10.4037/ajcc2015274

LaMarche, K., & Tullai-McGuinness, S. (2009). Canadian nurse practitioner job satisfaction. *Nursing Leadership (Toronto, Ontario), 22*(2), 41–57. https://doi.org/10.12927/cjnl.2009.20797

Masum, A. K., Azad, M. A., Hoque, K. E., Beh, L. S., Wanke, P., & Arslan, Ö. (2016). Job satisfaction and intention to quit: An empirical analysis of nurses in Turkey. *PeerJ, 4*, Article e1896. https://doi.org/10.7717/peerj.1896

Miller, K., Apold, S., Baas, L., Berner, B., & Levine-Brill, E. (2005). Job satisfaction among nurse practitioners. *The Journal for Nurse Practitioners, 1*(1), 30–33. https://doi.org/10.1016/j.nurpra.2005.06.011

Ministry of Health and Welfare, Taiwan, ROC. (2019). *National health insurance annual statistical report 2019*. https://www.nhi.gov.tw/English/Content_List.aspx?n=EFBE55E9A1FC16BB&topn=BCB2B0D2433F6491

Ministry of Health and Welfare, Taiwan, ROC. (2020). *List of the number of certified nurse practitioners from 1995 to 2020*. https://dep.mohw.gov.tw/DONAHC/cp-1044-43987-104.html (Original work published in Chinese)

Misener, T. R., & Cox, D. L. (2001). Development of the Misener Nurse Practitioner Job Satisfaction Scale. *Journal of Nursing Measurement, 9*(1), 91–108. https://doi.org/10.1891/1061-3749.9.1.91

Morioka, N., Tomio, J., Seto, T., & Kobayashi, Y. (2017). The association between higher nurse staffing standards in the fee schedules and the geographic distribution of hospital nurses: A cross-sectional study using nationwide administrative data. *BMC Nursing, 16*, Article 25. https://doi.org/10.1186/s12912-017-0219-1

National Health Insurance Administration, Ministry of Health and Welfare, Taiwan, ROC. (2020). *The statistics of nurse–patient ratios in Taiwan*. https://www.nhi.gov.tw/Content_List.aspx?n=4037A32CDEF1DDCF&topn=CDA985A80C0DE710

Poghosyan, L., Ghaffari, A., Liu, J., & Friedberg, M. W. (2020). Physician-nurse practitioner teamwork in primary care practices in New York: A cross-sectional survey. *Journal of General Internal Medicine, 35*(4), 1021–1028. https://doi.org/10.1007/s11606-019-05509-2

Poghosyan, L., Ghaffari, A., & Shaffer, J. (2019). Nurse Practitioner Primary Care Organizational Climate Questionnaire: Item response theory and differential item functioning. *Journal of Clinical Nursing, 28*(15–16), 2934–2945. https://doi.org/10.1111/jocn.14895

Poghosyan, L., Liu, J., Shang, J., & D'Aunno, T. (2017). Practice environments and job satisfaction and turnover intentions of nurse practitioners: Implications for primary care workforce capacity. *Health Care Management Review, 42*(2), 162–171. https://doi.org/10.1097/HMR.0000000000000094

Poghosyan, L., Nannini, A., & Clarke, S. (2013). Organizational climate in primary care settings: Implications for nurse practitioner practice. *Journal of the American Association of Nurse Practitioners, 25*(3), 134–140. https://doi.org/10.1111/j.1745-7599.2012.00765.x

Poghosyan, L., Nannini, A., Finkelstein, S. R., Mason, E., & Shaffer, J. A. (2013). Development and psychometric testing of the Nurse Practitioner Primary Care Organizational Climate

Questionnaire. *Nursing Research, 62*(5), 325–334. https://doi.org/10.1097/NNR.0b013e3182a131d2

Rambur, B., Palumbo, M. V., McIntosh, B., & Mongeon, J. (2003). A statewide analysis of RNs' intention to leave their position. *Nursing Outlook, 51*(4), 182–188. https://doi.org/10.1016/S0029-6554(03)00115-5

Ramoo, V., Abdullah, K. L., & Piaw, C. Y. (2013). The relationship between job satisfaction and intention to leave current employment among registered nurses in a teaching hospital. *Journal of Clinical Nursing, 22*(21–22), 3141–3152. https://doi.org/10.1111/jocn.12260

Rhoades, L., & Eisenberger, R. (2002). Perceived organizational support: A review of the literature. *Journal of Applied Psychology, 87*(4), 698–714. https://doi.org/10.1037/0021-9010.87.4.698

Ribelin, P. J. (2003). Retention reflects leadership style. *Nursing Management, 34*(8), 18–19. https://journals.lww.com/nursingmanagement/Fulltext/2003/08000/Retention_reflects_leadership_style.8.aspx

Running, A., Hoffman, L., & Mercer, V. (2008). Physician perceptions of nurse practitioners: A replication study. *Journal of the American Association of Nurse Practitioners, 20*(8), 429–433. https://doi.org/10.1111/j.1745-7599.2008.00339.x

Stanik-Hutt, J., Newhouse, R. P., White, K. M., Johantgen, M., Bass, E. B., Zangaro, G., Wilson, R., Fountain, L., Steinwachs, D. M., Heindel, L., & Weiner, J. P. (2013). The quality and effectiveness of care provided by nurse practitioners. *The Journal for Nurse Practitioners, 9*(8), 492–500.e413. https://doi.org/10.1016/j.nurpra.2013.07.004

Steinke, M. K., Rogers, M., Lehwaldt, D., & Lamarche, K. (2018). An examination of advanced practice nurses' job satisfaction internationally. *International Nursing Review, 65*(2), 162–172. https://doi.org/10.1111/inr.12389

Tsay, S.-L., Tsay, S.-F., Ke, C.-Y., Chen, C.-M., & Tung, H.-H. (2019). Analysis of nurse practitioner scope of practice in Taiwan using the longest policy cycle model. *Journal of the American Association of Nurse Practitioners, 31*(3), 198–205. https://doi.org/10.1097/JXX.0000000000000127

Watts, S. A. (2019). Advance your practice to include joy and reduce burnout. *The Journal for Nurse Practitioners, 15*(5), 389–390. https://doi.org/10.1016/j.nurpra.2019.02.002

21

Motivation to Care: A Qualitative Study on Iranian Nurses

Neda ASADI[1] • Robabeh MEMARIAN[2]* • Zohreh VANAKI[3]

ABSTRACT

Background: The performance of nurses, which is rooted in personal motivation, determines the quality of care. Therefore, it is important that nurses are motivated to provide high-quality care.

Purpose: The purpose of this study was to explore the factors that affect caring motivation from the perspectives of nurses in Iran.

Methods: This was a qualitative study. Seventeen nurses were interviewed using a semistructured, in-depth interview method. The interviews were recorded, transcribed verbatim, and analyzed using content analysis.

Results: Data analysis led to the identification of the two themes of (a) self-valuation and (b) providing beneficial care.

Conclusions/Implications for Practice: The findings of this study increase scholarly understanding of the caring motivations of nurses. These motivations may be used in related programs by senior nursing managers to improve the quality of nursing care.

Key Words:
nursing, motivation, quality care.

Introduction

Motivation helps persuade and guide people to perform a special activity (Tahrekhani & Sadeghian, 2015) and has been considered as a prerequisite for better organizational performance (Aduo-Adjei, Emmanuel, & Forster, 2016). Motivation has an essential role to play in addressing challenges in the health department (Aduo-Adjei et al., 2016), underscoring that achieving health goals is greatly dependent on motivated healthcare specialists providing effective, efficient, and high-quality services (Aduo-Adjei et al., 2016). Nurses are responsible for providing a large part of healthcare services (Jooste & Hamani, 2017). Their performance is rooted in personal motivation (Toode, Routasalo, & Suominen, 2011) and determines to a great extent the quality of patient care (Jooste & Hamani, 2017).

Because motivation is not an observable phenomenon, studies have focused on examining its effective factors and outcomes. Studies have proven the importance of motivation in nurse retention and job satisfaction and associated motivation with these factors (Bonenberger, Aikins, Akweongo, & Wyss, 2014). In a nationwide study, Iranian nurses reported having a median level of job satisfaction (Negarandeh, Dehghan-Nayeri, & Ghasemi, 2015), with only one third of the nurses reporting being satisfied with their jobs (Valizadeh et al., 2016). This matter suggests a potential threat to the quality of patient care, as one of the greatest challenges to the Iranian health system is the low care quality for patients, which has been strongly associated with the self-perceived motivation of nurses (Negarandeh et al., 2015).

Trying to fulfill the expectations of nurses and to maximize their performance is a challenging task for hospital managers (Oshvandi et al., 2008). Identifying nurses' motivators may help nurse managers better identify or develop strategies to motivate nursing staffs (Negarandeh et al., 2015). Most of the recent studies in this field have adopted quantitative approaches (Koch, Proynova, Paech, & Wetter, 2014; Ojakaa, Olango, & Jarvis, 2014), and a small number of qualitative studies have identified factors that affect caring motivation in nurses (Alhyas, Nielsen, Dawoud, & Majeed, 2013).

Generally, recent studies on factors that affect motivation in nurses have been few in number and inadequate in scope (Koch et al., 2014). Personal values (Koch et al., 2014) and the specific factors influencing the caring motivation of nurses (Moody & Pesut, 2006) remain unclear. However, the process of developing motivational strategies may be made easier by determining empirical evidence and applying information on motivation to care and on the forces working to enhance or suppress caring motivation (Toode et al., 2011).

Carter and Kulbok posited that qualitative studies are more appropriate for validating the meaning and multidimensional combinations of motivation (Carter & Kulbok, 2002). Applying a qualitative approach to assessing the caring motivation of nurses is necessary when the researcher intends to inquire about the behaviors and focus

[1]*RN, Doctoral Student, Faculty of Medical Sciences, Department of Nursing, Tarbiat Modares University, Tehran, Iran* • [2]*PhD, RN, Assistant Professor, Faculty of Medical Sciences, Department of Nursing, Tarbiat Modares University, Tehran, Iran* • [3]*PhD, RN, Associate Professor, Faculty of Medical Sciences, Department of Nursing, Tarbiat Modares University, Tehran, Iran.*

on the experiences of the participants. Descriptive qualitative studies allow researchers to describe or explore a phenomenon, problem, or issue and may encompass a broad range of questions relating to lived experiences, knowledge, attitudes, feelings, perceptions, and views. Descriptive qualitative studies are less interpretive than other qualitative approaches such as phenomenological studies and grounded theory (AllahBakhshian et al., 2017).

Therefore, considering the ability of the qualitative method to discover the factors affecting caring motivation in nurses and the lack of relevant qualitative studies in this field in an Iranian cultural context, this study was designed and conducted to achieve an in-depth, comprehensive view of the factors affecting the caring motivation of Iranian nurses from the perspective of these nurses.

Methods

This study presents the caring-motivation-related experiences of nurses in Iran. The sample consisted of 17 nurses (11 women and six men). Participants had worked as nurses for between 2 and 18 years. Two of the participants had master's degrees, and 15 had bachelor's degrees. Sampling was initially purposive, and then a theoretical sampling method was applied until data saturation was reached. The first two interviews were unstructured, and data analysis was used to extract relevant concepts. Afterward, the interviews were all semistructured. The interviews began with the general question: "Please explain a caring experience for which you were relatively more motivated." The interviews continued with the question "How would you maintain your motivation of care? Describe your experiences." The subsequent questions were guided based on the information provided by the participant and on the researcher's desire to clarify relevant issues.

Ethical Considerations

Ethical approval was obtained from Tarbiat Modares University (Approval no. 52d/3711). Before participation, the goals of the study were explained to the participants and the participants provided their consent to participate and to have their interview sessions recorded. Nurses were assured that their information would remain confidential.

Data Collection

Data were collected from June to November 2016 using semistructured interviews, which were performed and recorded in a quiet and calm room at the hospitals where the participants were working. The time and place of the interviews were determined by the participants. All of the interviews, which lasted between 30 and 60 minutes, were conducted by one researcher. The interviews were recorded and transcribed verbatim. In addition, in-field notes were taken to cover all aspects of the phenomenon.

Data Analysis

Data were analyzed using conventional qualitative content analysis. The qualitative content analysis is a method for describing the meaning of qualitative data systematically. This method is executed by allocating consecutive parts of the categories into a standardized code format that covers all aspects and features of the targeted phenomenon in terms of both description and interpretation and is used as a flexible and systematic approach to reduce the physical size of data sets (Schreier, 2014). Transcripts were divided into the smallest constituent meaning units, after repeated reviews. Reviewing and cycling between the codes continued until codes were assigned to subcategories and categories based on semantic similarity to gradually develop a new concept of caring motivation.

To validate the data, the interviews and the five primary codes were given to the first five participants for checking. Their subsequent suggestions for modification were considered (member check). Furthermore, sampling was conducted to maximize variety (e.g., age, gender, work experience, ward) in line with the suggestion of previous studies.

Results

Participants in this study related their experiences with regard to caring motivation. After data analysis, the two categories of "self-valuation" and "providing beneficial care" were extracted (Table 1).

Self-Valuation

Experiences and statements of the participants relevant to the "self-valuation" category were divided into three subcategories: forming the exterior effects of the profession, self-improvement in providing care, and value-based behaviors.

Forming the exterior effects of the profession

The participants discussed the efforts that they made to show the value of their work to others. Nurses consider patients as members of society who receive their services and who thus hold the potential to significantly affect the overall image of nursing in society. Moreover, in trying to avoid leaving a negative mental image of nursing, in addition to satisfying their patients, the participants described how they had worked to

TABLE 1.
Categories and Subcategories

Category	Subcategory
Self-valuation	• Forming the exterior effects of the profession • Self-improvement in providing care • Value-based behaviors
Providing beneficial care	• Providing quality care • Effective care • Individualized care

promote the exterior effects of their profession. Participant 11 (P11), a nurse from the gastroenterology ward, mentioned:

> *Each patient indicates a family. We should represent our competency so that society will accept us better. We should provide science-based nursing work.*

Paying attention to interpersonal relationships was one of the dimensions of promoting the exterior effects of the profession. This matter was so important to the participants that one stated the belief that it was rooted in the dignity of their profession and, in this regard, stated:

> *The dignity of our profession requires us to have ethical and professional relations with collaborative groups so that they will better recognize nurses and their abilities.* (P3)

Nurses also emphasized the importance of maintaining a face-to-face relationship with their patients. In this regard, one of the participants said:

> *A nurse should not look at the serum and the device first, but should first pay attention to the patient so that the patient feels that the nurse is there for helping them, and not for checking the devices.* (P1)

Advocating the importance of nursing to others was another example of promoting the exterior effects of the profession identified in this study. In this regard, one of the participants mentioned:

> *In some cases, I have talked to the doctors and persuaded them that there are better methods, and we have agreed on a patient and their treatment method. This way, they better understand my responsibilities and duties and recognize what I am doing here and the importance of what I am doing.* (P9)

Self-improvement in providing care

The participants reflected the presumption that self-improvement is one of the most effective methods to provide care, and they worked diligently to improve their practical and scientific competencies. The participants took responsibility for their own learning. Most expressed that, to develop their abilities, they took personal initiative to update their knowledge and that, although their organizations typically ignore retraining, they participated in workshops to gain scientific information motivated by their own personal interests:

> *Most of the time I attend workshops but earn no certificate for it. But sometimes these workshops have been so useful that I wanted to go again. I am interested in learning about up-to-date information.* (P8)

In addition, participants mentioned the importance of constant learning in the field of care provision, which may affect their actual care provision practices. One of the participants said:

> *Despite being tired, many times I would search new subjects. Sometimes I will search past midnight and continue studying.* (P16)

Echoing the above sentiment, P9 mentioned:

> *The fact is, many of the issues in our work are elusive and must constantly be reviewed. I keep summaries of articles in my locker at the hospital to review whenever I can. I have never severed my relationship with my pamphlets and books.*

Furthermore, the participants related that they regularly worked to improve their communication skills. One of them noted:

> *I tried to learn many things from caring, and I owe this to my profession. When I started working, through my daily communications with the patients and the colleagues, my communication techniques have changed for the better, which is natural, as long as you are willing to try.* (P12)

Value-based behaviors

Value-based behaviors was the third subcategory of self-valuation. Disregarding the negative aspects of the caring environment, the participants worked to separate themselves from the environment and negative environmental factors. They tried to focus their attention on their patients and to not let workplace issues affect their care provision efforts. In this regard, one of the participants said:

> *I have never let my work problems interfere with my patient care. I have never thought about working less for the patients. I perform my care completely and correctly.* (P7)

Moreover, the participants expressed that they do not limit themselves to their official, expected duties and have experienced a new view toward caring to care for the patient with no expectations from others. P5 said:

> *Sometimes, I would get up at 2 a.m. and perform gavage for the patient so that I would be reassured that the patient has eaten. I dedicate my break time to my patients. I do not expect anything from anybody in return.* (P5)

In addition, the participants who were in self-perceived economic need shared that they focused on their patients despite their own financial hardships. Many of the participants mentioned this matter:

> *For me, low income has never made me work less than my duties require. I see no relationship*

between providing care and my income. If our salaries are low or delayed, it is not our patients' fault. They are innocent. The problem lies with the system. (P9)

Providing Beneficial Care

Experiences and statements of the participants regarding providing beneficial care were distinguished into three subcategories, which are discussed below.

Providing quality care

From the point of view of many participants, the most desirable manner for providing care indicated quality care. This means that care is offered safely and based on relevant nursing standards without discriminatory behaviors during the caring process. The following reflects participant experiences in this subcategory:

> *When you adopt a specific format, you must abide by its standards. The standards should not be omitted. I have always tried to make the standards flexible in order to provide better-quality care.* (P4)

Most of the participants expressed the belief that quality of nursing care depended on patient satisfaction. In this regard, one of the participants stated:

> *I always put my patient's satisfaction first and, therefore, provide the best care that I can. If my patient is poor or illiterate, this does not change my behavior toward him or her. I always try to provide quality care for all of my patients.* (P14)

In addition, one participant mentioned the observance of safety in providing care as another dimension of providing quality care, stating:

> *You should be very accurate in all of these concerns and duties. You should not forget your patient's medication or mistakenly give their medication twice.* (P1)

Effective care

The participants reported that they try to provide effective care in ways that reduce patient pain and improve their condition to achieve desirable caring outcomes. In this regard, the participants mentioned:

> *On days that I am working, I will do my best to ensure that my patient feels less pain, so that my care is effective for them. I help my patients, even those who are about to pass away, so that they will pass more comfortably and in less pain.* (P9)

Helping patients be discharged sooner was another standard that the participants considered in providing effective care. One stated:

> *The most important thing that I can do is to provide high quality care so that my patient can be discharged sooner and go back to his/her work and life.* (P3)

In addition, the participants mentioned that they would attend to the mental condition of their patients during care and that they would try to reduce patients' concerns and raise their spirits. One of the participants said:

> *I do as much as I can for my patient to reduce their concerns. It is important for me as a nurse to be able to relieve my patients' concerns.* (P5)

The lived experiences and remarks of the participants in this regard indicated that the morale of nurses may be improved by the recovery of their patients. One of the participants mentioned:

> *Not adding to their problems is the best help for the patient. This also has a positive effect on the nurse's spirit too.* (P4)

Individualized care

Avoiding routine-based work and paying attention to the personal differences of patients were some of the measures used by the participants. In this regard, participants mentioned:

> *Each patient is different from the others in my eyes. It never becomes repetitious for me. I mean, I do not believe that caring is just physical work. One patient is interested in reading, so I suggest to his/her companions to bring some books or magazines. Another one likes music, so I play music.* (P9)

The experiences of participants in this subcategory indicated that, by paying attention to the needs of their patients, they were working to avoid providing only routine care:

> *One thing that I consider really important is evaluating the needs of patients. I mean, the patient's needs must be the basis for our work. The routines are not applicable for everyone.* (P3)

Discussion

This study described the self-perceived caring motivations of Iranian nurses. One motivation was promoting the exterior effects of the nursing profession by showing the importance of their work to others and creating a positive image in the minds of the patients. Studies have shown that the public image of nurses does not always match their professional image (ten Hoeve, Jansen, & Roodbol, 2014). In Iran, many people think of nurses merely as physicians' assistants (Nasrabadi & Emami, 2006) and the public image of nurses is weak (Alilu, Valizadeh, Zamanzadeh, Habibzadeh, & Gillespie, 2016). According to participants in Iran in the study by Nasrabadi and Emami, nurses are the healthcare workers who are least respected by the general public. A contributing factor for this is the hierarchical relationship between doctors and nurses. This originates from differences in education and from the historical role of nurses and physicians (Nasrabadi & Emami, 2006). The negative and incorrect attitude of people toward nurses is considered as one of the important factors that decreases the motivation of nurses to provide clinical care (Alilu et al., 2016). To modify the reputation of the nursing profession, it is necessary to replace the traditional viewpoint with a more realistic and correct viewpoint. In highlighting the abilities of nurses, the nursing profession is trying to adjust the social position of the nursing profession.

Participants in this study mentioned that professional self-improvement was another concept that motivated them to provide care. Concepts such as self-improvement are in accordance with nursing goals, which include providing care and maintaining internal motivation. Empowerment in the workplace could allow staffs to explore their creativity and provide appropriate solutions in situations that may even lie outside their area of responsibility (Papathanasiou et al., 2014). In Atefi, Abdullah, and Wong (2016), Malaysian nurses mentioned that professional development was one of the most important factors affecting motivation and was critical in improving their knowledge and skills to handle complicated patient needs. These results are all in line with the results of this study, which identified that nurses updating their information by participating in workshops and constant learning was necessary to maintaining motivation to provide care.

According to the results of this study, improving communication skills through professional interactions and providing care was a factor affecting care motivation. Nursing is a combination of knowledge, clinical practice, and interpersonal communications, and as a healthcare science, its performance requires not only scientific knowledge but also interpersonal skills and abilities (Kourkouta & Papathanasiou, 2014). Zhu, Chen, Shi, Liang, and Liu (2016) emphasized that, in addition to revealing the professional values of nurses, this competency should lead to improved nursing care quality and improved nurse–patient relations.

As mentioned earlier, the participants applied value-based behaviors that were beyond their role requirements and were not acknowledged or rewarded directly or publicly by the organization. Studies have revealed that these behaviors not only provide the basis for positive acts and participation but also prepare the ground for tolerating irregular costs, discomforts, and minor frustrations, which are frequently associated with organizational jobs (Lin & Hsiao, 2014) and are considered one of the most important factors affecting the quality of service provision (Hadjali & Salimi, 2012). Furthermore, Osman, Othman, Rana, Solaiman, and Lal (2015) showed that work motivation is strongly associated with these behaviors.

The willingness of nurses to provide beneficial care was a significant finding of this study. In talking about their overall experiences and perceptions of caring motivations, the participants described their work as humane. Helping others, they felt, was based on a humanistic perspective and a desire to help care for sick people. Newton, Kelly, Kremser, Jolly, and Billett (2009) identified four core motivations for individuals to choose a career in nursing: (a) a desire to help, (b) caring, (c) sense of achievement, and (d) self-validation. Newton et al.'s descriptions of the first and second themes are consistent with the findings of this study, in which caring was the dominant theme identified. Nurse participants in the study of Isfahan, Hosseini, Khoshknab, Peyrovi, and Khanke (2015) stated that a deep understanding of patients' clinical conditions and realizing the problems of patients and their families facilitated the emergence of ideas and new solutions that effectively reduced patient/patient–family problems and helped both the patients and hospital colleagues. Nurses have stated that they cannot be indifferent toward the pains and the physical, mental, and financial problems of hospitalized patients and that they would be willing to provide more and better services to the patients (Shahsavari Isfahani, Hosseini, Fallahi Khoshknab, Peyrovi, & Khanke, 2015). Results of this study found that the participants intended to provide safe, standardized nursing care so that they would be able to provide a good quality of care. In Kieft, de Brouwer, Francke, and Delnoij (2014), participants considered technical skills to be an aspect of nursing expertise and critical to providing care that is both effective and safe.

In most previous studies addressing level of motivation in individuals, working conditions were shown to relate positively to both quality of care and the enforcement of safety standards for patients. This indicates the need to incorporate motivation promotion strategies into quality improvement programs at healthcare centers (Alhassan et al., 2013).

Conclusions

In light of the key role played by nurses in improving patient outcomes, the healthcare system should encourage nurses to think and act beyond their usual roles and to engage in constant learning to maximize healthcare system outcomes in terms of both care outcomes and patient-perceived care quality. The findings and recommendations of this study may be used by senior nursing managers in programs that are designed to improve the quality of nursing care.

Limitations

The data for this study were gathered from only one healthcare facility and university and thus may not be representative of nurses in other organizations. Although the sample size was substantial and was sufficient in terms of qualitative research standards, the results may not be widely generalizable beyond the study population and sufficiently analogous settings.

Acknowledgments

Special thanks to the participants in this study for sharing their time and experiences. This study was funded by Tarbiat Modares University (52d/3711).

References

Aduo-Adjei, K., Emmanuel, O., & Forster, O. M. (2016). The impact of motivation on the work performance of health workers (Korle Bu Teachi1g Hospital): Evidence from Ghana. *Hospital Practices and Research, 1*(2), 47–52. https://doi.org/10.20286/HPR-010245

Alhassan, R. K., Spieker, N., van Ostenberg, P., Ogink, A., Nketiah-Amponsah, E., & de Wit, T. F. (2013). Association between health worker motivation and healthcare quality efforts in Ghana. *Human Resources for Health, 11*(1), 37. https://doi.org/10.1186/1478-4491-11-37

Alhyas, L., Nielsen, J. D. J., Dawoud, D., & Majeed, A. (2013). Factors affecting the motivation of healthcare professionals providing care to Emiratis with type 2 diabetes. *Journal of the Royal Society of Medicine Short Reports, 4*(2), 14. https://doi.org/10.1177/2042533313476419

Alilu, L., Valizadeh, L., Zamanzadeh, V., Habibzadeh, H., & Gillespie, M. (2016). A qualitative exploration of facilitators and inhibitors influencing nurses' intention to leave clinical nursing. *University of São Paulo Nursing School Journal, 50*(6), 982–989. https://doi.org/10.1590/s0080-623420160000700015

AllahBakhshian, M., Alimohammadi, N., Taleghani, F., Nik, A. Y., Abbasi, S., & Gholizadeh, L. (2017). Barriers to intensive care unit nurses' autonomy in Iran: A qualitative study. *Nursing Outlook, 65*(4), 392–399. https://doi.org/10.1016/j.outlook.2016.12.004

Atefi, N., Abdullah, K. L., & Wong, L. P. (2016). Job satisfaction of Malaysian registered nurses: A qualitative study. *Nursing in Critical Care, 21*(1), 8–17. https://doi.org/10.1111/nicc.12100

Bonenberger, M., Aikins, M., Akweongo, P., & Wyss, K. (2014). The effects of health worker motivation and job satisfaction on turnover intention in Ghana: A cross-sectional study. *Human Resources for Health, 12*(1), 43. https://doi.org/10.1186/1478-4491-12-43

Carter, K. F., & Kulbok, P. A. (2002). Motivation for health behaviours: A systematic review of the nursing literature. *Journal of Advanced Nursing, 40*(3), 316–330. https://doi.org/10.1046/j.1365-2648.2002.02373.x

Hadjali, H. R., & Salimi, M. (2012). An investigation on the effect of organizational citizenship behaviors (OCB) toward customer-orientation: A case of nursing home. *Procedia-Social and Behavioral Sciences, 57*, 524–532. https://doi.org/10.1016/j.sbspro.2012.09.1220

Jooste, K., & Hamani, M. (2017). The motivational needs of primary health care nurses to acquire power as leaders in a mine clinic setting. *Health SA Gesondheid, 22*, 43–51. https://doi.org/10.1016/j.hsag.2016.09.005

Kieft, R. A., de Brouwer, B. B., Francke, A. L., & Delnoij, D. M. (2014). How nurses and their work environment affect patient experiences of the quality of care: A qualitative study. *BMC Health Services Research, 14*(1), 249. https://doi.org/10.1186/1472-6963-14-249

Koch, S. H., Proynova, R., Paech, B., & Wetter, T. (2014). The perfectly motivated nurse and the others: Workplace and personal characteristics impact preference of nursing tasks. *Journal of Nursing Management, 22*(8), 1054–1064. https://doi.org/10.1111/jonm.12083

Kourkouta, L., & Papathanasiou, I. V. (2014). Communication in nursing practice. *Materia Socio-Medica, 26*(1), 65–67. https://doi.org/10.5455/msm.2014.26.65-67

Lin, R. S. J., & Hsiao, J. K. (2014). The relationships between transformational leadership, knowledge sharing, trust and organizational citizenship behavior. *International Journal of Innovation, Management and Technology, 5*(3), 171–174. https://doi.org/10.7763/IJIMT.2014.V5.508

Moody, R. C., & Pesut, D. J. (2006). The motivation to care: Application and extension of motivation theory to professional nursing work. *Journal of Health Organization and Management, 20*(1), 15–48.

Nasrabadi, A. N., & Emami, A. (2006). Perceptions of nursing practice in Iran. *Nursing Outlook, 54*(6), 320–327. https://doi.org/10.1016/j.outlook.2006.06.001

Negarandeh, R., Dehghan-Nayeri, N., & Ghasemi, E. (2015). Motivating factors among Iranian nurses. *Iranian Journal of Nursing and Midwifery Research, 20*(4), 436–441. https://doi.org/10.4103/1735-9066.161011

Newton, J. M., Kelly, C. M., Kremser, A. K., Jolly, B., & Billett, S. (2009). The motivations to nurse: An exploration of factors amongst undergraduate students, registered nurses and nurse managers. *Journal of Nursing Management, 17*(3), 392–400. https://doi.org/10.1111/j.1365-2834.2008.00945.x

Ojakaa, D., Olango, S., & Jarvis, J. (2014). Factors affecting motivation and retention of primary health care workers in three disparate regions in Kenya. *Human Resources for Health, 12*(1), 33. https://doi.org/10.1186/1478-4491-12-33

Oshvandi, K., Zamanzadeh, V., Ahmadi, F., Fathi-Azar, E., Anthony, D. M., & Harris, T. (2008). Barriers to nursing job motivation. *Research Journal of Biological Sciences, 3*(4), 426–434.

Osman, A., Othman, Y. H., Rana, S. M. S., Solaiman, M., & Lal, B. (2015). The influence of job satisfaction, job motivation & perceived organizational support towards organizational citizenship behavior (OCB): A perspective of American-based organization in Kulim, Malaysia. *Asian Social Science, 11*(21), 174–182. https://doi.org/10.5539/ass.v11n21p174

Papathanasiou, I. V., Fradelos, E. C., Kleisiaris, C. F., Tsaras, K., Kalota, M. A., & Kourkouta, L. (2014). Motivation, leadership, empowerment and confidence: Their relation with nurses' burnout. *Materia Socio-Medica, 26*(6), 405–410. https://doi.org/10.5455/msm.2014.26.405-410

Schreier, M. (2014). Qualitative content analysis. In U. Flick (Ed.), *The SAGE handbook of qualitative data analysis* (1st ed., pp. 170–183). Los Angeles, CA: Sage. https://doi.org/10.4135/9781446282243.n12

Shahsavari Isfahani, S., Hosseini, M. A., Fallahi Khoshknab, M. F., Peyrovi, H., & Khanke, H. R. (2015). What really motivates Iranian nurses to be creative in clinical settings?: A qualitative study. *Global Journal of Health Science*, *7*(5), 132–142. https://doi.org/10.5539/gjhs.v7n5p132

Tahrekhani, M., & Sadeghian, Z. (2015). Intrinsic motivation comparative investigation between nursery, midwifery, and medicine students during internship in Iran. *Procedia-Social and Behavioral Sciences*, *185*, 185–189. https://doi.org/10.1016/j.sbspro.2015.03.447

ten Hoeve, Y., Jansen, G., & Roodbol, P. (2014). The nursing profession: Public image, self-concept and professional identity. A discussion paper. *Journal of Advanced Nursing*, *70*(2), 295–309. https://doi.org/10.1111/jan.12177

Toode, K., Routasalo, P., & Suominen, T. (2011). Work motivation of nurses: A literature review. *International Journal of Nursing Studies*, *48*(2), 246–257. https://doi.org/10.1016/j.ijnurstu.2010.09.013

Valizadeh, L., Zamanzadeh, V., Habibzadeh, H., Alilu, L., Gillespie, M., & Shakibi, A. (2016). Experiences of Iranian nurses that intent to leave the clinical nursing: A content analysis. *Journal of Caring Sciences*, *5*(2), 169–178. https://doi.org/10.15171/jcs.2016.018

Zhu, B., Chen, C. R., Shi, Z. Y., Liang, H. X., & Liu, B. (2016). Mediating effect of self-efficacy in relationship between emotional intelligence and clinical communication competency of nurses. *International Journal of Nursing Sciences*, *3*(2), 162–168. https://doi.org/10.1016/j.ijnss.2016.04.003

The Development and Evaluation of an Analytical Framework to Explore Student Nurses' Cultural Beliefs of Dementia

Omorogieva OJO[1]* • Joanne BROOKE[2] • Camille CRONIN[3]

ABSTRACT

Background: People diagnosed with dementia need culturally sensitive, person-centered care to promote their health and well-being. Therefore, healthcare professionals should be able to provide culturally competent care, of which an element is the understanding of their own cultural heritage and how this impacts on their beliefs regarding dementia, as cultural norms and values provide meanings and understanding of chronic conditions such as dementia. This study used focus groups to explore the cultural beliefs of student nurses regarding dementia, generating a large set of qualitative data that required structure and a framework to analyze.

Purpose: One purpose of this article was to present the methodological analysis, which encompasses the analytical framework. The second purpose was to apply the framework to elicit the cultural beliefs regarding dementia among student nurses from multiple national backgrounds.

Methods: Focus groups with student nurses from five higher education institutes in England, the Philippines, Slovenia, and New Zealand were conducted, audiotaped, and transcribed verbatim. The qualitative data were analyzed using the framework method of analysis. Data from the focus groups conducted at the two higher education institutes in England were analyzed by encompassed synthesizing, refining, and agreeing on the codes, categories, and themes that were established separately by four researchers. The developed analytical framework was then tested on the qualitative data obtained from the focus groups conducted in Slovenia, the Philippines, and New Zealand.

Results: The results were presented in three parts: the cultural analytical framework, the process of developing the initial categories/themes, and the final themes that emerged from the data obtained from the focus groups.

Conclusions: An analytical framework was developed and applied to understand student nurses' cultural values and beliefs of dementia.

KEY WORDS:
framework analysis, dementia, culture, student nurses, qualitative analysis.

Introduction

Globally, it is estimated that 135.5 million people will be living with dementia by 2050, with an estimated 10 million new cases identified every year (World Health Organization, 2015). Dementia is a progressive terminal syndrome that affects memory, thinking, behavior, and activities of daily living (World Health Organization, 2017). The needs of people with dementia are unique to each individual as well as complex and dynamic, requiring culturally appropriate and responsive health and social care services (Alzheimer's Society, 2014; Dilworth-Anderson & Gibson, 2002).

Culture has been defined as a set of shared symbols, beliefs, and customs that define individual and/or group behavior (Dilworth-Anderson & Gibson, 2002). Culture includes shared patterns of behaviors and interactions as well as understandings that are learned through socialization. Culture may be seen as the growth of a group identity fostered by social patterns that are unique to that group and that change over time (Spencer-Oatey, 2012). Furthermore, some cultural norms and values provide meanings and understanding of syndromes such as dementia and enable collective knowledge within a group (Ow Yong & Manthorpe, 2016).

The need to consider the experiences of people with dementia from diverse cultural backgrounds and the need to provide culturally competent care have been widely acknowledged (Mullay, Schofield, Clarke, & Primrose, 2011). Cultural competence, the capacity of healthcare workers to provide culturally appropriate care to people with diverse values and

[1]*PhD, Senior Lecturer, Faculty of Education and Health, University of Greenwich, London, UK*• [2]*Professional Doctorate, Professor, Faculty of Health, Education & Life Sciences, Birmingham City University, Birmingham, UK*• [3]*PhD, Senior Lecturer, School of Health and Social Care, Southend Campus, University of Essex, Essex, UK.*

beliefs, is essential to providing person-centered care to people with dementia (Mullay et al., 2011).

Ethnicity and culture may affect the care that nurses provide to people with dementia (Ow Yong & Manthorpe, 2016) through the influence of underlying cultural assumptions and perspectives (Mullay et al., 2011) as well as dementia-related stigmas and shame and beliefs that dementia is a normal part of aging (Flaskerud, 2009). Consequently, nurses must understand their own cultural beliefs and values to provide culturally competent care to people with dementia (Brooke, Cronin, Stiell, & Ojo, 2018). Furthermore, this understanding will help nurses apply the concepts of person-centered care from the cultural perspective of the person with dementia (Doyle & Rubinstein, 2014; Johnston & Narayanasamy, 2016).

In many European countries, the nursing workforce has become culturally diverse because of the recruitment of nurses from Asian, African, and other European countries (Egede-Nissen, Sellevold, Jakobsen, & Sørlie, 2017). Moreover, the student nurse population is becoming increasingly culturally diverse. Therefore, the factors that may influence their beliefs, perceptions, and understandings about dementia must be evaluated and addressed to develop a culturally sensitive workforce (McKenzie & Brown, 2014).

One purpose of this article was to present the methodological analysis, which encompasses the analytical framework. The second purpose was to apply the framework to elicit the cultural beliefs regarding dementia among student nurses from England, Slovenia, the Philippines, and New Zealand.

Methods

This article draws on the framework method of data analysis defined by Gale, Heath, Cameron, Rashid, and Redwood (2013). Therefore, a cultural analytical framework was developed and then applied to support the interpretation of nursing students' cultural beliefs regarding dementia. The data will be discussed in a separate article.

The data were collected via focus groups, which allowed students to be recruited from naturally occurring groups, where existing relationships and social context support a deeper conversation on cultural beliefs regarding dementia (Brown, 2015; Githaiga, 2014). All focus groups were audio recorded and transcribed verbatim. The framework method of data analysis defined by Gale et al. (2013) was applied.

The Framework Method of Data Analysis

The framework method of analysis is one of many approaches to thematic analysis and qualitative content analysis (Gale et al., 2013). Framework analysis was first conceptualized in the 1980s by the National Centre for Social Research to support the analysis of qualitative data in applied policy research (Dixon-Woods, 2011). This approach to analysis entails the development of a matrix of thematic categories into which data may then be coded (Dixon-Woods, 2011). Moreover, this approach ensures that themes and concepts identified through knowledge or reasoning can be combined with other new themes or concepts that may emerge (Dixon-Woods, 2011).

Framework analysis is used widely in healthcare research, as it enables flexibility and team work while providing a rigorous and systematic method for conducting qualitative data analysis (Dixon-Woods, 2011; Ward, Furber, Tierney, & Swallow, 2013). Despite the use of framework analysis as an approach to qualitative data analysis in fields such as psychology, social policy, and nursing research (Parkinson, Eatough, Holmes, Stapley, & Midgley, 2016), this approach has rarely been used to explore cultural beliefs and values regarding dementia across different student nurse populations.

Gale et al. (2013) described seven stages of framework analysis, as follows:

Stage 1: Transcription – involves a good audio recording and a word-for-word transcription of the focus group interviews.

Stage 2: Familiarization – enables the researchers to know the data extensively by immersing themselves in the transcript and being able to gain a sense of the focus groups before coding and identifying recurring themes.

Stage 3: Coding – in this stage, the researcher reads every line of the transcript carefully and applies labels, codes, or paraphrasing that provides a description of what they have read in the transcript.

Stage 4: Developing a working analytical framework – all of the researchers meet to organize the data meaningfully to identify recurring and important themes.

Stage 5: Applying the analytical framework – this involves indexing subsequent transcripts by applying the conceptual framework that was developed in Stage 4. This enables the extraction of data into theoretical themes and subthemes.

Stage 6: Charting data into the framework matrix – involves organizing and summarizing the data in chart form to make the data more manageable. A spreadsheet may be used for the matrix, and the data are charted into the matrix.

Stage 7: Interpreting the data – involves synthesizing and interpreting the data, allowing refinement of the themes and subthemes, which enables the overall development of a conceptual framework. This stage involves the comparison of themes and subthemes and checking against the original transcripts and audio recordings to ensure appropriate context.

Development of the Cultural Analytical Framework

The cultural analytical framework was developed from data acquired during a multicenter and multinational study involving focus groups (n = 23) with nursing students from five higher education institutes (HEIs), including two institutes in England (n = 81 nursing students) and one institution each in the Philippines (n = 53), Slovenia (n = 41), and New Zealand (n = 6). Data were collected between November 2016 and December 2017.

The development and preliminary testing of the cultural analytical framework encompassed a review of the framework method of analysis of qualitative research described by Gale et al. (2013) and Spencer, Ritchie, Ormston, O'Connor, and Barnard (2014; Figure 1). The focus groups were then facilitated and audio recorded at two HEIs in England. Focus groups were transcribed and analyzed separately by four researchers using framework analysis (Gale et al., 2013; Parveen, Peltier, & Oyebode, 2017; Robertshaw & Cross, 2017). To ensure transparency and reflexivity, all of the stages (Gale et al., 2013; Spencer et al., 2014) were carefully followed by the researchers.

Familiarization, coding, and categorization of data

The data from the focus groups that were conducted at the two HEIs in England were analyzed independently by four experienced researchers using a process that included familiarization, coding, and categorization (Table 1). The researchers read and reread the transcripts to become familiar with the data, analyzed and reanalyzed the data, and checked and rechecked the data at different stages. The codes were developed independently by the four researchers, who used labels or paraphrases to denote their interpretations of passages in the transcripts. The four researchers then met multiple times to discuss the respective codes, agree on a common set of codes for the data, and categorize the codes into themes (Table 1). Codes with similar meanings or concepts were aggregated into the same category.

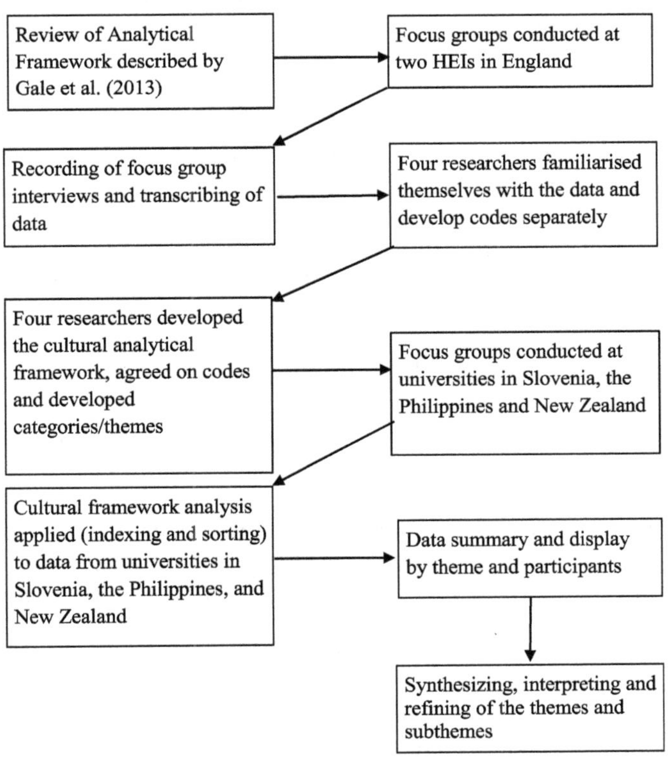

Figure 1. Process of developing the cultural analytical framework and its use in evaluating the dementia care experiences of nursing students.

TABLE 1.
Coding and Categorization

Category/Theme	Code
Defining dementia	1. Biological dementia
	2. Social and emotional dementia (impact on patient and family)
	3. Cultural and religious dementia
	4. Types of dementia
Experience and education	5. Experience
	6. Family
	7. Moving countries
	8. Carer to student
	9. First to third year
	10. Knowledge and awareness
Dementia language	11. Dementia as other
	12. Aggression
	13. Avoiding discussion
	14. Fear
	15. Stigma
	16. Media
Care setting	17. Family/own homes
	18. Care homes
	19. Acute hospitals
Care roles	20. Family
	21. Cultural
	22. Specialized
	23. Nursing
Ethical issues	24. Control
	25. Trust/honesty
	26. Capacity
	27. Institutionalization
	28. Resource/impact
Cultural perceptions	29. Growing up with dementia (in and out of the United Kingdom)
	30. Different generations
	31. Labeling
	32. Different cultural approaches to care

The cultural analytical framework was further developed by drawing on, synthesizing, and refining the codes and categories/themes that were established by the four researchers based on the data obtained from the two participating universities (Palmer et al., 2018; Roberts & Goodhand, 2018). This process involved the four researchers working together and having lengthy discussions to resolve disagreements and later to reach agreement regarding the themes that had emerged. Each stage of the framework was discussed exhaustively, and agreement on the final set of themes was achieved through consensus.

Preliminary testing of the cultural analytical framework

The cultural analytical framework was tested on the qualitative data that had been obtained from focus groups conducted in Slovenia, the Philippines, and New Zealand. Familiarization with the data was achieved by reading and rereading the transcripts. The codes and categories that had been identified from the framework developed using the two HEIs in England were used to analyze the qualitative data obtained from the three participating non-English HEIs. The data were analyzed one institution at a time, and the framework was developed to support the integration of the analysis of data from each HEI. This process included indexing and sorting all of the qualitative data (Akinlua, Meakin, & Freemantle, 2017; Spencer et al., 2014). Themes and subthemes were developed from all of the data and then revised and recategorized until the four researchers agreed on all of the final themes and subthemes (Sedekia, Jones, Nathan, Schellenberg, & Marchant, 2017; Smith et al., 2017). The four researchers worked cooperatively until all disagreements had been harmoniously resolved and full agreement had been achieved.

Whereas the four researchers analyzed the data from the Philippines and New Zealand, the Slovenian data were analyzed by researchers from Slovenia using the original framework, with direct quotes provided and included in the analysis.

Ethical Considerations

Ethical approval was sought and obtained from the Ethical Committee of the University of Greenwich (UREC/15.5.5.16). All of the students who had expressed interest in participating were briefed using the same information sheet, signed a consent form, and agreed to participate before being enrolled as participants.

Results

The results of this study are presented in the following three parts: cultural analytical framework (Table 1), the process of developing the initial categories/themes (Table 2), and the final themes (Table 3).

The Cultural Analytical Framework

In Table 1, the first conceptual analytical framework, a table of themes and codes, shows 32 codes ranging from biological dementia to aggression, family/own homes, capacity, and different cultural approaches to care. The first column of the framework enabled the categorization of the codes into themes. Thus, seven categories are shown.

Development of Themes and Subthemes

The seven themes/categories identified in this study included "defining dementia," "experience and education," "dementia language," "care setting," "care roles," "ethical issues," and "cultural perceptions." These themes were further associated with 29 subthemes (Table 2) that had emerged from the final data analysis. After further refinement, "cultural and religious dementia" was upgraded from a subtheme of "defining dementia" to the theme "religion and spirituality," and the "experience and education" theme was renamed and amalgamated with the original theme of "cultural perceptions," which was renamed "dementia over generations." Furthermore, "care settings" and "care roles" were amalgamated, and a range of subthemes, including "experience," "family," "moving countries," and "carer to student" were also moved to other themes (Table 2). The decisions for each stage of the analytical process were achieved through the cooperative efforts, rigorous discussions, disagreements, and agreements among the researchers, with resolutions reached through consensus.

The abovementioned process of refinement resulted in a final set of six themes (defining dementia, dementia language, care settings and roles, ethical issues, dementia over generations, and religion and spirituality) and 22 subthemes (Table 3). Further refinement of the themes to ensure a clear focus on cultural beliefs regarding dementia occurred, resulting in two major themes, "familial piety" and "dementia discourse," with the former encompassing five subthemes (familial experience, growing up, intergenerational, cultural view of aging, and family/own home) and the latter encompassing only three subthemes (aggression, stigma, and patience; Table 3). Selected quotes from nursing student participants at the participating HEIs are presented in the findings article (Brooke et al., 2019).

Discussion

This cultural analytical framework was established based on the principles of framework analysis (Gale et al., 2013) and developed using the cultural beliefs regarding dementia of student nurses from four different countries. Qualitative data must be analyzed using a set of principles (Smith & Firth, 2011). The principles underlying the analysis conducted in this article include transcribing the focus group interviews, gaining detailed insights into the phenomena under study using data review, coding the data, and linking the codes or units of data to form broad categories or themes that may guide the theory development process (Dixon-Woods, 2011; Smith & Firth, 2011).

This study applied the seven stages of framework analysis (Gale et al., 2013) to develop a cultural analytical framework that may be used to analyze the cultural beliefs of student nurses regarding dementia.

The processes used in the framework approach to analyze data involve numerous stages that enable researchers to move across the data in different directions until they develop an understanding of the essence of the data and the emerging themes (Smith & Firth, 2011). The constant refinement of themes in this study presented in Tables 1–3 led to the development of a conceptual framework.

TABLE 2.
Development and Change of Themes and Subthemes

Theme	Subtheme
Defining dementia	- Biological dementia - Social and emotional dementia - Cultural and religious dementia → moved to become a new theme "religion and spirituality" - Types of dementia
Experience and education → renamed and amalgamated with "cultural perceptions"	- Experience of dementia → moved to theme "defining dementia" - Family → moved to "care roles" or "care settings" (depending on each quote) - Moving countries → moved to new theme "dementia over generations" - Career to student → moved to "nursing" in "care roles"
Dementia language	- Dementia as other - Aggression - Avoiding discussion - Fear - Stigma - Media
Care settings → amalgamated with "care roles"	- Family/own homes - Care homes - Acute hospital
Care roles → amalgamated with "care settings"	- Family - Cultural → removed as now an overarching theme - Specialized - Nursing
Ethical issues	- Control - Trust and honesty → changed to "trust and therapeutic lying" - Capacity - Institutionalization → moved to "care homes" in "care settings"
Cultural perceptions → renamed "dementia over generations"	- Growing up with - Different generations - Labeling → moved to dementia as other in "dementia language" - Different cultural approaches to care

Limitations to the framework analysis approach have been discussed in the literature (Akinlua et al., 2017; Robertshaw & Cross, 2017; Ward et al., 2013). Ward et al. (2013) used a worked example and highlighted that framework analysis may be excessively time consuming. A review of other studies noted that, although Parveen et al. (2017) had used framework analysis to evaluate the perceptions of dementia and use of services among minority ethnic communities in the United Kingdom, participants were recruited at community events rather than purposively sampled, and no ethnic Whites were included in the sample. Moreover, the analysis relied on notes made by the research facilitator rather than on recordings and transcripts.

Similarly, Robertshaw, and Cross (2017) applied framework analysis to study the experiences of integrated dementia care from the perspectives of patient family members and care providers. Although the study relied on an open online course, which made the course accessible to a wide range of participants, including hard-to-reach groups, the study did not hold follow-up activities or probe further to clarify/resolve outstanding questions. Furthermore, the study lacked the rigor and depth of more traditional qualitative research studies and did not provide participants the opportunity to review the responses of other participants.

Data management often involves immersion in the data through reading and rereading, identifying the initial themes/categories, developing a coding matrix, and assigning data to the themes and categories in the coding matrix (Smith & Firth, 2011). According to Spencer, Ritchie, and O'Connor (2003), the data management stage involves generating a set of themes and concepts from which data are labeled, sorted, and synthesized.

Moreover, the process of qualitative data analysis involves obtaining descriptive accounts that summarize and synthesize the range of coded data by refining initial themes and categories, identifying the associations among the themes until the "whole picture" emerges, and developing more abstract concepts (Smith & Firth, 2011). This process typically involves

TABLE 3.
Further Development and Refining of Themes and Subthemes

Refined Theme	Initial Subtheme	Final Theme	Final Subtheme	Selected Quote
Defining dementia	Biological dementia Social and emotional dementia Types of dementia Experience of dementia	Familial piety	Familial experience	GFG1, P1 (Black British, Caribbean), p4, 87–89: *"So, just being able to deal with people with dementia. I was able to deal with my granddad and that made the difference because I understand what is like living with dementia."*
Care settings and roles	Family/own homes Care homes Acute hospital Specialized Nursing		Growing up	SFG1, P2 (Filipino), p14, 311–315: *"So, growing up I see my mother taking care of relatives, so I would never send my parents to a nursing home. For me it is because they have devoted their lives to me to take care of me, so I would also do the same for them. So that is just me, that is what I have seen, what my Mum has done, so I think that relates to my culture."*
Dementia over generations	Growing up with dementia Different generations Different cultural approaches Moving countries		Intergenerational	EFG2, P1 (White British), p17, 386–390: *"I think me and my sister have a better understanding, well maybe not a better understanding, but a different attitude towards it maybe, more understanding of it and using less stigmatic words, so we would never say demented or senile, we wouldn't say he was mad, but I don't really know why that is...."*
			Cultural view of aging	SFG3, P5 (Filipino), p6, 124–126: *"Aging is when adults get old they forget things, it is normal, so that is why they don't seek medical care because it is just a normal part of aging, it is normal, they just ignore it."*
			Family/own home	GFG1, P1 (Black British, Caribbean), p15, 337–338: *"So, as a family, we will deal with this at home. We will try our best to work with what they have and what we have got as resources to help them."*
Dementia language	Dementia as other Aggression Avoiding discussion Fear Stigma Media	Dementia discourse	Aggression	GFG2, P2 (White British), p5, 141–144: *"I didn't really realize that only, that patients with dementia could get aggressive, but it didn't really come into my head, I didn't think that they would and that was on my experience when I was on hospital placement and saw a dementia patient come in aggressive and I was like gosh. I didn't realize that it could go to that level."*
Ethical issues	Control Trust and therapeutic lying Capacity		Stigma	GFG2, P5 (White British), p2, 39: *"One of the beliefs that I have is, is that dementia can be a label."*
			Patience	SFG1, P3 (Filipino), 70–72: *"That is true I think these people need extra care, so as nurses we need to be extra patient as well."*
Religion and spirituality	No subthemes identified	Dropped from analysis, as a weak theme from only a couple of focus groups from England		

Note. G = Greenwich; S = Silliman; E = Essex; FG = focus group number; P = participant number; p = page number, lines.

using synthesized data to prepare descriptive accounts, identifying key dimensions, and mapping the range and diversity of each phenomenon (Spencer et al., 2003).

The explanatory accounts relate to developing associations/patterns within the concepts and themes and then reflecting on the original data and analytical stages to ensure that participant accounts are correctly presented (Smith & Firth, 2011). This process aims to reduce the risk of misinterpretation (Smith & Firth, 2011). Although these processes are useful, the authors of this article have shown further fidelity with respect to the approach that was used to develop the framework, the application of this framework in qualitative data analysis, and the clarity of the methods used. The stepwise approach used in this study was transparent, making it easy for researchers from institutions in different geographical areas to interpret and follow. In addition, the framework method of analysis is not tied to any theoretical approach, which helps ensure flexibility.

Implications for Practice

One of the goals of using framework analysis in the study of dementia is enabling the evaluation of the experiences of student nurses from different cultural backgrounds to address any significant gaps in knowledge and understanding. In addition, areas identified as inadequate may be referenced by nursing educators and added to or reinforced in the nursing curriculum. Finally, this approach facilitates the continued professional development of nursing students in terms of promoting culturally sensitive, person-centered dementia care.

Conclusions

In this study, a cultural analytical framework was developed and applied to elicit and clarify the cultural values and beliefs of student nurses regarding dementia. Despite the many qualitative approaches available to study this topic, researchers who clearly and transparently use framework analysis through the steps of transcription, familiarization, coding, developing a working analytical framework, applying the analytical framework, charting data into the framework matrix, and interpreting the data will be able to present their work in a valid and reliable framework matrix. This study applied framework analysis to develop a cultural analytical framework that was used to analyze data obtained from student nurses. However, further work is required to define and refine this framework to consider cultures that were not included in the original study.

Author Contributions

Study conception and design: All authors
Data collection: All authors
Data analysis and interpretation: All authors
Drafting of the article: OO
Critical revision of the article: All authors.

References

Akinlua, J. T., Meakin, R., & Freemantle, N. (2017). Beliefs about hypertension among Nigerian immigrants to the United Kingdom: A qualitative study. *PLOS ONE, 12*(7), e0181909. https://doi.org/10.1371/journal.pone.0181909

Alzheimer's Society. (2014). *Dementia UK update.* Retrieved from https://www.alzheimers.org.uk/sites/default/files/migrate/downloads/dementia_uk_update.pdf

Brooke, J., Cronin, C., Stiell, M., Ojo, O., Belcina, M. T. Jr., Smajlović, S. K., & Slark, J. (2019). Nursing students' cultural beliefs and understanding of dementia: A phenomenological study across three continents. *Nurse Education Today, 77,* 6–11. https://doi.org/10.1016/j.nedt.2019.02.007

Brooke, J. M., Cronin, C., Stiell, M., & Ojo, O. (2018). The intersection of culture in the provision of dementia care: A systematic review. *Journal of Clinical Nursing, 27*(17–18), 3241–3253. https://doi.org/10.1111/jocn.13999

Brown, S. (2015). Using focus groups in naturally occurring settings. *Qualitative Research Journal, 15*(1), 86–97. https://doi.org/10.1108/QRJ-11-2013-0068

Dilworth-Anderson, P., & Gibson, B. E. (2002). The cultural influence of values, norms, meanings, and perceptions in understanding dementia in ethnic minorities. *Alzheimer Disease and Associated Disorders, 16*(2, Suppl.), S56–S63. https://doi.org/10.1097/00002093-200200002-00005

Dixon-Woods, M. (2011). Using framework-based synthesis for conducting reviews of qualitative studies. *BMC Medicine, 9*(1), 39–40. https://doi.org/10.1186/1741-7015-9-39

Doyle, P. J., & Rubinstein, R. L. (2014). Person-centered dementia care and the cultural matrix of othering. *The Gerontologist, 54*(6), 952–963. https://doi.org/10.1093/geront/gnt081

Egede-Nissen, V., Sellevold, G. S., Jakobsen, R., & Sørlie, V. (2017). Ethical and cultural striving: Lived experiences of minority nurses in dementia care. *Nursing Ethics, 24*(6), 752–766. https://doi.org/10.1177/0969733015624489

Flaskerud, J. H. (2009). Dementia, ethnicity, and culture. *Issues in Mental Health Nursing, 30*(8), 522–523. https://doi.org/10.1080/01612840903039433

Gale, N. K., Heath, G., Cameron, E., Rashid, S., & Redwood, S. (2013). Using the framework method for the analysis of qualitative data in multi-disciplinary health research. *BMC Medical Research Methodology, 13,* 117. https://doi.org/10.1186/1471-2288-13-117

Githaiga, J. N. (2014). Methodological considerations in utilization of focus groups in an IPA study of bereaved parental cancer caregivers in Nairobi. *Qualitative Research in Psychology, 11*(4), 400–419. https://doi.org/10.1080/14780887.2014.933918

Johnston, B., & Narayanasamy, M. (2016). Exploring psychosocial interventions for people with dementia that enhance personhood and relate to legacy—An integrative review. *BMC Geriatrics, 16*, 77. https://doi.org/10.1186/s12877-016-0250-1

McKenzie, E. L., & Brown, P. M. (2014). Nursing students' intentions to work in dementia care: Influence of age, ageism, and perceived barriers. *Educational Gerontology, 40*(8), 618–633. https://doi.org/10.1080/03601277.2013.863545

Mullay, S., Schofield, P., Clarke, A., & Primrose, W. (2011). Cultural diversity and dementia in Scottish care homes. *British Journal of Nursing, 20*(12), 716–720. https://doi.org/10.12968/bjon.2011.20.12.716

Ow Yong, B., & Manthorpe, J. (2016). The experiences of Indian migrant care home staff working with people with dementia: A pilot study exploring cultural perspectives. *Working With Older People: Community Care Policy & Practice, 20*(1), 3–13. https://doi.org/10.1108/WWOP-07-2015-0012

Palmer, K. S., Brown, A. D., Evans, J. M., Marani, H., Russell, K. K., Martin, D., & Ivers, N. M. (2018). Qualitative analysis of the dynamics of policy design and implementation in hospital funding reform. *PLOS ONE, 13*(1), e0191996. https://doi.org/10.1371/journal.pone.0191996

Parkinson, S., Eatough, V., Holmes, J., Stapley, E., & Midgley, N. (2016). Framework analysis: A worked example of a study exploring young people's experiences of depression. *Qualitative Research in Psychology, 13*(2), 109–129. https://doi.org/10.1080/14780887.2015.1119228

Parveen, S., Peltier, C., & Oyebode, J. R. (2017). Perceptions of dementia and use of services in minority ethnic communities: A scoping exercise. *Health & Social Care in the Community, 25*(2), 734–742. https://doi.org/10.1111/hsc.12363

Roberts, F. E., & Goodhand, K. (2018). Scottish healthcare student's perceptions of an interprofessional ward simulation: An exploratory, descriptive study. *Nursing & Health Sciences, 20*(1), 107–115. https://doi.org/10.1111/nhs.12393

Robertshaw, D., & Cross, A. (2017). Experiences of integrated care for dementia from family and carer perspectives: A framework analysis of massive open online course discussion board posts. *Dementia, 18*(4), 1492–1506. https://doi.org/10.1177/1471301217719991

Sedekia, Y., Jones, C., Nathan, R., Schellenberg, J., & Marchant, T. (2017). Using contraceptives to delay first birth: A qualitative study of individual, community and health provider perceptions in southern Tanzania. *BMC Public Health, 17*(1), 768. https://doi.org/10.1186/s12889-017-4759-9

Smith, J., & Firth, J. (2011). Qualitative data analysis: The framework approach. *Nurse Researcher, 18*(2), 52–62. https://doi.org/10.7748/nr2011.01.18.2.52.c8284

Smith, S. A., Visram, S., O'Malley, C., Summerbell, C., Araujo-Soares, V., Hillier-Brown, F., & Lake, A. A. (2017). Designing equitable workplace dietary interventions: Perceptions of intervention deliverers. *BMC Public Health, 17*(1), 808. https://doi.org/10.1186/s12889-017-4810-x

Spencer, L., Ritchie, J., & O'Connor, W. (2003). Analysis: Practices, principles and processes. In J. Ritchie & J. Lewis (Eds.), *Qualitative research practice: A guide for social science students and researchers* (pp. 199–218). London, England: Sage. (Original work published 2003)

Spencer, L., Ritchie, J., Ormston, R., O'Connor, W., & Barnard, M. (2014). Analysis: Principles and processes. In J. Ritchie, J. Lewis, C. M. Nicholls, & R. Ormston (Eds.), *Qualitative research practice A guide for social science students and researchers* (ed., pp. 269–293). London, England: Sage. (Original work published 2003)

Spencer-Oatey, H. (2012). *What is culture? A compilation of quotations. GlobalPeople Core Concept Compilations.* Retrieved from http://www.go.warwick.ac.uk/globalknowledge

Ward, D. J., Furber, C., Tierney, S., & Swallow, V. (2013). Using framework analysis in nursing research: A worked example. *Journal of Advanced Nursing, 69*(11), 2423–2431. https://doi.org/10.1111/jan.12127

World Health Organization. (2015). *Dementia—A public health priority.* Retrieved from http://www.who.int/mental_health/neurology/dementia/dementia_thematicbrief_executivesummary.pdf

World Health Organization. (2017). *Dementia.* Retrieved from http://www.who.int/news-room/fact-sheets/detail/dementia

23

The Relationship Between Positive Perceptions Toward Organizational Politics and the Work-Related Outcomes of Nurses

Ali MOVAHEDI[1]* • Mohammad BIDKHORI[2] • Tajmohammad ARAZI[3] • Mostafa KHALEGHIPOUR[4] • Fatemeh AMINI[5]

ABSTRACT

Background: Organizational politics (OP) exists to varying degrees in all organizations. OP plays an important role in creating synergy between employees and the goals of the organization.

Purpose: We aimed to investigate the relationship between positive perceptions toward OP and work-related outcomes in nurses, including stress level, burnout level, turnover intention, and job satisfaction.

Methods: This descriptive, analytical study was conducted from April to June 2018 on nurses at Neyshabur University of Medical Sciences Hospitals in Neyshabur, northeastern Iran. The study included 280 nurses working in two teaching hospitals. Five standardized tools were used, including the Perception of Organizational Politics Scale, the Nursing Stress Scale, the Burnout Measure Scale, the Turnover Intention Inventory Scale, and the Minnesota Satisfaction Questionnaire.

Results: The results indicate that the participants did not hold positive perceptions toward OP. The mean Perception of Organizational Politics Scale score was 2.63 ± 0.55. Multiple linear regression analyses showed a significant and positive relationship between positive perception toward OP and job satisfaction and a negative relationship between positive perception toward OP and turnover intention, burnout, and job stress.

Conclusions: Nurses who perceive the work environment to be political will experience greater levels of stress, turnover intention, and burnout and lower levels of job satisfaction. Politics is an issue that should be handled by all levels of management. Managers should use supportive, nonpolitical workplace strategies to improve the work-related outcomes of employees.

Key Words:
organizational politics, job burnout, nurses' stress, nursing satisfaction, turnover intention.

Introduction

Organizational politics (OP) exists to varying degrees in all organizations (Faye & Long, 2014). Politics is a part of the organizational environment. OP is important because it creates a perception of the informal processes of conflicts in organizations and impact on the performance of employees (Vigoda-Gadot & Drory, 2006). OP plays an important role in promoting synergy between employees and organizational goals (Sparrow & Gaston, 1996). Moreover, positive OP may lead to competitive advantage, especially in the presence of appropriately politically skilled employees. A politically skilled management may lead to the successful management of organizational environments that are under stress and may also foster feelings of confidence, trust, and sincerity (Drory & Vigoda-Gadot, 2010). OP may be functional or dysfunctional depending on the workplace circumstances (Cropanzano, Howes, Grandey, & Toth, 1997). OP is commonly defined as activities that are illegitimate, self-serving, and probably harmful to an organization or its employees (Rosen, Chang, Johnson, & Levy, 2009). OP is a consequence of diverse interests, competitions, conflicts, and, most importantly, the need for personal survival, power, or advancement (Cacciattolo, 2015). OP is a challenge that employees must deal with daily (Labrague et al., 2017). OP may mute the voices and opinions of staffs as well as facts and may, as a result, promote uncertainty (Vince, 2001).

Organizational Politics and Work-Related Outcomes

Perceptions toward OP may affect the work-related outcomes of employees such as stress, job burnout, turnover intention, and job satisfaction. Stress occurs when demands exceed an

[1]MSN, RN, Instructor of Critical Care Nursing, Department of Anesthesia and Operating Room Nursing, Neyshabur University of Medical Sciences, Neyshabur, Iran • [2]MS, Doctoral Student, Department of Epidemiology, School of Public Health, Tehran University of Medical Sciences, Tehran, Iran • [3] MSN, RN, Instructor of Medical Surgical Nursing, Department of Anesthesia and Operating Room Nursing, Neyshabur University of Medical Sciences, Neyshabur, Iran • [4]PhD, MD, Assistant Professor of Anesthesiology, Department of Anesthesia and Operating Room Nursing, Neyshabur University of Medical Sciences, Neyshabur, Iran • [5]BSN, RN, Instructor of Anesthesia Nursing, Department of Anesthesia and Operating Room Nursing, Neyshabur University of Medical Sciences, Neyshabur, Iran.

individual's abilities. Responses to occupational stress in nurses may affect the physical, mental, emotional, or psychological dimensions (Gulavani & Shinde, 2014). Job burnout is the psychological response to job-related stress and affects the dimensions of fatigue, cynicism, and professional inefficacy (Rotenstein et al., 2018). Burnout is a chronic job-related disorder and an occupational hazard for healthcare professionals. Approximately 38% of healthcare professionals have chronic occupational complications such as job burnout and low health status levels, which have been shown to decrease the quality of patient care (Dolan et al., 2015). Turnover intention means thinking of resigning from one's current job and doing research to find another job (Apostel, Syrek, & Antoni, 2018). Replacing staffs is a costly process for companies in terms of conducting recruitment and training (Collins & Smith, 2006). Job satisfaction refers to the general attitude of the person toward his or her job. Individuals with higher levels of job satisfaction hold more positive attitudes toward their profession (Robbins, 2001).

Several studies have shown OP to affect job satisfaction negatively (Atinga, Domfeh, Kayi, Abuosi, & Dzansi, 2014). OP may lead to negative perceptions and negligent behaviors such as turnover intention (Basar & Basim, 2016). Perceptions toward OP may have negative effects on emotional workplace states such as job stress (Abbas, Raja, Darr, & Bouckenooghe, 2014). Hospitals are an organization in which human resources play a key role in providing services to individuals. Nurses play an important role in these organizations.

In Iran, most nurses hold a bachelor's degree and work in public or private hospitals on a permanent, casual, or contractual basis. The entry-level salary for nurses in Iran is usually less than $1,000 per month, which is better than most other entry-level salaries for bachelor-prepared individuals.

Nursing is a stressful job, and this stress may impact the delivery and quality of healthcare negatively (Johnston, Jones, Charles, McCann, & McKee, 2013). Working in a politically charged environment may increase stress and impact the work-related outcomes of nurses. Therefore, an understanding of nurses' perceptions of OP is essential to guiding related research projects and quality initiatives. As OP may differ from country to country, this study was designed to investigate the relationship between positive perceptions toward OP and work-related outcomes of nurses including stress level, burnout level, turnover intention, and job satisfaction.

Methods

Design

This descriptive, analytical study was conducted from April to June 2018 on 280 nurses in two teaching hospitals at Neyshabur University of Medical Sciences in Neyshabur, northeastern Iran. Licensed registered nurses with at least 1 year of work experience who were a permanent, casual, or contractual employee and who consented to participate were included as participants. Three hundred questionnaires were distributed, and 280 completed questionnaires were received (response rate: 93.3%). Participants were selected using a stratified random sampling technique based on the number of nurses in the hospitals and wards.

Instruments

A paper-based, self-report questionnaire with six sections was used to collect the study data.

Section 1

This section includes demographic information, including age, gender, institution, ward, level of education, and work experience.

Section 2

The main tool in this study was the 12-item version of Perception of Organizational Politics Scale (POPS) by Ferris, Adams, Kolodinsky, Hochwarter, and Ammeter (2002). The tool was designed to measure three aspects of OP: "general political behavior" (Items 1 and 2), "go along to get ahead" (Items 3–7), and "pay and promotion policies" (Items 8–12). The participants were asked to give their opinion on each item using a 5-point Likert scale ranging from *strongly disagree* (1) to *strongly agree* (5). A reverse code was used for the seven negative items on the scale. A higher total score was associated with a more positive perception toward OP. The questionnaire earned a Cronbach's alpha of .79 in a previous study (Ferris et al., 2002) and earned a Cronbach's alpha of .83 in this study.

Section 3

The Nursing Stress Scale was used to assess the perceived stress of the participants (Gray-Toft & Anderson, 1981). This tool consists of 34 items that describe stressful workplace situations for nurses and is scored using a Likert-type scale (1 = *never*, 2 = *occasionally*, 3 = *frequently*, and 4 = *very frequently*), with a higher total score associated with a higher level of stress.

Section 4

The 10-item version of the Burnout Measure Scale (Malach-Pines, 2005) was used to measure job burnout. This scale uses a 7-point Likert scale ranging from 1 = *never* to 7 = *always*, with a higher mean score reflecting a higher level of burnout.

Section 5

Turnover intention was quantified using the six-item Turnover Intention Inventory Scale (Bothma & Roodt, 2013), which was developed to measure turnover intention using a 5-point Likert scale ranging from 1 = *never* to 5 = *always*. Two of the items on this scale were reverse coded. A higher mean score on this scale is associated with higher turnover intention.

Section 6

The job satisfaction of the participants was measured using the 20-item version of the Minnesota Satisfaction Questionnaire (Weiss, Dawis, England, & Lofquist, 1977), which was developed to measure job satisfaction using a 5-point Likert scale ranging from 1 = *very dissatisfied* to 5 = *very satisfied*. A higher mean score on this scale is associated with a higher level of job satisfaction.

The content validities of these five questionnaires were assessed. Eight nursing school faculty members reviewed the cultural perspectives of all the items on the translated questionnaires. Relevancy, clarity, and comprehensiveness were assessed for the content validity of each questionnaire using the item content validity index, scale content validity index, and comprehensiveness index. The content validity ratios for all of the items were greater than .8.

Statistical Analysis

Data analysis was performed using SPSS Version 16.0 for Windows (SPSS, Inc., Chicago, IL, USA). Descriptive statistics were used to describe the demographic and clinical characteristics of the participants by calculating frequencies, mean scores, and standard deviations. For data analysis, independent *t* test, linear regression, and multiple comparisons were used. *P* values less than .05 were considered statistically significant in all of the statistical analyses.

Ethical Considerations

This study was approved by the ethics committee of Neyshabur University of Medical Sciences (Ethical Approval Number: IR.NUMS.REC.1396.17), which also issued an official letter to the hospitals to obtain their permission and cooperation for the study. Verbal consent was obtained from the participants, who were assured that all of their data would be treated anonymously and kept confidential and that they could withdraw from the study at any time during the study.

TABLE 1.
Sociodemographic Characteristics of the Participants (N = 280)

Characteristic	*n*	%
Age (*M* and *SD*)	28.1	5.0
23–28 years	180	64.3
29–34 years	69	24.6
≥ 35	31	11.1
Gender		
Female	160	57.2
Male	120	42.8
Marital status		
Single	90	32.2
Married	190	67.8
Institution		
22 Bahman	212	75.7
Hakim	68	24.3
Level of education		
Bachelor's degree	268	95.7
Master's degree	12	4.3
Working experience (*M* and *SD*)	4.3	4.5
< 5 years	208	75.0
5–10 years	40	14.0
> 10 years	32	11.0
Nursing subgroup		
Nurse	188	67.1
Operating room nurse	50	17.8
Anesthesia nurse	42	15.1
Ward		
Medical	46	16.4
Surgical	64	22.9
Emergency department	84	30.0
Operating room	86	30.7

Results

Two hundred eighty questionnaires were returned. Over half (57.2%) of the participants were female, and 67.8% were married. The mean (*SD*) age of the participants was 28.1 (5.0) years (range: 23–50 years), and their mean work experience was 4.3 ± 4.5 years. The demographic characteristics of the participants are displayed in Table 1.

The mean POPS score of the nurses was 2.63 ± 0.55 (minimum score was 1.5 and maximum score was 3.92). Item 5 earned the highest mean score (3.7 ± 1.0), with 65.0% of the participants either disagreeing or strongly disagreeing on this item. In addition, over 69% of the participants either agreed or strongly agree with Item 7, and 66.4% and 65.0% of the participants, respectively, either disagreed or strongly disagreed with Items 4 and 3. The frequency of the perceptions of the participants toward OP is displayed in Table 2, with the POPS dimensions ranked by mean score. The participants held a more positive perception of "pay and promotion policies" (2.67 ± 0.73) than either "go along to get ahead" (2.65 ± 0.58) or "general political behavior" (2.51 ± 1.09).

Multiple linear regression analyses showed a significant and positive relationship between POPS score and job satisfaction ($p < .001$, $r = .46$). The participants who held more positive perceptions toward OP had higher levels of job satisfaction. In addition, a negative relationship was found between positive perception toward OP and turnover intention ($p < .001$, $r = -.27$), burnout ($p < .001$, $r = -.28$), and job stress ($p < .001$, $r = -.47$; Table 3). A significant relationship was found between the POPS score and gender ($p < .001$, $r = -.27$). The perceptions toward OP of female participants were more positive than those of their male counterparts. In addition, a significant relationship was found between the POPS score and the number of the participants' work shifts ($p < .01$, $r = .21$), with those holding more positive perceptions toward OP working more work shifts per month. Multiple comparisons between the POPS score and nursing subgroups (nurses, operating room nurses, and anesthesia nurses) and wards (medical, surgical, emergency department, and operating room) showed no significant relationship ($p < .47$ and $p < .53$, respectively). No other

TABLE 2.

Frequency of Perceptions of the Nurses Toward Organizational Politics

Item	Agree or Strongly Agree		Disagree or Strongly Disagree			
	n	%	*n*	%	Mean	*SD*
1. People in this organization attempt to build themselves up by tearing others down.[a]	151	53.9	61	21.8	2.5	1.1
2. There has always been an influential group in this organization that no one ever crosses.[a]	156	55.7	67	23.9	2.5	1.2
3. Employees are encouraged to speak out frankly even when they are critical of well-established ideas.	53	18.9	169	60.4	2.3	1.1
4. There is no place for yes-men around here: good ideas are desired even when it means disagreeing with superiors.	28	10.0	186	66.4	2.2	0.8
5. If coworkers offer to lend some assistance, it is because they expect to get something out of it, not because they really care.[a]	40	14.2	182	65.0	3.7	1.0
6. People here usually do not speak up for fear of retaliation by others.[a]	141	50.4	103	36.8	2.6	1.3
7. There is a group of people in my organization who always get things their way because no one wants to challenge them.[a]	194	69.2	42	15.0	2.2	1.0
8. I have seen changes made in policies here that only serve the purposes of a few individuals, not the work unit or the organization.[a]	152	54.2	54	19.3	2.6	1.0
9. Favoritism rather than merit determines who gets ahead around here.[a]	172	61.4	56	20.0	2.4	1.0
10. Rewards come only to those who work hard in this organization.	106	37.9	119	42.5	3.0	1.2
11. Since I have worked in this department, I have never seen the pay and promotion policies applied politically	78	27.9	122	43.5	2.6	1.2
12. Promotions in this department generally go to top performers	84	30.0	145	51.8	2.6	1.2

[a]Reversed item.

significant relationship between the POPS score and other demographic and job-related factors (such as age, marital status, or work experience) was found.

Discussion

The total POPS score of the participants in this study was lower than that reported in other recent studies (Danish, Humayon, Aslam, Usman, & Tariq, 2014; Daskin & Tezer, 2012; Faye & Long, 2014). The POPS score of the nurses in the study of Labrague et al. (2017) was 2.80 ± 0.59. The participants in this study held the highest positive perception of the "pay and promotion policies" dimension. These results may be explained by this study having been performed in government hospitals that follow national payment policies.

Perception of OP is a predictor of work outcomes. Perception of OP in this study was examined in terms of its relationships to job satisfaction, turnover intention, burnout, and job stress. In other related studies, perceptions of OP among nurses and nonnursing employees were found to be associated with job satisfaction, turnover intention, burnout, and job stress (Abbas et al., 2014; Cropanzano et al., 1997; Ferris et al., 2002; Labrague et al., 2017). In this study, perceiving the work environment to be political was shown to be associated with greater levels of stress, turnover intention, and burnout and a lower level of job satisfaction. More than 60% of the participants in this

TABLE 3.

Linear Regression Results of the Perception of Organizational Politics Scale (Independent Variable) on Work Outcomes (Dependent Variables)

Work Outcome	R^2	Constant α	*SE*	Coefficient β	95% CI	*p*
Job satisfaction	.219	2.083	0.060	0.375	[0.25, 0.49]	< .001
Job stress	.225	3.466	0.061	−0.384	[−0.50, −0.26]	< .001
Turnover intention	.077	3.743	0.095	−0.322	[−0.51, −0.13]	< .001
Burnout	.080	4.787	0.014	−0.506	[−0.79, −0.21]	< .001

study perceived favoritism as being more important than merit in determining who gets ahead in their organization. These results may indicate that, in highly politicized environments, employees feel that their efforts will not be recognized or rewarded. Politics in the work environment may lead to undesirable workplace conditions such as stress, burnout, and turnover intention. In this study, politics was found to be a better predictor of stress and satisfaction than of turnover intention and burnout (Table 3).

Organizational Politics and Work-Related Outcomes

Stress is a common problem in the workplaces, and nursing is an inherently stressful occupation. Hospital environments easily become tense because of the stresses involved with caring for patients and dealing with patient families. A positive perception toward OP may make managing these stresses and crises easier and lead to improved job performance. Implementing clear and supportive policies will make nurses more confident in stressful situations. On the other hand, punitive policies or discriminatory behaviors will increase nurses' stress.

Job satisfaction depends on organizational expectations. Autonomy and pay are regarded as the two most important factors affecting job satisfaction. The job satisfaction of hospital nurses is closely related to organizational commitment and job stress (Lu, Zhao, & While, 2019). Supportive, nonpolitical workplace strategies have the potential to increase job satisfaction. Promotion policies within organizations should be clear and based on merit.

In this study, the participants who held a more-positive perception toward OP had a lower level of burnout. Burnout is associated with job stress in nurses and impacts negatively on their quality of life. Moreover, the job support resources available to nurses have always been insufficient to meet their emotional demand (Wu, Zhu, Wang, Wang, & Lan, 2007). However, although burnout is related to multiple social, psychological, and environmental factors, OP is one factor that is controllable. To reduce burnout, OP should be adjusted so that the OP burden of nurses does not exceed their abilities to handle. Hospital managers should reduce OP, promote a friendly work environment, and build trust among employees.

A strong relationship was identified in this study between OP and turnover intention. One previous study did not identify a significant relationship between these two variables (Chang, Rosen, & Levy, 2009), whereas others did (Abbas et al., 2014; Daskin & Tezer, 2012; Javed, Abrar, Bashir, & Shabir, 2014; Labrague et al., 2017). When nurses hold negative perceptions toward OP, they may be encouraged to quit their job. Turnover leads to the loss of experienced nurses, which is detrimental to hospitals and decreases the quality of patient care. Moreover, the participants in this study who held more-positive perceptions toward OP worked more shifts per month than their peers. Enforcing non-politically-based compensation policies, encouraging employees to speak out frankly, and providing rewards and promotions based solely on performance may decrease the turnover intention of nurses.

In this study, the female participants held a more positive perception toward OP than their male peers. In Danish et al., no gender difference was found for perception of OP in the educational sector in Pakistan (Danish et al., 2014).

In Iran, although nurses are hired by government hospitals based on their performance on recruitment tests, no standard mechanism is used to select hospital managers. Thus, promotion to management is often based on personal biases and preferences. This process may foster negative attitudes among employees toward OP and negatively affect job outcomes.

The positive and negative aspects of the perceptions of OP and the impact of the dimensions of OP on different work-related outcomes should be examined in future studies. Qualitative studies may provide richer insights into OP outcomes. Finally, the differences in perceptions of OP between management and employees should be examined and compared.

Study Limitations

The data used in this study were obtained from self-report questionnaires and thus may be affected by reporting bias. In addition, the work-related outcome levels may have been underestimated or overestimated by the participants. Furthermore, the participants were from one city in Iran only, and a national survey may yield different results. Finally, no similar studies have been conducted in Iran, so no direct comparison of results is possible.

Conclusions

Politics exists in every organization and cannot be eliminated completely. OP is not purely a negative factor for organizations, and its consequences include positive effects such as enhanced employee commitment and organization-citizenship behaviors. However, in overly politicized environments, employees may feel their efforts will not be recognized or rewarded. Therefore, managers should use politics as a positive tool to enhance the performance of employees. The results of this study support that holding a positive perception toward OP increases job satisfaction and decreases job stress, burnout level, and turnover intention in nurses.

Implications for Practice

The findings of this study give nursing managers and policymakers valuable information regarding the positive and negative aspects of the OP perceptions of nurses. Nursing managers and leaders should be aware of the harmful effects of politics in their organization. Politics is an issue that should be handled effectively by all levels of management. Managers should use supportive, nonpolitical workplace strategies to improve employee work-related outcomes such as job stress, burnout, turnover intention, and job satisfaction. Clear and consistent policies can foster trust between employees and managers within an organization. Supportive policies will make nurses more confident in stressful situations. On the other hand, punitive policies or discriminatory behaviors will increase nurses' stress. Finally, organization policies related to employee promotion should be clear and merit-based.

Acknowledgments

This study was funded by Neyshabur University of Medical Sciences. We would like to thank the hospital managers, data collectors, and all of the staff nurses who participated in this study.

Author Contributions

Study conception and design: AM
Data collection: FA
Data analysis and interpretation: MB, AM
Drafting of the article: AM
Critical revision of the article: AM, TA, MK

References

Abbas, M., Raja, U., Darr, W., & Bouckenooghe, D. (2014). Combined effects of perceived politics and psychological capital on job satisfaction, turnover intentions, and performance. *Journal of Management, 40*(7), 1813–1830. https://doi.org/10.1177/0149206312455243

Apostel, E., Syrek, C. J., & Antoni, C. H. (2018). Turnover intention as a response to illegitimate tasks: The moderating role of appreciative leadership. *International Journal of Stress Management, 25*(3), 234–249. https://doi.org/10.1037/str0000061

Atinga, R. A., Domfeh, K. A., Kayi, E., Abuosi, A., & Dzansi, G. (2014). Effects of perceived workplace politics in hospitals on nurses' behavioural intentions in Ghana. *Journal of Nursing Management, 22*(2), 159–169. https://doi.org/10.1111/jonm.12178

Basar, U., & Basim, N. (2016). A cross-sectional survey on consequences of nurses' burnout: Moderating role of organizational politics. *Journal of Advanced Nursing, 72*(8), 1838–1850. https://doi.org/10.1111/jan.12958

Bothma, C. F. C., & Roodt, G. (2013). The validation of the turnover intention scale. *SA Journal of Human Resource Management, 11*(1), 1–12. https://doi.org/10.4102/sajhrm.v11i1.507

Cacciattolo, K. (2015). Organisational politics: The positive & negative sides. *ESJ: European Scientific Journal, 11*(1), 121–129.

Chang, C.-H., Rosen, C. C., & Levy, P. E. (2009). The relationship between perceptions of organizational politics and employee attitudes, strain, and behavior: A meta-analytic examination. *Academy of Management Journal, 52*(4), 779–801. https://doi.org/10.5465/amj.2009.43670894

Collins, C. J., & Smith, K. G. (2006). Knowledge exchange and combination: The role of human resource practices in the performance of high-technology firms. *Academy of Management Journal, 49*(3), 544–560. https://doi.org/10.5465/amj.2006.21794671

Cropanzano, R., Howes, J. C., Grandey, A. A., & Toth, P. (1997). The relationship of organizational politics and support to work behaviors, attitudes, and stress. *Journal of Organizational Behavior, 18*(2), 159–180. https://doi.org/10.1002/(SICI)1099-1379(199703)18:2<159::AID-JOB795>3.0.CO;2-D

Danish, R. Q., Humayon, A. A., Aslam, N., Usman, A., & Tariq, M. I. (2014). Employee's perceptions of organizational politics and stress at workplace: A comparative study of public and private sector universities. *Research Journal of Recent Sciences, 3*(7), 44–52.

Daskin, M., & Tezer, M. (2012). Organizational politics and turnover: An empirical research from hospitality industry. *Tourism, 60*(3), 273–291.

Dolan, E. D., Mohr, D., Lempa, M., Joos, S., Fihn, S. D., Nelson, K. M., & Helfrich, C. D. (2015). Using a single item to measure burnout in primary care staff: A psychometric evaluation. *Journal of General Internal Medicine, 30*(5), 582–587. https://doi.org/10.1007/s11606-014-3112-6

Drory, A., & Vigoda-Gadot, E. (2010). Organizational politics and human resource management: A typology and the Israeli experience. *Human Resource Management Review, 20*(3), 194–202. https://doi.org/10.1016/j.hrmr.2009.08.005

Faye, K., & Long, Y. (2014). The impact of job satisfaction in the relationships between workplace politics and work related outcomes and attitudes: Evidence from organizations in Senegal. *International Journal of Business and Management, 9*(5), 160–168. https://doi.org/0.5539/ijbm.v9n5p160

Ferris, G. R., Adams, G., Kolodinsky, R. W., Hochwarter, W. A., & Ammeter, A. P. (2002). Perceptions of organizational politics: Theory and research directions. In F. J. Yammarino & F. Dansereau (Eds.), *Research in multi-level issues, Vol. 1. The many faces of multi-level issues* (pp. 179–254). West Yorkshire, England: Emerald Group Publishing Limited. https://doi.org/10.1016/S1475-9144(02)01034-2

Gray-Toft, P., & Anderson, J. G. (1981). The nursing stress scale: Development of an instrument. *Journal of Behavioral Assessment, 3*(1), 11–23. https://doi.org/10.1007/BF01321348

Gulavani, A., & Shinde, M. (2014). Occupational stress and job satisfaction among nurses. *International Journal of Science and Research (IJSR), 3*(4), 733–740.

Javed, M., Abrar, M., Bashir, M., & Shabir, M. (2014). Effect of perceived organizational politics and core self evaluation on turnover intention: A South Asian perspective. *International Journal of Human Resource Studies, 4*(2), 33–49. https://doi.org/10.5296/ijhrs.v4i2.5791

Johnston, D. W., Jones, M. C., Charles, K., McCann, S. K., & McKee, L. (2013). Stress in nurses: Stress-related affect and its determinants examined over the nursing day. *Annals of Behavioral Medicine, 45*(3), 348–356. https://doi.org/10.1007/s12160-012-9458-2

Labrague, L. J., McEnroe-Petitte, D. M., Gloe, D., Tsaras, K., Arteche, D. L., & Maldia, F. (2017). Organizational politics, nurses' stress, burnout levels, turnover intention and job satisfaction. *International Nursing Review, 64*(1), 109–116. https://doi.org/10.1111/inr.12347

Lu, H., Zhao, Y., & While, A. (2019). Job satisfaction among hospital nurses: A literature review. *International Journal of Nursing Studies, 94*, 21–31. https://doi.org/10.1016/j.ijnurstu.2019.01.011

Malach-Pines, A. (2005). The burnout measure, short version. *International Journal of Stress Management, 12*(1), 78–88. https://doi.org/10.1037/1072-5245.12.1.78

Robbins, S. P. (2001). *Organisational behaviour: Global and Southern African perspectives*. Cape Town, South Africa: Pearson Education.

Rosen, C. C., Chang, C.-H., Johnson, R. E., & Levy, P. E. (2009). Perceptions of the organizational context and psychological contract breach: Assessing competing perspectives. *Organizational Behavior and Human Decision Processes, 108*(2), 202–217. https://doi.org/10.1016/j.obhdp.2008.07.003

Rotenstein, L. S., Torre, M., Ramos, M. A., Rosales, R. C., Guille, C., Sen, S., & Mata, D. A. (2018). Prevalence of burnout among physicians: A systematic review. *JAMA, 320*(11), 1131–1150. https://doi.org/10.1001/jama.2018.12777

Sparrow, P. R., & Gaston, K. (1996). Generic climate maps: A strategic application of climate survey data? *Journal of Organizational Behavior, 17*(6), 679–698. https://doi.org/10.1002/(sici)1099-1379(199611)17:6<679::aid-job786>3.0.co;2-m

Vigoda-Gadot, E., & Drory, A. (Eds.). (2006). *Handbook of organizational politics*. Northampton, MA: Edward Elgar.

Vince, R. (2001). Power and emotion in organizational learning. *Human Relations, 54*(10), 1325–1351. https://doi.org/10.1177/a019197

Weiss, D., Dawis, R., England, G., & Lofquist, L. (1977). *Manual for the Minnesota Satisfaction questionnaire (short form). Minnesota Studies in Vocational Rehabilitation*. Minneapolis, MN: University of Minnesota.

Wu, S., Zhu, W., Wang, Z., Wang, M., & Lan, Y. (2007). Relationship between burnout and occupational stress among nurses in China. *Journal of Advanced Nursing, 59*(3), 233–239. https://doi.org/10.1111/j.1365-2648.2007.04301.x

24

Relationship Between the Problem-Solving Skills and Empathy Skills of Operating Room Nurses

Fatma AY[1]* • Şehrinaz POLAT[2] • Tennur KASHIMI[3]

ABSTRACT

Background: The use of empathy in problem solving and communication is a focus of nursing practice and is of great significance in raising the quality of patient care.

Purpose: The purposes of this study are to investigate the relationship between problem solving and empathy among operating room nurses and to explore the factors that relate to these two competencies.

Methods: This is a cross-sectional, descriptive study. Study data were gathered using a personal information form, the Interpersonal Problem Solving Inventory, and the Basic Empathy Scale ($N = 80$). Descriptive and comparative statistics were employed to evaluate the study data.

Results: Age, marital status, and career length were not found to affect the subscale scores of cognitive empathy ($p > .05$). A negative correlation was found between the subscale scores for "diffidence" and "cognitive empathy." Moreover, the emotional empathy scores of the graduate nurses were higher than those of the master's/doctorate degree nurses to a degree that approached significance ($p = .078$). Furthermore, emotional empathy levels were found to decrease as the scores for insistent/persistent approach, lack of self-confidence, and educational level increased ($p < .05$). The descriptive characteristics of the participating nurses were found not to affect their problem-solving skills.

Conclusions/Implications for Practice: Problem solving is a focus of nursing practice and of great importance for raising the quality of patient care. Constructive problem-solving skills affect cognitive empathy skills. Educational level and career length were found to relate negatively and level of self-confidence was found to relate positively with level of cognitive empathy. Finally, lower empathy scores were associated with difficult working conditions in operating rooms, intense stress, and high levels of potential stress-driven conflicts between workers in work settings.

KEY WORDS:
operating room, critical thinking, surgery, cognitive, emotional.

Introduction

Healthcare institutions are where individuals seek remedies to their health problems. These institutions face problems, which relate to both employees and care recipients. These problems may occur spontaneously and require immediate solution. Moreover, these problems require that the preferred remedies be adapted to address the unique nature of both organizational circumstances and individual requirements. Therefore, it is important that nurses, who are a major component of the healthcare system, have problem-solving skills.

Operating rooms are complex, high-risk environments with intense levels of stress that require rapid judgment making and fast implementation of appropriate decisions to increase patients' chances of survival (Kanan, 2011; Jeon, Lakanmaa, Meretoja, & Leino-Kilpi, 2017). Furthermore, aseptic principles may never be compromised, and a high level of coordination and cooperation among team members should be maintained in these areas (Kanan, 2011; Sandelin & Gustafsson, 2015). The members of a surgical team may vary in the operating room (Sandelin & Gustafsson, 2015; Sonoda, Onozuka, & Hagihara, 2018). Under these difficult conditions, time management and workload are important stress factors for nurses (Happell et al., 2013; Suresh, Matthews, & Coyne, 2013). At the same time, operating room nurses are legally responsible for the nature and quality of the healthcare service received by patients before, during, and after their surgical intervention (Kanan, 2011). The American Nurses Association defines a nurse as "the healthcare professional establishing, coordinating and administering the care while applying the nursing process in an aim to meet the identified physiological, psychological, sociocultural and spiritual needs of patients who are potentially at the risk of jeopardized protective reflexes or self-care ability because of surgery or invasive intervention" (Association of periOperative Registered Nurses, 2015).

Problem solving is the most critical aspect of the nursing practice. The fact that nursing requires mental and abstract

[1]*PhD, RN, Assistant Professor, Faculty of Health Sciences, Department of Midwifery, Istanbul University-Cerrahpaşa, Turkey* • [2]*PhD, RN, Directorate of Nursing Services, Hospital of Faculty of Medicine, Istanbul University, Turkey* • [3]*MS, RN, Director, Operating Room, Hospital of Faculty of Medicine, Istanbul University, Turkey.*

skills, such as identifying individual needs and finding appropriate remedies, was first stated in 1960s. In 1960s, the nursing theorists Abdellah, Orem, and Levin emphasized the mental aspect of nursing. They argued that the most critical requirement of nurses in the clinical field is the ability to decide on and plan the right action and that nursing care should be founded on a sound knowledge base (Taşcı, 2005).

The World Health Organization has stated that "taking measures and applying a problem-solving approach to provide appropriate care is one of the compulsory competencies of nurses" (Taşcı, 2005). Thus, enhancing the problem-solving skills of nurses is of great importance in raising the quality of patient care (Taylor, 2000; Yu & Kirk, 2008). On the other hand, Bagnal (1981) argued that people with problem-solving skills need to be equipped with personal traits including innovation, clear manifestation of preferences and decisions, having a sense of responsibility, flexible thinking, courage and adventurousness, ability to show distinct ideas, self-confidence, a broad area of interest, acting rationally and objectively, creativity, productivity, and critical perspective (as cited in Çam & Tümkaya, 2008).

To provide the best surgical care to a patient, team members must work together effectively (Sonoda et al., 2018). One of the most important factors affecting the quality of healthcare service delivery is effective communication between healthcare professionals and healthcare recipients, with empathy forming the basis for effective communication.

Because of the intrinsic nature of the nursing profession, nurses should have empathy skills. Thus, empathy is the essence of the nursing profession (Fields et al., 2004; Vioulac, Aubree, Massy, & Untas, 2016). A review of resources in the literature on problem solving reveals that gathering problem-related data is the first major step toward determining the root causes of a problem. In this respect, empathy is an important skill that helps properly identify a problem. On the basis of the definition of empathy, sensing another person's feelings and thoughts and placing oneself in his or her position or feeling from within his or her frame of reference should work to improve one's problem-solving skills, particularly those skills related to social problem solving (Taşcı, 2005; Topçu, Baker, & Aydın, 2010; Vioulac et al., 2016). It is possible to explain empathic content emotionally as well as cognitively. Emotional empathy (EE) means feeling the emotions of another person and providing the most appropriate response based on his or her emotional state. This is very important in patient–nurse communications. Cognitive empathy (CE) is the ability to recognize the feelings of another without experiencing those feelings yourself (de Kemp, Overbeek, de Wied, Engels, & Scholte, 2007).

Gender, age, level of education, marital status, years of work, duration working at current institution, and problem-solving situations have been shown in the literature not to affect the problem-solving or empathy skills of nurses (Abaan & Altıntoprak, 2005; Kelleci & Gölbaşı, 2004; Yu & Kirk, 2008). Empathy is especially critical to the quality of nursing care and is an essential component of any form of caring relationship. The findings in the literature regarding empathy among nurses are inconsistent (Yu & Kirk, 2008), and no findings in the literature address the relationship between problem-solving skills and empathy skills in operating room nurses.

Today, the healthcare system demands that nurses use their professional knowledge to handle patient problems and needs in flexible and creative ways. Problem solving is a primary focus of the nursing practice and is of great importance to raising the quality of patient care (Kelleci & Gölbaşı, 2004; Yu & Kirk, 2008). Enhancing the problem-solving and empathy skills of nurses may be expected to facilitate their identification of the sources of problems encountered during the delivery of healthcare services and their resolution of these problems.

The purposes of this study are to investigate the relationship between problem solving and empathy in operating room nurses and to explore the factors related to these two competencies.

Methods

Study Model and Hypotheses

This study is a cross-sectional and descriptive study. The three hypotheses regarding the relationships between the independent variables are as follows:

- H1: Sociodemographic characteristics affect problem-solving skills.
- H2: Sociodemographic characteristics affect level of empathy.
- H3: Problem-solving skills are positively and significantly correlated with empathy.

Study Population and Sample

The study was conducted during the period of May–June 2015 at three hospitals affiliated with Istanbul University. The study population consisted of 121 nurses who were currently working in the operating rooms of these hospitals. The study sample consisted of the 80 nurses who volunteered to participate and answered all of the questions on the inventory.

Data Collection Tool

Study data were gathered using a personal information form, the Interpersonal Problem Solving Inventory (IPSI), and the Basic Empathy Scale.

Personal information form

This questionnaire, created by the researchers, is composed of 10 questions on the age, gender, educational background, organization and department, position, and organizational and professional functions of the respondent.

Interpersonal problem solving inventory

The IPSI, developed and validated by Çam and Tümkaya (2008), was used in this study. The Cronbach's α internal consistency coefficients of the IPSI subscales were previously evaluated at between .67 and .91. The IPSI includes 50 items, all of which are scored on a 5-point Likert scale, with 1 = *strictly inappropriate* and 5 = *fully appropriate*. The lack of self-confidence (LSC) subscale assesses lack of confidence in problem solving. The constructive problem solving (CPS) subscale assesses emotions, thoughts, and behaviors that contribute to the effective and constructive solution of interpersonal problems. The negative approach to the problem subscale assesses intensely the negative emotions and thoughts such as helplessness, pessimism, and disappointment that are experienced when an interpersonal problem is encountered. The abstaining from responsibility subscale assesses failure to take responsibility for solving the problem. The persistent approach (PA) subscale assesses self-assertive/persistent thoughts and behaviors in solving problems encountered in interpersonal relationships. A high score on a subscale indicates a high interpersonal-problem-solving capability for that subscale category (Çam & Tümkaya, 2008). A high score on the negative approach to the problem subscale indicates a higher likelihood of experiencing intense negative feelings and thoughts such as helplessness, pessimism, and sadness when encountering a problem. A high score on CPS indicates that the respondent will show more of the emotions, thoughts, and behaviors that contribute to the problem in an effective and constructive way. A low level of self-confidence indicates that the respondent will exhibit low self-confidence toward effectively resolving a problem. A high score on the abstaining from responsibility subscale indicates a high inclination to assume responsibility to resolve a problem (Table 1). The high level of insistent approach indicates that the participant is more willing to solve problems (Çam & Tümkaya, 2008). In this study, the Cronbach's α reliability coefficients were .901, .899, .763, .679, and .810, respectively.

Basic empathy skill scale

The Basic Empathy Skill Scale was developed by Jolliffe and Farrington (2006) and validated by Topçu et al. (2010) in Turkish. It is a 5-Likert scale (1 = *strictly disagree* and 5 = *strictly agree*) consisting of 20 items, of which nine measure CE and 11 measure EE. The Cronbach's α coefficients that were calculated for the reliability study range between .76 and .80. The lowest possible scores are 9 and 45 and the highest possible scores are 11 and 55 for the CE and EE subscales, respectively. A high score on the CE subscale indicates that the CE level is high, and a high score on the EE subscale indicates that the EE level is high (Topçu et al., 2010). The two subscales of the Basic Empathy Skill Scale have been found to be highly reliable. The Cronbach's α reliability coefficients in this study were .782 for the CE subscale and .649 for the EE subscale.

Data Collection

The study was conducted between May and June 2015 at three hospitals affiliated with Istanbul University. The researcher explained the study to those nurses who agreed to participate. The questionnaire form was distributed to the participants, the purpose of the investigation was clarified, and permission to use participant data was obtained. The participants completed the questionnaire on their own, and the completed questionnaires were collected afterward. The time required to complete the questionnaire was 15–20 minutes in total.

Evaluation of Data

Number Cruncher Statistical System 2007 (Kaysville, UT, USA) software was used to perform statistical analysis. To compare the quantitative data, in addition to using descriptive statistical methods (mean, standard deviation, median, frequency, ratio, minimum, maximum), the Student *t* test was used to compare the parameters with the regular distribution in the two groups and the Mann–Whitney *U* test was used to compare the parameters without normal distribution in the two groups. In addition, a one-way analysis of variance test was used to compare three or more groups with normal distribution, and a Kruskal–Wallis test was used to compare three or more groups without normal distribution. Pearson's correlation analysis and Spearman's correlation analysis were used to evaluate the relationships among the parameters. Finally, linear regression analysis was employed

TABLE 1.
Score Distribution for Interpersonal Problem-Solving Skills and Basic Empathy Skills

Subdimension of the scale	Min–Max	Median	Mean	*SD*
Interpersonal Problem-Solving Skills				
Negative approach to the problem	18–62	33.0	35.69	10.95
Constructive problem solving	36–77	48.5	51.66	8.99
Lack of self-confidence	7–26	12.0	13.19	4.17
Abstaining from responsibility	5–20	12.0	11.28	3.44
Persistent approach	10–29	19.5	19.87	4.21
Basic Empathy Skills				
Cognitive empathy	27–45	36.0	35.77	4.34
Emotional empathy	31–53	39.5	39.95	5.25

TABLE 2.
Distribution of Descriptive Characteristics

Characteristic	*n*	%
Age (*M* and *SD*; years)	37.56	8.12
≤ 35	33	41.2
> 36	47	58.8
Gender		
Female	78	97.5
Male	2	2.5
Marital status		
Married	64	80.0
Single	16	20.0
Duration working as a nurse (years; *M* and *SD*)	15.84	8.30
1–10	23	28.7
11–20	35	43.8
≥ 21	22	27.5
Duration working at current hospital (years)		
1–10	42	52.4
11–20	21	26.3
≥ 21	17	21.3
Educational level		
High school	5	6.3
Associate degree	8	10.0
Undergraduate	54	67.5
Master's/doctorate degree	13	16.2

to evaluate multivariate data. Significance was determined by a p value of $< .05$.

Ethical Considerations

Ethical conformity approval was obtained from the Non-Interventional Clinical Research Ethics Board at Istanbul Medipol University (108400987-165, issued on March 30, 2015). Written consent was obtained from the administrations of the participating hospitals. Furthermore, the informed consent of nurses who volunteered to participate was obtained. Permission to use the abovementioned scales that were used in this study as data collection tools was obtained via e-mail from their original authors.

Results

Eighty nurses (97.5% female, $n = 78$; 2.5% male, $n = 2$) were enrolled as participants. The age of participants ranged between 24 and 64 (mean = 37.56 ± 8.12) years, mean years of professional nursing experience was 15.84 ± 8.30, and mean years working in the current hospital was 13.19 ± 8.23. Other descriptive characteristics for the participants are provided in Table 2.

A comparison of scale subdimension scores revealed a negative and statistically significant correlation at a level of 22.3%. Statistical significance was reached only between the LSC subscale and the CE subscale ($r = -.223$, $p = .047$; Table 3). Thus, a higher LSC score was associated with a lower CE score.

Comparisons between participants' descriptive characteristics and subdimension scores on the problem-solving skill scale revealed no significant differences. Thus, demographic characteristics such as age, educational background, and career length were found to have no influence on problem-solving skills ($p > .05$; Table 4).

Age, marital status, and professional career length were not found to affect the CE and EE subscale scores, with no statistically significant correlations found between the two subscales ($p > .05$; Table 4). However, the EE scores of undergraduate nurses were found to be higher than those of postgraduate nurses, at a level that approached statistical significance ($p = .078$). In addition, the average CE scores of nurses who had worked for 1–10 and 11–20 years were higher than those of nurses who had worked for 21 years or more, at a level that approached statistical significance ($p = .066$).

A statistically significant difference was found between mean years working in the current hospital and educational background, respectively, and CE scores ($p = .027$ and $p = .013$; Table 4). On the basis of paired comparison analysis, the CE scores of participants with 1–10 years of working experience at their current hospital were higher than those with ≥ 21 years of working experience at their current hospital ($p = .027$). Also on the basis of paired comparison analysis, the CE score of participants educated to the undergraduate level was found to be higher at a statistically significant level than those educated to the master's/doctorate degree level ($p = .013$).

The comparison of problem-solving skill scores by descriptive characteristics revealed no statistically significant difference between subscale scores and the variables of age, marital status, length of professional and organizational career, or educational background ($p > .05$). Thus, the descriptive characteristics of the participants did not affect their problem-solving skills.

TABLE 3.
Correlation Between Basic Empathy Skills and Problem-Solving Skills

	Basic Empathic Skill			
	Cognitive Empathy		Emotional Empathy	
Problem-Solving Skill	*r*	*p*	*r*	*p*
Negative approach to the problem	−.092	.418	.113	.320
Constructive problem solving	.200[a]	.075	.036	.749
Lack of self-confidence	−.223[a]	.047*	−.211	.060
Abstaining from responsibility	−.037	.742	−.071	.533
Persistent approach	.118	.296	.189	.093

Note. r = Pearson correlation test.
[a]Spearman's correlation test.
*$p < .05$.

Regression Analysis of Risk Factors Affecting Cognitive and Empathy Skills

Variables found after univariate analysis to have significance levels of $p < .01$ were subsequently modeled and evaluated. A regression analysis was conducted to determine the effect on CE skills of educational level, duration of institutional work, CPS level, and self-insecurity level. The explanatory power of this model was 29.9% ($R^2 = .299$), and the model was significant ($p < .001$). As a result of the analysis, CPS ($p = .006$), educational status of graduate ($p < .001$), and working for the current hospital for a period of more than 20 years ($p = .004$) were found to have a significant and positive influence on the CE score.

A 1-unit increase in the CPS score was found to increase CE skills by 0.139 points ($\beta = 0.139$, 95% CI [0.041, 0.237], $p < .01$). For education, graduate education was found to decrease the CE score by 4.520 points ($\beta = -4.520$, 95% CI [−6.986, −2.054], $p < .001$). For duration working for the current hospital, working for the same institution for a period exceeding 20 years was found to decrease the CE score by 3.429 points ($\beta = -3.429$, 95% CI [−5.756, −1.102], $p < .05$). In addition, a 1-unit increase in the LSC score was found to decrease the CE score by 0.114 points, which did not achieve statistical significance ($\beta = 0.114$, 95% CI [−0.325, 0.096], $p > .05$).

Regression analysis was used to evaluate the effects of education, PA, and LSC on the risk factors affecting EE. As a result of this evaluation, the explanatory power of the model was determined as 15.3% ($R^2 = .153$), which was significant despite the low level ($F = 3.388, p = .001$). The effects of PA ($p = .021$) and educational status ($p = .015$) on the EE score were shown through analysis to be statistically significant (Table 5). A 1-unit increase in PA score was found to increase the EE score by 0.323 points ($\beta = 0.323$, 95% CI [0.049, 0.596], $p < .05$). For education, having a graduate education was found to decrease the EE score by 3.989 points ($\beta = -3.989$, 95% CI [−7.193, −0.786], $p < .05$). Moreover, the LSC score was found to be 0.119 points lower than the EE score. However, this result was not statistically significant ($\beta = -0.193$, 95% CI [−0.467, 0.080], $p > .05$). Dummy variables were used in the regression analysis of sociodemographic characteristics (educational status and years working for the current hospital).

Discussion

This study found that age, marital status, educational background, years of professional working experience, and years working for the current hospital did not affect the problem-solving skills of the participants. In the literature, the findings of several studies indicate that characteristics such as age, educational background, department of service, and career length do not affect the problem-solving skills of nurses (Abaan & Altıntoprak, 2005; Kelleci & Gölbaşı, 2004; Yu & Kirk, 2008), whereas other studies indicate that these variables do affect these skills (Ançel, 2006; Watt-Watson, Garfinkel, Gallop, Stevens, & Streiner, 2000; Yu & Kirk, 2008). However, beyond these characteristics, some studies have reported a positive correlation between the problem-solving skills of nurses and their educational level, with this correlation mediated by the physical conditions of the workplace, good relationships with colleagues, and educational background (Yıldız & Güven, 2009). These findings suggest that factors affecting the empathy and problem-solving skills of nurses working in operating rooms differ from known and expected factors.

Operating room nurses deliver dynamic nursing care that requires attention and close observation because of the fast turnover of patients. In addition to the problem-solving skills that they use during the patient care process, these nurses must use or operate a myriad of lifesaving technological devices and equipment (AbuAlRub, 2004; Özgür, Yıldırım, & Aktaş, 2008). The circumstances in which nurses employ their problem-solving skills are generally near-death critical conditions and emergencies. Furthermore, operating rooms are more isolated than other areas of the hospital, which affects nurses who work in operating rooms and intensive care units (AbuAlRub, 2004; Özgür et al., 2008).

Communication is a critical factor that affects the delivery of healthcare services. Communication does not only take place between a service recipient and a provider. To establish a teamwork philosophy between employees, it is essential to build effective communication (Sandelin & Gustafsson, 2015). Empathic communication helps enhance the problem-solving skills of nurses as they work to learn about individual experiences (Kumcağız, Yılmaz, Çelik, & Avcı, 2011). Studies in the literature have found that nurses who are satisfied with their relationships with colleagues, physicians, and supervisors have a high level of problem-solving skills (Abaan & Altıntoprak, 2005; Kumcağız et al., 2011) and that higher problem-solving skills are associated with a higher level of individual achievement (Abaan & Altıntoprak, 2005; Chan, 2001). Another finding of this study is that CPS increases the cognitive emphatic level. This may be attributed to constructive problem-solving skills increasing CE, as these skills are associated with feelings, thoughts, and behaviors that contribute to problem resolution.

A review of the literature on empathy and communication skills revealed, as expected, that these skills increased with level of education (Kumcağız et al., 2011; Vioulac et al., 2016). However, a number of studies have reported no significant correlation between age, marital status, and professional working experience and empathy skills or communication abilities in nurses (Kumcağız et al., 2011; Yu & Kirk, 2008).

EE is assumed to be a more intuitive reaction to emotions. Factors that affect EE are nurses working with small patient groups, frequent contact with patient groups, and long periods spent accompanying or being in close contact with patient groups (Vioulac et al., 2016). Studies in the literature have reported no correlation between the empathy skills of nurses and demographic characteristics (Vioulac et al., 2016). This study supports this finding, with the empathy

TABLE 4.

Evaluation of Problem-Solving Skills Score, by Descriptive Characteristics

	Basic Empathy Skill					
	Cognitive Empathy		Emotional Empathy		Negative Approach to the Problem	
	M	*SD*	*M*	*SD*	*M*	*SD*
Characteristic	Median		Median		Median	
Age (years)						
≤ 35	36.52	4.53	39.45	5.76	34.45	11.01
	36		38		31	
≥ 36	35.26	4.17	40.30	4.90	36.55	10.94
	35		40		33	
p	.203[a]		.483[a]		.402[a]	
Marital status						
Married	35.50	4.52	39.75	4.75	35.48	1.14
	35		40		33	
Single	36.88	3.42	40.75	7.06	36.50	10.46
	37		40		37	
p	.260[a]		.598[a]		.742[a]	
Duration working as a nurse (years)						
1–10	36.61	4.58	40.52	6.02	34.48	9.26
	37		40		31	
11–20	36.37	3.99	39.34	5.13	36.34	12.50
	36		39		34	
≥ 21	33.95	4.27	40.32	4.71	35.91	10.29
	34		40		33	
p	.066[c]		.660[c]		.817[c]	
Duration working at current hospital (years)						
1–10	36.45	4.26	39.88	5.76	34.36	10.38
	37		38		33	
11–20	36.43	4.04	39.52	4.56	37.86	13.16
	36		40		33	
≥ 21	33.29	4.22	40.65	4.97	36.29	9.41
	33		40		38	
p	.027*[c]		.805[c]		.479[c]	
Educational level						
High school and associate degree	35.31	5.11	38.92	3.71	35.54	9.27
	36		39		33	
Undergraduate	36.61	3.83	40.81	5.22	35.93	10.97
	37		40		35	
Master's/doctorate degree	32.77	4.48	37.38	6.02	34.85	13.07
	33		36		31	
p	.013*[c]		.078[c]		.950[c]	

[a]Student *t* test. [b]Mann–Whitney *U* test. [c]One-way analysis of variance test. [d]Kruskal–Wallis test.
*$p < .05$.

skills of operating room nurses found to be close to the peak value of the scale.

Studies in the literature reveal a positive correlation between empathy and career length (Watt-Watson et al., 2000; Yu & Kirk, 2008) as well as a correlation between increased professional experience and lower empathy (Yu & Kirk, 2008). This study found an association between longer periods working for the same hospital and higher levels of education with lower empathy scores. This may be attributed to the difficult working conditions in operating rooms, intense stress, and high level of potential stress-driven conflicts between employees in work settings.

Problem-Solving Skill											
Constructive Problem Solving			Lack of Self-Confidence			Abstaining From Responsibility			Persistent Approach		
M	*SD*	Median	*M*	*SD*	Median	*M*	*SD*	Median	*M*	*SD*	Median
52.52	10.51	49	13.30	4.30	12	11.79	3.31	12	19.45	4.94	18
51.06	7.82	48	13.11	4.12	12	10.91	3.51	11	20.17	3.64	20
		.573[b]			.898[b]			.266[a]			.458[a]
51.59	8.96	49	13.33	4.22	13	11.14	3.43	11	19.73	4.12	19
51.94	9.40	50	12.63	4.06	12	11.81	3.53	13	20.44	4.66	21
		.890[b]			.574[b]			.488[a]			.554[a]
52.52	10.99	48	12.65	3.31	12	11.78	2.54	12	20.04	4.76	19
51.83	8.19	51	13.31	4.64	12	11.29	3.94	11	19.80	3.98	19
50.50	8.16	48	13.55	4.31	14	10.73	3.47	11	19.82	4.15	20
		.621[d]			.817[d]			.594[c]			.975[c]
52.55	10.10	49	12.83	3.89	12	11.36	3.19	12	20.02	4.80	19
50.52	7.19	48	13.52	4.26	13	11.67	4.05	12	19.90	3.40	20
50.88	8.30	50	13.65	4.86	13	10.59	3.32	10	19.47	3.73	20
		.668[d]			.696[d]			.620[c]			.902[c]
50.15	6.38	48	14.54	5.16	12	11.54	3.31	12	20.08	3.07	21
50.91	8.98	49	12.56	3.43	12	11.07	3.46	12	19.28	4.26	19
56.31	10.32	55	14.46	5.50	13	11.85	3.67	11	22.15	4.45	23
		.251[d]			.435[d]			.739[c]			.084[c]

Stress is a major factor that affects the empathy skills and relationship-building abilities of nurses (Vioulac et al., 2016). Nurses are exposed to a wide variety of stressors such as quality of the service, duration of shifts, workload, time pressures, and limited decision-making authority (Patrick & Lavery, 2007; Shimizutani et al., 2008; Vioulac et al., 2016). In particular, environments evoking a sense of death (e.g., operating rooms) is another factor known to elevate perceived stress (Ashker, Penprase, & Salman, 2012). High stress may lead to negative consequences such as reduced problem-solving abilities (Zhao, Lei, He, Gu, & Li, 2015). Both having a long nursing career and working in stressful environments such as operating

TABLE 5.
Regression Model of Risk Factors Affecting Cognitive and Emotional Empathy

Model	β	*SE*	*t*	*p*	95% CI
Model A					
(Constant)	31.707	3.049	10.398	< .001**	[25.630, 37.784]
Constructive problem solving	0.139	0.049	2.825	.006**	[0.041, 0.237]
Lack of self-confidence	−0.114	0.106	−1.084	.282	[−0.325, 0.096]
Education (high school)	0.154	1.273	0.121	.904	[−2.384, 2.691]
Education (postgraduate)	−4.520	1.237	−3,653	< .001**	[−6.986, −2.054]
Duration working as a nurse (≥ 21 years)	−3.429	1.168	−2.937	.004**	[−5.756, −1.102]
Duration working at current hospital (11–20 years)	−0.565	1.081	−0.523	.603	[−2.719, 1.589]
Model B					
(Constant)	37.024	3.302	11.212	< .001**	[30.446, 43.602]
Persistent approach	0.323	0.137	2.352	.021*	[0.049, 0.596]
Lack of self-confidence	−0.193	0.137	−1.408	.163	[−0.467, 0.080]
Education (high school)	−1.766	1.562	−1.130	.262	[−4.878, 1.346]
Education (postgraduate)	−3.989	1.608	−2.481	.015*	[−7.193, −0.786]

[a]Dependent variable: cognitive empathy (R^2 = .299). [b]Dependent variable: emotional empathy (R^2 = .153).
*$p < .05$. **$p < .01$.

rooms may negatively affect empathy and problem-solving skills. However, this study revealed that working for a long period at the current hospital had no influence on problem-solving skills. The low reliability of the scales means that the variance may be high in other samples that are drawn from the same main sample, with the resultant data thus not reflecting the truth.

Low reliability coefficients reduce the significance and value of the results obtained by increasing the standard error of the data (Şencan, 2005). The Cronbach's α of the EE scale used in the study was between .60 and .80 and is highly trustworthy. However, the Cronbach's α value is close to .60 (i.e., .649). This result may elicit suspicion in regression analysis estimates that are done to determine the variables that affect EE. In the correlation analysis, a statistically significant weak correlation was found only between the LSC subdimension and CE. However, the fact that the subscales of empathy and problem-solving skills are significantly related to the regression models may also be related to the reliability levels of the scales.

According to the results of the regression analysis, all of the variables remaining in Model A affected level of low for the CE (R^2 = 299). Having constructive problem-solving skills (p = .006), having a high level of education (p < .001), and working for the current hospital for over 20 years (p = .004) were found to be significantly related to CE.

Other variables were found to have no significant effect. According to the results of the regression analysis, all of the remaining variables in Model B accounted for a relatively low portion of the EE (R^2 = .153). When the *t* test results for the significance of the regression coefficients were examined, it was determined that PA (p = .021) and educational status (p = .015) were significant predictors of EE. Other variables had no significant effect (Table 5). The increase in the level of education of nurses may have increased their cognitive and emotional development. Thus, working in the same hospital for over 20 years was found to increase the levels of CE and EE. This result may be because of greater professional experience and regular experience handling numerous, different problems. In addition, the low explanatory power of the models may also be because of the fact that many other arguments that may affect empathy were not modeled. When constant values are fixed and the value of the independent variables entering the regression formula is zero, constant value is the estimated value of the dependent variable. According to findings of this study, sociodemographic characteristics and problem-solving abilities did not affect empathy level, although the CE value was 31.707 and the EE value was 37.024. Repeating this research in larger and different nurse groups may be useful to verify these research results.

Conclusions

The following results were derived from this study: First, constructive problem-solving skills affect CE skills. EE is adversely affected by the PA and LSC. Second, no correlation was found between the demographic characteristics of nurses and their problem-solving skills. Third, as level of education increases, cognitive and emotional levels of empathy decrease.

Duration of time spent working at one's current healthcare institution and educational level were both found to correlate negatively with the CE score. The higher the educational level and PA and the lower the self-confidence of the participants, the lower their EE levels. Finally, higher constructive problem-solving scores were associated with higher CE skills.

Limitations

The major limitation of the study is that it was conducted in the affiliated hospitals of one healthcare organization. The study data were obtained from operating room nurses who currently worked in these hospitals and who volunteered to participate. The conditions of nurses who did not participate in the study cannot be ascertained. A second important limitation is that the data reflect the subjective perceptions and statements of the participants. A third important limitation is that participant characteristics such as trust in management, trust in the institution, burnout, and communication skills were not assessed. For this reason, the effects of these variables on problem-solving and empathy skills remain unknown.

Author Contributions

Study conception and design: SP
Data collection: TK
Data analysis and interpretation: FA, SP
Drafting of the article: FA
Critical revision of the article: FA

References

Abaan, S., & Altıntoprak, A. (2005). Nurses' perceptions of their problem solving ability: Analysis of self apprasials. *Journal of School Nursing, 12*(1), 62–76. (Original work published in Turkish)

AbuAlRub, R. F. (2004). Job stress, job performance, and social support among hospital nurses. *Journal of Nursing Scholarship, 36*(1), 73–78. https://doi.org/10.1111/j.1547-5069.2004.04016.x

Ançel, G. (2006). Developing empathy in nurses: An inservice training program. *Archives of Psychiatric Nursing, 20*(6), 249–257. https://doi.org/10.1016/j.apnu.2006.05.002

Ashker, V. E., Penprase, B., & Salman, A. (2012). Work-related emotional stressors and coping strategies that affect the well-being of nurses working in hemodialysis units. *Journal of the American Nephrology Nurses' Association, 39*(3), 231–236.

Association of periOperative Registered Nurses. (2015). *Guidelines for perioperative practice* (p. 694). Denver, CO: Author.

Çam, S., & Tümkaya, S. (2008). Developing the interpersonal problem solving inventory for high school students: The validity and reliability process. *Turkish Psychological Counseling and Guidance Journal, 3*(28), 95–111. (Original work published in Turkish)

Chan, D. W. (2001). Dimensionality and correlates of problem solving: The use of the problem solving inventory in the Chinese context. *Behaviour Research and Therapy, 39*(7), 859–875. https://doi.org/10.1016/S0005-7967(00)00082-6

de Kemp, R. A., Overbeek, G., de Wied, M., Engels, R. C., & Scholte, R. H. (2007). Early adolescent empathy, parental support, and antisocial behavior. *The Journal of Genetic Psychology, 168*(1), 5–18. https://doi.org/10.3200/GNTP.168.1.5-18

Fields, S. K., Hojat, M., Gonnella, J. S., Mangione, S., Kane, G., & Magee, M. (2004). Comparisons of nurses and physicians on an operational measure of empathy. *Evaluation & the Health Professions, 27*(1), 80–94. https://doi.org/10.1177/0163278703261206

Happell, B., Dwyer, T., Reid-Searl, K., Burke, K. J., Caperchione, C. M., & Gaskin, C. J. (2013). Nurses and stress: Recognizing causes and seeking solutions. *Journal of Nursing Management, 21*(4), 638–647. https://doi.org/10.1111/jonm.12037

Jeon, Y., Lakanmaa, R. L., Meretoja, R., & Leino-Kilpi, H. (2017). Competence assessment instruments in perianesthesia nursing care: A scoping review of the literature. *Journal of Perianesthesia Nursing, 32*(6), 542–556. https://doi.org/10.1016/j.jopan.2016.09.008

Jolliffe, D., & Farrington, D. P. (2006). Development and validation of the basic empathy scale. *Journal of Adolescence, 29*(4), 589–611. https://doi.org/10.1016/j.adolescence.2005.08.010

Kanan, N. (2011). Neurosurgical operating room nurse's roles and responsibilities. *Florence Nightingale Journal of Nursing, 19*(3), 179–186. (Original work published in Turkish)

Kelleci, M., & Gölbaşı, Z. (2004). Determining the problem solving skills and some related factors of nurses who work in a university hospital. *Cumhuriyet Nursing Journal, 8*(2), 1–8. (Original work published in Turkish)

Kumcağız, H., Yılmaz, M., Çelik, S. B., & Avcı, İ. A. (2011). Communication skills of nurses: Samsun sample. *Dicle Medical Journal, 38*(1), 49–56. (Original work published in Turkish)

Özgür, G., Yıldırım, S., & Aktaş, N. (2008). Determination of operating room and critical care nurses' mental health in the university hospital. *Cumhuriyet Nursing Journal, 12*(2), 21–30. (Original work published in Turkish)

Patrick, K., & Lavery, J. F. (2007). Burnout in nursing. *The Australian Journal of Advanced Nursing, 24*(3), 43–48.

Sandelin, A., & Gustafsson, B. Å. (2015). Operating theatre nurses' experiences of teamwork for safe surgery. *Nordic Journal of Nursing Research, 35*(3), 179–185. https://doi.org/10.1177/0107408315591337

Şencan, H. (2005). *Reliability and validity of the social and behavioral measures* (1st ed., p. 172). Ankara, Turkey: Seçkin. (Original work published in Turkish)

Shimizutani, M., Odagiri, Y., Ohya, Y., Shimomitsu, T., Kristensen, T. S., Maruta, T., & Iimori, M. (2008). Relationship of nurse burnout with personality characteristics and coping behaviors. *Industrial Health, 46*(4), 326–335. https://doi.org/10.2486/indhealth.46.326

Sonoda, Y., Onozuka, D., & Hagihara, A. (2018). Factors related to teamwork performance and stress of operating room nurses. *Journal of Nursing Management, 26*(1), 66–73. https://doi.org/10.1111/jonm.12522

Suresh, P., Matthews, A., & Coyne, I. (2013). Stress and stressors in the clinical environment: A comparative study of fourth-year student nurses and newly qualified general nurses in Ireland. *Journal of Clinical Nursing, 22*(5–6), 770–779. https://doi.org/10.1111/j.1365-2702.2012.04145.x

Taşcı, S. (2005). The problem solving process in nursing. *Journal of Health Sciences, 14*(Suppl.), 73–78. (Original work published in Turkish)

Taylor, C. (2000). Clinical problem-solving in nursing: Insights from the literature. *Journal of Advanced Nursing, 31*(4), 842–849. https://doi.org/10.1046/j.1365-2648.2000.01342.x

Topçu, Ç., Baker, Ö. E., & Aydın, Y. A. (2010). Turkish adaptation of basic empathy scale: Validity and reliability study. *Turkish Psychological Counseling and Guidance Journal, 4*(34), 174–182. (Original work published in Turkish)

Vioulac, C., Aubree, C., Massy, Z. A., & Untas, A. (2016). Empathy and stress in nurses working in haemodialysis: A qualitative study. *Journal of Advanced Nursing, 72*(5), 1075–1085. https://doi.org/10.1111/jan.12899

Watt-Watson, J., Garfinkel, P., Gallop, R., Stevens, B., & Streiner, D. (2000). The impact of nurses' empathic responses on patients' pain management in acute care. *Nursing Research, 49*(4), 191–200. https://doi.org/10.1097/00006199-200007000-00002

Yıldız, H., & Güven, M. (2009). Research on burnout level of nurses and their problem solving skills. *Life Sciences, 4*(4), 1–20. (Original work published in Turkish)

Yu, J., & Kirk, M. (2008). Measurement of empathy in nursing research: Systematic review. *Journal of Advanced Nursing, 64*(5), 440–454. https://doi.org/10.1111/j.1365-2648.2008.04831.x

Zhao, F. F., Lei, X. L., He, W., Gu, Y. H., & Li, D. W. (2015). The study of perceived stress, coping strategy and self-efficacy of Chinese undergraduate nursing students in clinical practice. *International Journal of Nursing Practice, 21*(4), 401–409. https://doi.org/10.1111/ijn.12273

25

Evaluating the Effectiveness of Interventions on Increasing Participation in Cervical Cancer Screening

Gonul KURT[1]* • Aygul AKYUZ[2]

ABSTRACT

Background: Although cervical cancer is highly preventable through regular screenings using Pap smear or human papillomavirus–deoxyribonucleic acid tests, cervical cancer remains a prevalent women's health issue across the world. Therefore, encouraging women to screen for cervical cancer is very important for the early detection of cervical cancer.

Purpose: The purposes of this study were to (1) assess the effectiveness of three interventions that are typically used to increase the uptake of cervical cancer screening during home visits and (2) determine the participation rate in cervical cancer screenings after invitation, the health promotion perceptions, and the cervical cancer and screening-related knowledge of women. The three interventions noted in Purpose 1 were one-on-one training accompanied by an educational brochure, providing the educational brochure only, and giving an invitation without any relevant information.

Methods: This interventional study was conducted on women who were between the ages of 30 and 65 years in three Turkish provinces (Ankara, Malatya, and Trabzon). Five hundred twenty home visits were made, and 356 women who did not have a Pap smear test within the previous year were invited for cervical cancer screening. Women were randomized into one of three intervention groups, and the participants in each group were invited to attend a national cervical cancer screening program and to undergo a cervical cancer screening using the related intervention type.

Results: The results showed that the interventions used during home visits and knowledge were effective in encouraging women to participate in cervical cancer screening. It was determined that the participants who had received one-on-one training accompanied by an educational brochure had a higher cervical cancer screening rate than their peers who were offered a brochure only or a verbal invitation only.

Conclusions: Invitations to screenings that are made by providing training accompanied with a brochure were found to be effective in increasing the participation of women in cervical cancer screening.

KEY WORDS:
cervical cancer screening, home visit, invitation, cervical cancer, Pap smear test.

Introduction

Cervical cancer is the second leading cause of cancer mortality among women worldwide, with approximately 530,000 new cases of invasive cervical carcinoma and approximately 280,000 related deaths reported each year. About 95% of the cases occur in less developed countries. The incidence of this disease is reportedly increasing, particularly in developing countries (Globocan, 2018; Visanuyothin, Chompikul, & Mongkolchati, 2015; World Health Organization [WHO], 2018). In Turkey, cervical cancer is the third most common type of cancer among gynecologic malignancies, with an incidence of 4.5 cases per 100,000 (Public Health Institute of Turkey, Cancer Control Center, 2018). According to Globocan (2018), in Turkey, an estimated 2,733 new cases will be found and approximately 1,553 related deaths will occur because of cervical cancer by 2025 (Globocan, 2018).

Cervical cancer is highly preventable through regular and appropriate, timely screenings (Bassal, Schejter, Cohen, & Keinan-Boker, 2017; Visanuyothin et al., 2015). Thus, cervical cancer is included among the cancers for which screening programs are recommended by the WHO. The most common technique recommended by WHO for the screening and early diagnosis of this disease is Pap smear or human papillomavirus–deoxyribonucleic acid tests (American Cancer Society, 2015; Gücük, Alkan, Arıca, & Ateş, 2011; Lu, 2014; Wright & Kuhn, 2012). Cervical cancer screening (CCS) programs with Pap smear or human papillomavirus–deoxyribonucleic acid tests have been shown to decrease the incidence of cervical cancer by 34%–80% and the related mortality rate in many developed countries (DeGregorio et al., 2017; Kitchener et al., 2018; Visanuyothin et al., 2015). A wide variety of Pap smear tests and uptake of CCS procedures exist around the world. According to the results of studies conducted in various countries, the ratio of women who have received at least one CCS with Pap smear test varies widely, with rates of 52.6% in Taiwan, 66% in Mexico, 72% in Botswana, 93% in the United States, 30.5% in Malaysia, 23.1% in China, 5.3% in India, and 4.1% in Morocco (Gakidou, Nordhagen,

[1]*PhD, RN, Assistant Professor, Faculty of Health Sciences, Department of Midwifery, Sakarya University, Sakarya, Turkey* • [2]*PhD, RN, Professor, Department of Obstetrics and Gynecology Nursing, Florence Nightingale Hospital School of Nursing, Demiroglu Bilim University, Istanbul, Turkey.*

& Obermeyer, 2008; Lee & Wang, 2011; Lee-Lin et al., 2007; Mingo et al., 2012). The CCS participation rate in domestic Cancer Early Diagnosis, Screening and Education Centers (KETEMs), which are the only facilities that conduct community-based cancer screening in Turkey, was reported to be only 11.3% in 2008 (Özgül, 2010; Tuncer, Özgül, Özen Olcayto, Gültekin, & Erdin, 2009). Studies conducted in various regions and on various groups in Turkey have also reported low participation rates for CCS (varying between 11% and 56%; Babacan Gümüş & Çam, 2011; Güvenç, Akyuz, & Yenen, 2013; Uluocak & Bekar, 2012). These results show that the participation rate for CCS in Turkey remains below desired levels and below the levels that are prevalent in developed countries.

The participation of women in CCS is known to be inadequate in many developing countries. The sociodemographic and cultural characteristics of the women, health beliefs, their knowledge about cervical cancer and the Pap smear test, and the lack of available screening programs were all found to influence the participation rates of women in CCS (Güvenç et al., 2013; Lee, 2018; Lu, 2014; Uluocak & Bekar, 2012). In different areas and in light of the results of various studies across Turkey, reasons why women do not participate in CCS include lack of knowledge about CCS and national screening program services, health beliefs (i.e., believing CCS is not necessary if there are no symptoms, ignoring the necessity of CCS, and fear that the Pap smear test is painful), perceived barriers related to CCS (i.e., fear of results and embarrassment), and environmental factors (i.e., difficulties in accessing healthcare units; cost, quality, and continuation of the service; and long waits at the healthcare center; Babacan Gümüş & Çam, 2011; Güvenç et al., 2013; Uluocak & Bekar, 2012; Yücel, Çeber, & Özentürk, 2009). In addition, sociocultural norms and religious beliefs affect the willingness of women in Turkey to participate in CCS. CCS-related examinations cause embarrassment for women, who prefer that a female physician conduct the procedure. One study conducted in Turkey reported that the women who had never undergone a Pap smear test had significantly higher perceived barriers to CCS than women who had. The same study reported that gynecologic-examination-related embarrassment and preference for a female physician affected women's decisions to participate in CCS (Güvenç et al., 2013). Similarly, another study showed that women who found the Pap smear test painful and did not know where they could go to have a Pap smear test were more likely to avoid having this test (Esin, Bulduk, & Ardic, 2011). As these results show, it may be argued that the most important determinants of participation in CCS are knowledge, awareness, and perceived barriers about this subject. Several studies have noted that removing the perceived barriers to and fostering awareness of cervical cancer, risk factors, and the CCS program, as well as using interventions to provide information about CCS and to develop health protection behaviors, have all been reported to be important steps in increasing the participation of women in CCS programs (Boonpongmanee & Jittanoon, 2007; Güvenç et al., 2013; Kitchener et al., 2018; Lu, 2014). Bowles, Gao, Brandzel, Bradford, and Buist (2016) reported that sending out Pap-specific letters containing reminders of the availability of multiple preventive services was effective at promoting CCS (Bowles et al., 2016). In a study that was conducted to increase participation in CCS, 200 women were given one-on-one education and 200 were trained using a video produced by a national television channel. They found the 3-month posttest screening rate (after the one-on-one education) was higher in women who were educated using the video (Lam et al., 2003).

Nurses play a critical role in providing preventive healthcare services. Moreover, nurses who are trained in early diagnosis cancer programs in developed countries play an essential role in public health screenings and educational programs by cooperating with other healthcare professionals (Anttila & Nieminen, 2007; Güvenç et al., 2013; Vokó et al., 2012). The responsibility of nurses include meeting the information needs of women by giving them healthcare training, encouraging women to participate in screening, implementing Pap smear tests, collecting and evaluating screening data, and directing women to healthcare services for early diagnosis and/or cervical cancer prevention based on their diagnosis (Güvenç et al., 2013).

Taking into consideration that the CCS rates of women in Turkey are below the desired level and that the most important reason that women do not participate in CCS is lack of knowledge or awareness of CCS, studies that are designed to identify activities that will increase the participation of women in CCS are genuinely needed. Therefore, this study was designed to inform women about cervical cancer, the related risk factors, and the CCS program's role in both building awareness about the services of the national cancer screening program and removing perceived barriers using various interventions. The findings of this study are hoped to help increase the participation of women in CCS.

In view of the above, the primary purpose of this study was to assess the effectiveness of the three different interventions (training accompanied by a brochure, giving a brochure only, and giving an invitation without any information only) in terms of increasing awareness about cervical cancer, related risk factors, and the CCS as well as of removing the perceived barriers of women during home visits to increase the participation of women in national CCS and the uptake of CCS. Secondarily, the level of participation in CCS after invitation, health promotion perceptions, and providing knowledge related to cervical cancer and the Pap smear test was assessed.

Methods

Study Design and Participants

This interventional study was performed in the three Turkish provinces of Ankara, Malatya, and Trabzon between August 2011 and April 2012. Formal approvals were obtained from the Ministry of Health of Turkey (approval number: 10990335).

The target population consisted of women living in the regions served by the three KETEMs—Ankara Etlik Zübeyde Hanım Women's Hospital, Malatya State Hospital, and Trabzon Fatih State Hospital.

Home visits were made by the principal investigator to the women who met the inclusion criteria in each province. Those women who agreed to participate were randomly assigned to the three different interventions:

(i) One-on-one training accompanied by an educational brochure (education + brochure group)
(ii) An educational brochure only (brochure-only group)
(iii) An invitation only, without additional information (invitation-only group)

After the intervention, all participants were invited to the KETEMs for CCS. During the screening, all participants were informed about the role of the national CCS program in increasing awareness about services at the KETEMs. The principal investigator made only one home visit to each woman.

Inclusion and Exclusion Criteria

The criteria for inclusion in this study were as follows: 30–65 years old (based on the age range of the national CCS); being or having been sexually active; able to speak, read, and understand the Turkish language; and providing informed consent.

Subjects were excluded from participation if they

- had gynecologic cancer;
- had received a hysterectomy;
- had received a Pap smear test during the previous year; and
- were pregnant or in the 3-month postpartum period.

Study Sample and Intervention Groups

Convenience sampling was used to select the target provinces of Ankara, Malatya, and Trabzon, which were respectively located in the northern, eastern, and middle regions to provide representative social and cultural diversity.

After identifying the provinces, the sampling was made for groups that would be made available for home visits. Accordingly, a two-staged stratification sampling method was used to determine the study sample. A total of 134,704 women between the ages of 30–65 years resided in the three target provinces. Five hundred twenty women from each were calculated to be needed for the first-stage stratification. The total sample size was then stratified to each region for the second-stage stratification sampling. For this stage, it was assumed that the rate of Pap smear tests for each region was 25%, 5%, and 10%, respectively (these are the official rates estimated by the Republic of Turkey Ministry of Health's Cancer General Office). The sample size was calculated for each region as 96 in Ankara, 147 in Malatya, and 277 in Trabzon, with a 2.5% error rate and a 97.5% confidence interval. To stratify these women by province, Equation 1 was used:

$$n_h = \frac{N_h\sqrt{P_hQ_h}}{\sum N_h\sqrt{P_hQ_h}}n$$

After determining the sample size, the contact information for the women was obtained from the KETEM registry. The contact information of the women was numbered and ordered and then was classified by block randomization into one of the three interventions. The investigator made one home visit to each randomly selected woman to determine if they met the eligibility criteria.

Developing the Educational Brochure

An educational brochure was developed to invite the women for CCS at the KETEMs and to impart knowledge of and awareness about cervical cancer, CCS with Pap smear test, and the services provided at the KETEMs. In developing the educational brochure, the key concepts to be included to inform the participants about CCS were determined and then the content relevant to these concepts were developed. A comprehensive literature review was undertaken to design the brochure (Güvenç et al., 2013; Kög et al., 2012; Yücel et al., 2009). In addition, existing educational brochures were analyzed, and professionals in the field were consulted.

The tagline "Give yourself a chance, get regularly screened for cervical cancer" was used in the brochure to draw participants' attention. The educational brochure provided information related to "What is cervical cancer?", "What are the causes and symptoms of cervical cancer?", "What is a Pap smear test?", "Why is the Pap smear test done?", "When should the Pap smear test be done?", and "Information about KETEMs." In addition, the brochure invited women to participate in free CCS with Pap smear test at the KETEM in their area.

Content experts included a gynecologist and a senior nurse lecturer with expertise in women's health, both of whom were consulted during the prepublication evaluation of the brochure. These individuals participated in the evaluation of the brochures before printing. The brochure content was also reviewed by KETEM management for cultural sensitivity and education level appropriateness, and modifications were made based on KETEM's feedback.

The completed educational brochure was first administered by the investigator to 15 women as a pilot study to ascertain whether the content could be easily understood. The women in the pilot study were excluded from the main study.

Instruments

Outcome data were obtained using the following surveys: "Participant Description Questionnaire," "Knowledge Questionnaire about Cervical Cancer and Pap Smear Test," and "Health Belief Model Scale for Cervical Cancer and the Pap Smear Test."

Participant description questionnaire

The investigators developed this form based on a review of the literature. The form consists of questions that are used to determine the sociodemographic, obstetric, and gynecologic features of the women as well as Pap smear history and awareness of the available services at the KETEMs.

Knowledge questionnaire about cervical cancer and Pap smear test

This form consists of 10 questions that are designed to measure the basic knowledge related to cervical cancer and the Pap smear test. The questions were systemically prepared by the investigators using the same literature that was consulted in preparing the brochures. Participants were asked to mark the statements as either "true" or "false." In the evaluation of the statements, a score of 1 was given for correct answers and 0 was given for incorrect answers. The range of total possible scores was 0–10, with higher scores indicating higher knowledge of cervical cancer and of the Pap smear test. The reliability of this questionnaire was calculated using the Kuder–Richardson 20 formula, which found a reliability coefficient of .80.

Health belief model scale for cervical cancer and the Pap smear test

The Health Belief Model (HBM) was developed by Güvenç, Akyüz, and Açıkel in 2011 to measure the health beliefs of women in relation to cervical cancer and the Pap smear test. This scale includes 35 items, with all items scored on a 5-point Likert scale. The HBM includes five subscales: seriousness, susceptibility, Pap smear benefits, Pap smear barriers, and health motivation. The Pap smear barriers subscale is negatively associated and the other subscales are positively associated with screening behavior. As each scale was evaluated separately and not combined into a single total score, each participant obtained points for each subscale. In the original testing, Cronbach's alpha coefficients for the five subscales were .78, .78, .86, .82, and .62, respectively (Güvenç et al., 2011). In this study, Cronbach's alpha coefficients were calculated to be .84 for seriousness, .97 for susceptibility, .83 for Pap smear benefits, .56 for health motivation, and .79 for Pap smear barriers.

Procedures and Data Collection

Consecutive home visits with the participants were made by the principal investigator. First, the compliance of women with the inclusion criteria was confirmed using the "Participant Description Questionnaire" during the home visit. Those who met the inclusion criteria for each group were then informed about the aim of the study and given the HBM and the "Knowledge Questionnaire about Cervical Cancer and Pap Smear Test" to complete. The participants in each intervention group were then invited to the KETEMs for CCS according to the interventions identified in the randomization table. In this regard:

(1) Brochure + education group: The principal investigator conducted one-on-one training regarding the importance of cervical cancer and the Pap smear test and distributed an educational brochure to the participants in this group. The training brochure was left with the women so that they could review it at their leisure. During the training session, the following information was explained to the women:

- Anatomical location of the cervix
- Prevalence, symptoms, and risk factors of cervical cancer
- Importance of the Pap smear test to the early diagnosis of cervical cancer
- Information about the Pap smear test
- How the Pap smear test is performed
- How frequently the Pap smear test should be performed
- Who should receive a Pap smear test
- Issues that need to be considered before getting a Pap smear test

(2) Brochure-only group: The participants in this group were asked to read the educational brochure.

(3) Invitation-only group: The participants in this group were invited to receive a CCS without receiving additional training or an educational brochure.

After the intervention, the women in each intervention group were informed about the CCS services that are regularly offered by KETEMs. Moreover, they were informed that these services are offered at no cost and without prior appointment or long wait times. In addition, they were told that treatment provided at the KETEMs is free when any problem is detected as a result of screening. The women were then invited to the KETEM in their region of residence for CCS.

By the end of the study, 520 home visits were made. However, only 500 women were interviewed, as 20 women were unreachable because of a change of address. Of the women who were contacted (n = 500), 71 were excluded because of reasons including having undergone a hysterectomy, being currently pregnant, having had cervical cancer, and not agreeing to the interview. Thus, 429 were interviewed. However, 73 cases were not invited to the KETEM for CCS, as they had undergone a Pap smear test within the previous year. Therefore, the final study was conducted with 356 participants, including 118 women in the education + brochure group, 119 in the brochure-only group, and 119 in the invitation-only group (Figure 1).

Cervical cancer screening and form completion at Cancer Early Diagnosis, Screening and Education Centers

During the home visit, the participants were informed that they could visit the KETEM for CCS on any date they wished. After the data collection had been completed in a province, the participants were given a 3-month period in which to visit the KETEMs for CCS (see Table 1). In most studies, screening

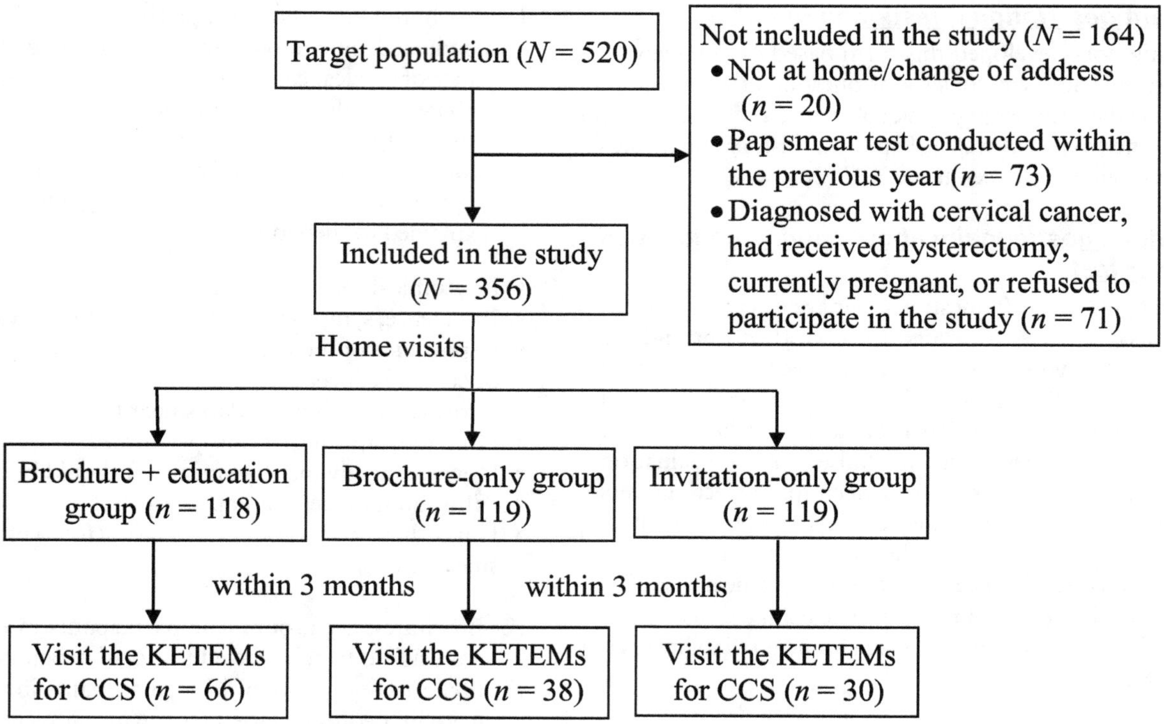

Figure 1. Flow chart of the study. CCS = cervical cancer screening; KETEMs = Cancer Early Diagnosis, Screening and Education Centers.

participation rates were calculated for a period ranging from 2 to 12 months after the invitation to receive a screening (Bowles et al., 2016; Kitchener et al., 2018; Taylor et al., 2002; Yücel et al., 2009).

The Pap smear samples of the women in each group who appeared at the screening after invitation were collected by the KETEM staff, who, without prior knowledge of the participants' grouping, also administered the HBM and "Knowledge Questionnaire about Cervical Cancer and Pap Smear Test." The completed data collection forms and cytology results of the women were sent by KETEM staff to the principal investigator via mail after the 3-month waiting period.

Data Analysis

The study data were analyzed using SPSS Version 15.0 (SPSS Inc., Chicago, IL, USA). The distribution of the data was expressed as counts and percentages, and descriptive statistics were presented with arithmetical mean and standard deviation (*SD*). The conformity of the normal distribution of data was assessed using the one-sample Kolmogorov–Smirnov test,

TABLE 1.
Time Points of Data Collection for Each Province

Stage/Province	Month								
	First	Second	Third	Fourth	Fifth	Sixth	Seventh	Eighth	Ninth
Home visit (pretest)									
Ankara	*	*							
Trabzon			*	*					
Malatya					*	*			
CCS at the KETEM (posttest) after home visit									
Ankara	*	*	*	*	*				
Trabzon			*	*	*	*	*		
Malatya					*	*	*	*	*

Note. CCS = cervical cancer screening; KETEM = Cancer Early Diagnosis, Screening and Education Center.

after which it was determined that the data were not indicators of a normal distribution. Because the data did not represent a normal distribution, the chi-square (χ^2), Kruskal–Wallis, and Mann–Whitney *U* tests were used to determine the differences among the groups. The source of differences are typically investigated using the Bonferroni-corrected Mann–Whitney *U* test when a difference is found using Kruskal–Wallis analysis.

The effect of independent variables on the dependent variable was evaluated using single and multiple logistic regression analyses. The variables found to be significant in single-variable logistic regression were evaluated using the multiple backward logistic regression model.

Row or column percentages were provided in the tables, and their interpretations according to the position of the dependent variable were investigated. An explanation was provided under each table when line percentages were used. A *p* value of less than .05 was accepted as statistically significant.

Results

In this study, 77.6% of the participants were between the ages of 30 and 49 years, with a mean age of 43.5 ± 8.13 years; 91.6% were married, 49% listed their highest level of education as primary school, and 89.3% were unemployed. No statistically significant differences in sociodemographic data were identified among the three groups.

Table 2 shows the distribution of the participants according to whether they participated in CCS after the interventions with home visit. The rates of participation for CCS with Pap smear test were 55.9%, 31.9%, and 25.2%, respectively, for the brochure + education, brochure-only, and invitation-only groups. The CCS rates were higher in the brochure + education group. The difference between the groups was highly significant ($p < .001$; Table 2).

Table 3 presents the distribution of the mean preintervention and postintervention knowledge scores, HBM subscores, and score differences among the intervention groups. A statistically significant difference was identified between the intervention groups in terms of preintervention knowledge scores ($p < .05$). The source of the difference was investigated using the Bonferroni-corrected Mann–Whitney *U* test. The preintervention knowledge scores of the brochure + education group was found to be lower than the invitation-only group ($z = 3.610$, $p < .001$).

Furthermore, a statistically significant difference was found between the intervention groups in terms of postintervention knowledge scores ($p < .05$). According to the pairwise comparisons, which were conducted to identify intervention-related differences between the groups, the postintervention knowledge scores in the brochure + education group were higher than in the invitation-only group ($z = 3.116$, $p = .002$). In addition, the postintervention knowledge scores in the brochure-only group were higher than in the invitation-only group ($z = 2.878$, $p = .004$).

When the change between the preintervention and postintervention knowledge was assessed by group, the difference in the brochure + education group was higher than in both the brochure-only group ($z = 7.099$, $p < .001$) and the invitation-only group ($z = 8.928$, $p < .001$). Furthermore, the knowledge increase in the brochure-only group was higher than in the invitation-only group ($z = 7.153$, $p < .001$). All of these differences were highly significant ($p < .001$).

No statistically significant difference was found among the intervention groups in terms of the preintervention and postintervention HBM subscale scores ($p > .05$).

The difference in the changes in score between the preintervention and postintervention HBM benefits and Pap smear barriers subscales was found to be significant across the intervention groups. The intergroup differences were found primarily between the brochure + education group and the brochure-only group ($z = 2.455$, $p = .014$) and the invitation-only group ($z = 3.040$, $p = .002$) in terms of the Pap smear benefits subscale scores and between the brochure + education group and brochure-only group ($z = 2.442$, $p = .015$) and between the brochure + education group and invitation-only group ($z = 2.712$, $p = .007$) in terms of the Pap smear barriers subscale scores. The perceived Pap smear benefits and the perceived Pap smear barriers among the brochure + education group participants respectively increased and decreased more than among their invitation-only group peers ($p < .05$; Table 3).

Univariate and multiple logistic regression analyses were performed to examine in a multifactorial manner the factors affecting postintervention CCS rates as well as to determine

TABLE 2.
The Distribution of Participants According to Participation in Cervical Cancer Screening Status After the Interventions With Home Visit (N = 356)

		Participated (n = 134)		Did Not Participate (n = 222)			
Intervention Group	N	n	%[a]	n	%[a]	χ^2	p
Brochure + education	118	66	55.9	52	44.1	26.305	< .001
Brochure only	119	38	31.9	81	68.1		
Invitation only	119	30	25.2	89	74.8		

[a]Row percentages.

TABLE 3.

The Distribution of Mean Preintervention and Postintervention Knowledge Scores, Health Belief Model (HBM) Subscores, and Score Differences of Participants, by Intervention Group

	Intervention Group							
	Brochure + Education		Brochure Only		Invitation Only			
Variable	*M*	*SD*	*M*	*SD*	*M*	*SD*	χ^{2a}	*p*
Knowledge scores[b]								
Before intervention	1.87	1.91	2.27	1.89	3.14	2.65	13.91	<.001[d]
After intervention	8.80	1.07	8.78	1.13	7.00	3.03	11.65	.003[d,e]
Knowledge scores' differences	7.63	1.37	5.49	1.30	2.24	1.84	114.70	<.001[c,d,e]
HBM subscale scores before the intervention (*n* = 356)								
Susceptibility	3.18	1.14	3.23	1.08	3.33	1.06	1.19	.552
Seriousness	3.63	1.02	3.81	1.00	3.82	0.93	2.76	.251
Pap smear benefits	3.69	0.58	3.62	0.62	3.65	0.59	0.47	.793
Health motivation	2.04	0.49	1.97	0.40	2.02	0.55	1.54	.464
Pap smear barriers	2.58	0.72	2.56	0.66	2.63	0.69	1.10	.590
HBM subscale scores after the intervention (*n* = 134)								
Susceptibility	3.16	0.82	3.17	0.85	3.00	0.72	1.80	.406
Seriousness	3.92	0.84	4.00	0.79	3.79	0.88	1.56	.458
Pap smear benefits	4.39	0.38	4.35	0.49	4.17	0.57	3.49	.175
Health motivation	2.63	0.53	2.61	0.67	2.50	0.70	1.18	.554
Pap smear barriers	2.09	0.51	2.14	0.63	2.26	0.73	1.08	.582
Differences in HBM subscale scores between preintervention and postintervention (*n* = 134)								
Susceptibility	0.11	1.10	0.07	0.94	−0.26	1.02	3.34	.188
Seriousness	0.17	1.02	0.14	0.87	0.01	0.95	0.22	.895
Pap smear benefits[b]	0.79	0.63	0.51	0.56	0.36	0.62	11.25	.004[c,d]
Health motivation	0.61	0.53	0.60	0.64	0.42	0.62	5.66	.059
Pap smear barriers[b]	−0.67	0.84	−0.30	0.80	−0.22	0.74	9.52	.009[c,d]

[a]Kruskal–Wallis test. [b]Bonferroni-corrected Mann–Whitney *U* test (level of Type 1 error was set at α = .017). [c]The statistically significant difference between the brochure + education group and the brochure-only group. [d]The statistically significant difference between the brochure + education group and the invitation-only group. [e]The statistically significant difference between the brochure-only group and the invitation-only group.

the relationship between these factors. Univariate logistic regression analysis found that the sociodemographic factors of the participants (age, education, occupational status), number of pregnancies, age at first marriage and at first childbirth, menopausal status, preintervention awareness of KETEM, family history of cancer, and health beliefs (except Pap smear benefits and health motivation) had no effect on screening rates. However, multiple logistic regression analysis showed that being invited with a brochure + education and a high knowledge score had a significant influence on participation in CCS after the intervention with home visit. The participation rate in CCS of the participants in the brochure + education group was 3.05 times higher than among those participants who were only given a brochure and 5.46 times higher than among those participants who were only given a personal invitation.

A positive relationship was found between the postintervention knowledge score and participation in CCS. Each unit increase in knowledge score was associated with an 0.83 times increase in the likelihood of participation in CCS (Table 4).

Discussion

In Turkey, as in many developing countries, the CCS rate is not yet at the desired level (Babacan Gümüş & Çam, 2011; Güvenç et al., 2013; Uluocak & Bekar, 2012; Yücel et al., 2009). This study assessed the effectiveness of three different interventions in increasing participation in the national CCS.

The sociodemographic characteristics of the women in the three groups were similar in this study, which is important in terms of showing the similarity among the groups being compared. In this study, 55.9% of the participants in the brochure + education group, 31.9% in the brochure-only group, and 25.2% in the invitation-only group went to KETEMs after the intervention and home visit to receive a CCS with Pap smear test. The participants in the brochure + education group had a higher Pap smear test rate

TABLE 4.
The Multivariable Investigation of the Factors Affecting Participation in Cervical Cancer Screening After the Interventions and the Results of Multiple Logistic Regression Analysis

Factor Affecting the CCS	*OR*	95% CI	Wald	*p*
Intervention groups				
Brochure + education	ref		30.71	< .001
Brochure only	3.05	[1.73, 5.37]	14.87	< .001
Invitation only	5.46	[2.92, 10.18]	28.40	< .001
Knowledge score	0.83	[0.74, 0.94]	9.53	.002
Constant	2.77		2.25	.133

Note. CCS = cervical cancer screening; ref = reference; *OR* = odds ratio; CI = confidence interval.

than the those in the other intervention groups (Table 2). This result supports educational training accompanied by a brochure during home visits as the most effective intervention for increasing the participation of women in CCS. In a study conducted by KETEM staff in the same region in which our study was conducted, 10,963 women were invited (through letters and phone calls) for cervical and breast cancer screenings between 2008 and 2010. Over the course of the study, 1,478 women (13.5%) visited the KETEM for screening (Kög et al., 2012). In another study, which was conducted to increase the participation in CCS of Chinese women living in North America, Taylor et al. left educational materials during home visits with one group of women who had not had a Pap smear test, sent educational materials by mail to another group, and implemented no intervention to the third group. They found women in the educational materials + home visit group to have a higher participation rate in CCS than their peers in the other two groups at 6 months postintervention. They also found providing the information during home visits to be an effective approach to educate women about participating in cancer screening programs and to increase participation in these programs (Taylor et al., 2002). Providing instructor-based training and educational materials has been found to be the most effective method to increase the participation of women in CCS in other similar studies (Güvenç et al., 2013; Lam et al., 2003; Nguyen et al., 2006; Yücel et al., 2009). On the basis of this and previous studies, screening programs alone are not sufficient to encourage the participation of women in CCS. Therefore, the organization and substructure of the health system should be reconstituted accordingly, and a service model for informing women about screening programs as well as for providing training and raising awareness should be developed.

In addition, the comparative effectiveness of providing a brochure + education and only giving a brochure was tested in terms of increasing knowledge of cervical cancer and the Pap smear test. Although the mean pretest knowledge score of the brochure + education group was the lowest of the three groups, the mean score for this group and the brochure-only group both significantly increased after the intervention. The highest difference in preintervention and postintervention knowledge scores was attained by the brochure + education group, whereas statistically significant increases were also found for the brochure-only and invitation-only groups (Table 3). Considering that the postintervention screening rate was higher in the brochure + education group, it may be argued that knowledge of cervical cancer and the Pap smear test affects participation rates in CCS. On the other hand, the presence of increased knowledge in the group given only a brochure may also indicate that the women read the brochure and followed its recommendations. Similarly, other studies that were conducted to increase the participation of women in CCS indicate that knowledge scores increase significantly after participants receive cervical cancer and the Pap smear test training (Damiani et al., 2015; Ferris, Hupman, Waller, Cudnik, & Watkins, 2009; Güvenç et al., 2013; Visanuyothin et al., 2015).

The cervical-cancer and Pap-smear-test-related health beliefs of women, including perceived susceptibility, perceived seriousness, and perceived barriers, strongly influence screening behavior and participation in CCS (Güvenç et al., 2011). In this study, the health beliefs of women related to cervical cancer and the Pap smear test were evaluated to determine the perceived barriers related to screening behavior. The preintervention mean HBM subscale scores of the participants in all of the three intervention groups were similar in this study, which is important in terms of showing the pretest similarity among the groups. Moreover, the HBM subscale scores of the three groups were similar after the intervention. However, when evaluated in terms of the changes between the preintervention and postintervention HBM subscores by intervention group, the participants in the brochure + education group who received Pap smear tests after being invited reflected significantly improved Pap smear benefit perceptions and significantly lower perceived barriers to receiving Pap smears than their peers in the other intervention groups. Using different intervention methods did not indicate a change in the seriousness, susceptibility, or health motivation perceptions of the participants (Table 3). A similar study conducted to increase the rate of screening showed that the Pap smear benefit perceptions of the group provided training on cervical cancer and the Pap smear test were significantly higher and that their Pap smear barrier perceptions were significantly lower (Park, Chang, & Chung, 2005). Similarly, another study that was conducted to increase the participation in CCS of women in Turkey reported that the perceived barriers of women toward the Pap smear test decreased after educational interventions (Güvenç et al., 2013). Another related study reported that the Pap smear barrier perceptions of women decreased after receiving interventions to increase participation in CCS (Boonpongmanee & Jittanoon, 2007). In this regard, it is likely that interventions to increase participation in CCS lead to a better understanding of the importance and benefits of the Pap smear test, potentially leading to earlier diagnoses of cervical cancer and reduced perceived barriers to receiving the test.

This study shows interventions and knowledge score to be effective in increasing the uptake of CCS after home visits, where the interventions that were used to increase the participation of women in CCS programs were evaluated. The most effective intervention for increasing participation in CCS was invitation using a brochure + education. The CCS participation rate among the participants in the brochure + education group was 3.05 times higher than among those who were only given a brochure and 5.46 times higher than among those who were only verbally invited. Moreover, a positive association was observed between knowledge scores and probability of CCS participation (Table 4). Similarly, other studies have shown that home visits and one-on-one training administered by an instructor are effective in encouraging the participation of women in national cervical cancer control programs and in increasing their knowledge on the subject (Albada, Ausems, Bensing, & van Dulmen, 2009; Spadea, Bellini, Kunst, Stirbu, & Costa, 2010; Studts et al., 2012).

Implications for Clinical Practice and Research

Women's knowledge of cervical cancer and CCS after education and raised awareness plays a significant role in influencing their decision to be screened. The use of training accompanied by a brochure during home visits, the active participation of nurses during screenings, and the distribution of necessary resources to current health organizations (qualified staff, vehicles to conduct home visits, etc.) are highly recommended to increase the participation of women in CCS, the uptake of cervical screening, and related awareness. Furthermore, all healthcare professionals should be educated regarding the current CCS recommendations for women and be made aware of available community-based screening programs.

In this study, women with high perceived barriers related to the Pap smear test (e.g., embarrassment about the gynecologic examination, fatalistic beliefs about healthcare behaviors) tended not to participate in CCS. Therefore, interventions that are aimed to increase participation in CCS should focus on the health beliefs and cultural norms that are specific to the women in each target community.

Conclusions

This study found providing training accompanied by a brochure to be the most effective intervention in terms of increasing participation in CCS. These results support that interventions that are conducted to increase knowledge and awareness of cervical cancer are effective in encouraging participation in CCS.

This study is affected by several limitations. First, the Cronbach's alpha value of one of the HBM subscales was lower than .70. Second, this study was limited to three provinces from three regions of Turkey. Moreover, only women currently residing in the main city in these provinces were interviewed. The effectiveness of the recommended methods in encouraging the participation of women in CCS across a broad range of areas (e.g., both urban and rural areas) should be evaluated in future studies.

Acknowledgments

We would like to thank Dr. Mufit Cemal Yenen and Dr. Murat Dede for their contributions as mentors and the healthcare staffs at the participating KETEMs for supporting us during the data collection period.

References

Albada, A., Ausems, M. G., Bensing, J. M., & van Dulmen, S. (2009). Tailored information about cancer risk and screening: A systematic review. *Patient Education and Counseling, 77*(2), 155–171. https://doi.org/10.1016/j.pec.2009.03.005

American Cancer Society. (2015). *Cancer facts & figures 2015.* Retrieved from http://www.cancer.org/acs/groups/content/@editorial/documents/document/acspc-044552.pdf

Anttila, A., & Nieminen, P. (2007). Cervical cancer screening programme in Finland with an example on implementing alternative screening methods. *Collegium Antropologicum, 31*(2, Suppl.), 17–22.

Babacan Gümüş, A., & Çam, O. (2011). Relationships between early diagnosis attitudes in cervical cancer of women and levels of self-esteem, body perception and hopelessness. *Nobel Medicus, 7*(3), 46–52. (Original work published in Turkish)

Bassal, R., Schejter, E., Cohen, D., & Keinan-Boker, L. (2017). Implementation of a national screening program for detection of malignant and pre-malignant cervical morbidity in Israel. *Harefuah, 156*(1), 51–53.

Boonpongmanee, C., & Jittanoon, P. (2007). Predictors of Papanicolaou testing in working women in Bangkok, Thailand. *Cancer Nursing, 30*(5), 384–389. https://doi.org/10.1097/01.NCC.0000290804.38335.32

Bowles, E. J., Gao, H., Brandzel, S., Bradford, S. C., & Buist, D. S. (2016). Comparative effectiveness of two outreach strategies for cervical cancer screening. *Preventive Medicine, 86*, 19–27. https://doi.org/10.1016/j.ypmed.2016.01.016

Damiani, G., Basso, D., Acampora, A., Bianchi, C. B., Silvestrini, G., Frisicale, E. M., ... Ricciardi, W. (2015). The impact of level of education on adherence to breast and cervical cancer screening: Evidence from a systematic review and meta-analysis. *Preventive Medicine, 81*, 281–289. https://doi.org/10.1016/j.ypmed.2015.09.011

DeGregorio, G., Manga, S., Kıyang, E., Manjuh, F., Bradford, L., Cholli, P., ... Ogembo, J. G. (2017). Implementing a fee-for-service cervical cancer screening and treatment program in Cameroon: Challenges and opportunities. *The Oncologist, 22*(7), 850–859. https://doi.org/10.1634/theoncologist.2016-0383

Esin, M. N., Bulduk, S., & Ardic, A. (2011). Beliefs about cervical cancer screening among Turkish married women. *Journal of Cancer Education, 26*(3), 510–515. https://doi.org/10.1007/s13187-011-0198-y

Ferris, D. G., Hupman, C., Waller, J. L., Cudnik, J., & Watkins, C. (2009). Assessment of the impact of cervical cancer prevention educational videos for Quechua- and Spanish-speaking Peruvian women. *Journal of Lower Genital Tract Disease, 13*(4), 244–251. https://doi.org/10.1097/LGT.0b013e318196785f

Gakidou, E., Nordhagen, S., & Obermeyer, Z. (2008). Coverage of cervical cancer screening in 57 countries: Low average levels and large inequalities. *PLoS Medicine, 5*(6), e132. https://doi.org/10.1371/journal.pmed.0050132

Globocan. (2018). International Agency for Research on Cancer, Global Cancer Observatory, *Cancer Tomorrow [Internet]*. Retrieved from https://gco.iarc.fr/tomorrow/

Gücük, S., Alkan, S., Arıca, S., & Ateş, A. (2011). Evaluation of Pap smear information among applicants of Van mother–child health and family planning center. *TAF Preventive Medicine Bulletin, 10*(5), 527–532. (Original work published in Turkish)

Güvenç, G., Akyüz, A., & Açıkel, C. H. (2011). Health Belief Model Scale for cervical cancer and Pap smear test: Psychometric testing. *Journal of Advanced Nursing, 67*(2), 428–437. https://doi.org/10.1111/j.1365-2648.2010.05450.x

Güvenç, G., Akyuz, A., & Yenen, M. C. (2013). Effectiveness of nursing interventions to increase Pap smear test screening. *Research in Nursing & Health, 36*(2), 146–157. https://doi.org/10.1002/nur.21526

Kitchener, H., Gittins, M., Cruickshank, M., Moseley, C., Fletcher, S., Albrow, R., ... Roberts, C. (2018). A cluster randomized trial of strategies to increase uptake amongst young women invited for their first cervical screen: The STRATEGIC trial. *Journal of Medical Screening, 25*(2), 88–98. https://doi.org/10.1177/0969141317696518

Kög, İ., Turan, T., Karabük, E., Karayünlü, B., Özgül, N., Demir, Ö. F., ... Köse, M. F. (2012). Cervical and breast cancer screening programme results of Etlik KETEM Group. *TAF Preventive Medicine Bulletin, 11*(2), 145–152. (Original work published in Turkish)

Lam, T. K., McPhee, S. J., Mock, J., Wong, C., Doan, H. T., Nguyen, T., ... Luong, T. N. (2003). Encouraging Vietnamese-American women to obtain Pap tests through lay health worker outreach and media education. *Journal of General Internal Medicine, 18*(7), 516–524. https://doi.org/10.1046/j.1525-1497.2003.21043.x

Lee, F. H. (2018). Intention to receive breast cancer screening and related factors of influence among Vietnamese women in transnational marriages. *The Journal of Nursing Research, 26*(2), 112–122. https://doi.org/10.1097/jnr.0000000000000210

Lee, F. H., & Wang, H. H. (2011). The utilization of Pap test services of women: A nationwide study in Taiwan. *Cancer Nursing, 34*(6), 464–469. https://doi.org/10.1097/NCC.0b013e31820b7866

Lee-Lin, F., Pett, M., Menon, U., Lee, S., Nail, L., Mooney, K., & Itano, J. (2007). Cervical cancer beliefs and Pap test screening practices among Chinese American Immigrants. *Oncology Nursing Forum, 34*(6), 1203–1209. https://doi.org/10.1188/07.ONF.1203-1209

Lu, H. Y. (2014). Determinants of intentions among Taiwanese women to seek information regarding cervical cancer. *The Journal of Nursing Research, 22*(2), 101–110. https://doi.org/10.1097/jnr.0000000000000030

Mingo, A. M., Panozzo, C. A., DiAngi, Y. T., Smith, J. S., Steenhoff, A. P., Ramogola-Masire, D., & Brewer, N. T. (2012). Cervical cancer awareness and screening in Botswana. *International Journal of Gynecological Cancer, 22*(4), 638–644. https://doi.org/10.1097/IGC.0b013e318249470a

Nguyen, T. T., McPhee, S. J., Gildengorin, G., Nguyen, T., Wong, C., Lai, K. Q., ... Ha-Iaconis, T. (2006). Papanicolaou testing among Vietnamese Americans: Results of a multifaceted intervention. *American Journal of Preventive Medicine, 31*(1), 1–9. https://doi.org/10.1016/j.amepre.2006.03.005

Özgül, N. (2010). The state of cervical cancer in Turkey and cervical cancer screening studies. In A. M. Tuncer (Ed.), *Cancer control in Turkey* (pp. 379–384). Ankara, Turkey: Republic of Turkey Ministry of Health.

Park, S., Chang, S., & Chung, C. (2005). Effects of a cognition–emotion focused program to increase public participation in Papanicolaou smear screening. *Public Health Nursing, 22*(4), 289–298. https://doi.org/10.1111/j.0737-1209.2005.220404.x

Public Health Institute of Turkey, Cancer Control Center. (2018). *Statistics of cancer 2015*. Retrieved from https://hsgm.saglik.gov.tr/depo/birimler/kanser-db/istatistik/Turkiye_Kanser_Istatistikleri_2015.pdf (Original work published in Turkish)

Spadea, T., Bellini, S., Kunst, A., Stirbu, I., & Costa, G. (2010). The impact of interventions to improve attendance in female cancer screening among lower socioeconomic groups: A review. *Preventive Medicine, 50*(4), 159–164. https://doi.org/10.1016/j.ypmed.2010.01.007

Studts, C. R., Tarasenko, Y. N., Schoenberg, N. E., Shelton, B. J., Hatcher-Keller, J., & Dignan, M. B. (2012). A community-based randomized trial of a faith-placed intervention to reduce cervical cancer burden in Appalachia. *Preventive Medicine, 54*(6), 408–414. https://doi.org/10.1016/j.ypmed.2012.03.019

Taylor, V. M., Hislop, T. G., Jackson, J. C., Tu, S. P., Yasui, Y., Schwartz, S. M., ... Thompson, B. (2002). A randomized controlled trial of interventions to promote cervical cancer screening among Chinese women in North America. *Journal of the National Cancer Institute, 94*(9), 670–677. https://doi.org/10.1093/jnci/94.9.670

Tuncer, M., Özgül, N., Özen Olcayto, E., Gültekin, M., & Erdin, B. (2009). *National cancer control program 2009–2015*. Ankara, Turkey: T. C. Ministry of Health, Department of Cancer Control.

Uluocak, T., & Bekar, M. (2012). Determination of women who work in health sector knowledge and attitude about cervical cancer. *Turkish Journal of Gynecological Oncology, 15*(2), 50–57. (Original work published in Turkish)

Visanuyothin, S., Chompikul, J., & Mongkolchati, A. (2015). Determinants of cervical cancer screening adherence in urban areas of Nakhon Ratchasima Province, Thailand. *Journal of Infection and Public Health, 8*, 543–552. https://doi.org/10.1016/j.jiph.2015.04.018

Vokó, Z., Nagyjánosi, L., Margitai, B., Kövi, R., Tóth, Z., László, D., & Kaló, Z. (2012). Modeling cost-effectiveness of cervical cancer screening in Hungary. *Value in Health, 15*(1), 39–45. https://doi.org/10.1016/j.jval.2011.10.003

World Health Organization. (2018). *Sexual and reproductive health.* Retrieved from http://www.who.int/reproductivehealth/cervical-cancer-public-health-concern/en/

Wright, T. C. Jr., & Kuhn, L. (2012). Alternative approaches to cervical cancer screening for developing countries. *Best Practice & Research Clinical Obstetrics & Gynecology, 26*(2), 197–208. https://doi.org/10.1016/j.bpobgyn.2011.11.004

Yücel, U., Çeber, E., & Özentürk, G. (2009). Efficacy of a training course given by midwives concerning cervical cancer risk factors and prevention. *Asian Pacific Journal of Cancer Prevention, 10*(3), 437–442.

Permissions

All chapters in this book were first published by Wolters Kluwer; hereby published with permission under the Creative Commons Attribution License or equivalent. Every chapter published in this book has been scrutinized by our experts. Their significance has been extensively debated. The topics covered herein carry significant findings which will fuel the growth of the discipline. They may even be implemented as practical applications or may be referred to as a beginning point for another development.

The contributors of this book come from diverse backgrounds, making this book a truly international effort. This book will bring forth new frontiers with its revolutionizing research information and detailed analysis of the nascent developments around the world.

We would like to thank all the contributing authors for lending their expertise to make the book truly unique. They have played a crucial role in the development of this book. Without their invaluable contributions this book wouldn't have been possible. They have made vital efforts to compile up to date information on the varied aspects of this subject to make this book a valuable addition to the collection of many professionals and students.

This book was conceptualized with the vision of imparting up-to-date information and advanced data in this field. To ensure the same, a matchless editorial board was set up. Every individual on the board went through rigorous rounds of assessment to prove their worth. After which they invested a large part of their time researching and compiling the most relevant data for our readers.

The editorial board has been involved in producing this book since its inception. They have spent rigorous hours researching and exploring the diverse topics which have resulted in the successful publishing of this book. They have passed on their knowledge of decades through this book. To expedite this challenging task, the publisher supported the team at every step. A small team of assistant editors was also appointed to further simplify the editing procedure and attain best results for the readers.

Apart from the editorial board, the designing team has also invested a significant amount of their time in understanding the subject and creating the most relevant covers. They scrutinized every image to scout for the most suitable representation of the subject and create an appropriate cover for the book.

The publishing team has been an ardent support to the editorial, designing and production team. Their endless efforts to recruit the best for this project, has resulted in the accomplishment of this book. They are a veteran in the field of academics and their pool of knowledge is as vast as their experience in printing. Their expertise and guidance has proved useful at every step. Their uncompromising quality standards have made this book an exceptional effort. Their encouragement from time to time has been an inspiration for everyone.

The publisher and the editorial board hope that this book will prove to be a valuable piece of knowledge for researchers, students, practitioners and scholars across the globe.

List of Contributors

Yuqin PAN and Ruyi CHEN
Faculty of Jinhua Polytechnic, Zhejiang Province, China

Hsiu-Mei CHANG
Department of Nursing, National Taiwan University Hospital, Taiwan, ROC

Ean-Weng HUANG
Department of Information Management, National Taipei University of Nursing and Health Sciences, Taiwan, ROC

I-Ching HOU
Department of Nursing, National Yang Ming University, Taiwan, ROC

Hsiu-Yun LIU
Department of Nursing, National Taiwan University Hospital, Taiwan, ROC

Fang-Shan LI
Department of Nursing, National Taiwan University Hospital H sin-Chu Branch, Taiwan, ROC

Shwu-Fen CHIOU
School of Nursing, National Taipei University of Nursing and Health Sciences, Taiwan, ROC

Wen-Chih FANN
Department of Emergency Medicine, Chia-Yi Chang Gung Memorial Hospital, Taiwan

Chang-Chiao HUNG
Department of Nursing, Chang Gung University of Science and Technology and Associate Research Fellow, Department of Nursing, Chia-Yi Chang Gung Memorial Hospital, Taiwan

Wendy CHABOYER
School of Nursing and Midwifery, Menzies Health Institute Queensland, Griffith University, Queensland, Australia

Bih-O LEE
College of Nursing, Kaohsiung Medical University, Taiwan and Faculty of Nursing, Universitas Airlangga, Indonesia

Jaana SEITOVIRTA
Department of Nursing Science, University of Eastern Finland, Finland

Aku-Ville LEHTIM-KI
School of Business, Department of Information and Service Economy, Aalto University, Finland

Katri VEHVIL-INEN-JULKUNEN
Department of Nursing Science, University of Eastern Finland, Finland

Lasse MITRONEN
Department of Marketing, School of Business, Aalto University, Finland

Tarja KVIST
Department of Nursing Science, University of Eastern Finland, Finland

Ke-Hsin Chueh
Department of Nursing, Fu Jen Catholic University

Chia-Chuan Chang
Department of Nursing, Fu Jen Catholic University; and Deputy Director, Fu Jen Catholic University Hospital

Mei-Ling Yeh
Graduate Institute of Integration of Traditional Chinese Medicine with Western Nursing, National Taipei University of Nursing and Health Sciences

Min Sun PARK
Department of Nursing, Cheongju University, Cheongju, Republic of Korea

Su Jung LEE and Young Rim CHOI
College of Nursing, Korea University, Seoul, Republic of Korea

Sung Ok CHANG
College of Nursing and BK21 FOUR R&E Center for Learning Health Systems, Korea University, Seoul, Republic of Korea

Sergio RICO-MARTÍN
Department of Nursing, Nursing and Occupational Therapy College, University of Extremadura, Cáceres, Spain

Jorge M. DE NICOLÁS-JIMÉNEZ
Zona Centro Health Center, Extremadura Health Service, Cáceres, Spain

Mariana MARTÍNEZ-ÁLVAREZ
Department of Nursing, Faculty of Medicine, University of Extremadura, Badajoz, Spain

Sergio CORDOVILLA-GUARDIA, Esperanza SANTANO-MOGENA and Julián F. CALDERÓN-GARCÍA
Department of Nursing, Nursing and Occupational Therapy College, University of Extremadura, Cáceres, Spain

Chiou-Fen LIN
College of Nursing, School of Gerontology Health Management, Taipei Medical University and Adjunct Nursing Consultant, Department of Nursing, Shuang Ho Hospital, Taipei Medical University
School of Nursing, Taipei Medical University and Nursing Consultant, Department of Nursing, Shuang Ho Hospital, Taipei Medical University

Chung-I HUANG
Center for Management and Development and Adjunct Assistant Professor, School of Health Care Administration, Taipei Medical University

Che-Ming YANG
College of Management and College of Humanities and Social Sciences, Taipei Medical University and Director, Department of Nuclear Medicine, Taipei Medical University Shuang Ho Hospital

Meei-Shiow LU
College of Nursing, Taipei Medical University and Chairperson, Board of Controllers, Taiwan Union of Nurses Association

Masoumeh BARZEGAR SAFARI
Health Economics Policy Research Center, Tehran Medical Sciences Branch, Islamic Azad University, Tehran, Iran

Mohammadkarim BAHADORI
Health Management Research Center, Baqiyatallah University of Medical Sciences, Tehran, Iran

Khalil ALIMOHAMMADZADEH
Department of Healthcare Management, School of Management and Social Sciences, North Tehran Branch, Islamic Azad University, Health Economics policy Research Center, Tehran Medical Sciences Islamic Azad University, Tehran, Iran

Ayse DELIKTAS and Ruveyde AYDIN
Faculty of Nursing, Department of Obstetrics & Gynaecological Nursing, Akdeniz University, Turkey

Oznur KORUKCU
Faculty of Nursing, Department of Obstetrics & Gynaecological Nursing, Akdeniz University, Turkey

Kamile KABUKCUOGLU
Faculty of Nursing, Department of Obstetrics & Gynaecological Nursing, Akdeniz University, Turkey

Aysun BEKDEMİR
Home Health Services Coordination Center, Üsküdar State Hospital, Istanbul, Turkey

Nesrin İLHAN
Department of Nursing, Bezmialem Vakif University, Istanbul, Turkey

Fu-Chih LAI
College of Nursing, Taipei Medical University

Way-Ren HUANG
PhD, RN, Postdoctoral Research Fellow, Operations Center for Industry Collaboration, National Tsing Hua University

Chia-Jung HSIEH
School of Nursing, College of Nursing, National Taipei University of Nursing and Health Sciences

Ozge TAYFUR EKMEKCI
Faculty of Economics and Administrative Science, Department of Business Administration, Hacettepe University, Ankara, Turkey

Dorela XHAKO
Faculty of Economics and Administrative Science, Department of Business Administration, Hacettepe University, Ankara, Turkey

Selin METIN CAMGOZ
Faculty of Economics and Administrative Science, Department of Business Administration, Hacettepe University, Ankara, Turkey

Shu-Fen LO
Department of Nursing, Tzu Chi University of Science and Technology, Nursing Technology Innovation Service Research Center, Taiwan, ROC

Li-Jung CHANG
Department of Nursing, Tzu Chi University of Science and Technology, Taiwan, ROC

Mark HAYTER
Nursing and Health Research, Faculty of Health Sciences, University of Hull, England, UK

An-Chi O YANG
Department of Nursing, Tzu Chi University and Doctoral Program Student, School and Graduate Institute of Nursing, National Taiwan University, Taipei, Taiwan, ROC

Mashael Hasan ALAMRANI
Faculty of Applied Medical Science, Department of Nursing, University of Tabuk, Saudi Arabia

Kamila Ahmad ALAMMAR
Nursing Education Adminstration, King Fahad Medical City, Saudi Arabia

Sarah Saad ALQAHTANI
Nursing Education Department, AlAmal Complex for Mental Health and Master's Student, College of Nursing, King Saud University, Saudi Arabia

Olfat A. SALEM
Nursing Administration and Education Department, College of Nursing, King Saudi University, Saudi Arabia and Faculty of Nursing, Nursing Administration Department, Menoufiya University, Egypt

Alaa ALBASHAYREH
College of Nursing, University of Iowa, Iowa City, Iowa, USA

Omar M. AL-RAWAJFAH
College of Nursing, Sultan Qaboos University, Muscat, Oman and Adjunct Associate Professor, Faculty of Nursing, Al Al-Bayt University, Mafraq, Jordan

Huda AL-AWAISI
PhD, RN, Acting Head of Nursing Research, Directorate of Nursing, Sultan Qaboos University Hospital, Muscat, Oman

Suja KARKADA
Department of Fundamentals and Administration, College of Nursing, Sultan Qaboos University, Muscat, Oman

Sulaiman D. AL SABEI
Department of Fundamentals and Administration, College of Nursing, Sultan Qaboos University, Muscat, Oman

Ming-Yi Hsu
School of Nursing, Chung Shan Medical University and Adjunct Supervisor, Department of Nursing, Chung Shan Medical University Hospital

Shu-Fen Su
Department of Nursing, National Taichung University of Science and Technology

Lien-Ying Chiang
MSN, RN, Department of Nursing, Taichung Veterans General Hospital

Sou-Jen Shih
Department of Nursing, Taichung Veterans General Hospital

Yu-Chen Chen
Department of Nursing, Cheng-Ching General Hospital

Sheena RAMAZANU
MClin Res, RN, The Hong Kong Polytechnic University, Hong Kong; and Staff Nurse, Yishun Community Hospital, Singapore

Doris LEUNG and Vico Chung Lim CHIANG
School of Nursing, The Hong Kong Polytechnic University, Hong Kong

Zohreh HOSSEINI MARZNAKI
Amol Faculty of Nursing and Midwifery Sciences, Department of Nursing, Mazandaran University of Medical Sciences, Sari, Iran

Khatere KHANJANKHANI
Department of Health Policy, School of Public Health, Tehran University of Medical Sciences, Tehran, Iran

Waliu Jawula SALISU
Cambridge Liver Unit, Cambridge University Hospitals NHS Foundation Trust, Addenbrookes Hospital, Cambridge, United Kingdom

Fatemeh HAJIHOSSEINI
Amol Faculty of Nursing and Midwifery Sciences, Department of Nursing, Mazandaran University of Medical Sciences, Sari, Iran

Saeed BARZEGARI
Amol Faculty of Paramedical Sciences, Department of Health Information Technology, Mazandaran University of Medical Sciences, Sari, Iran

Li-Hui HO
MS, RN, NP, Department of Neurosurgery, China Medical Hospital, Taiwan, Republic of China

Shu-Chen CHANG
Department of Nursing, Chunghwa Christian Hospital , College of Nursing and Health Sciences, Da-Yeh University, Taiwan, Republic of China

Kevin KAU
Academic Writing Education Center, National Taiwan University, Taiwan, Republic of China

Shu-Ying SHIU
MS, RN, NP, Emergency Room, Department of Nursing, Chunghwa Christian Hospital, Taiwan, Republic of China

Sheng-Shiung HUANG
College of Nursing and Health Sciences, Da-Yeh University, Taiwan, Republic of China

Ya-Jung WANG
Department of Nursing, Da-Yeh University, Taiwan, Republic of China

Shiow-Luan TSAY
College of Nursing and Health Sciences, Da-Yeh University, Taiwan, Republic of China

Neda ASADI, Robabeh MEMARIAN and Zohreh VANAKI
Faculty of Medical Sciences, Department of Nursing, Tarbiat Modares University, Tehran, Iran

Omorogieva OJO
Faculty of Education and Health, University of Greenwich, London, UK

Joanne BROOKE
Faculty of Health, Education & Life Sciences, Birmingham City University, Birmingham, UK

Camille CRONIN
School of Health and Social Care, Southend Campus, University of Essex, Essex, UK

Ali MOVAHEDI
MSN, RN, Instructor of Critical Care Nursing, Department of Anesthesia and Operating Room Nursing, Neyshabur University of Medical Sciences, Neyshabur, Iran

Mohammad BIDKHORI
Department of Epidemiology, School of Public Health, Tehran University of Medical Sciences, Tehran, Iran

Tajmohammad ARAZI and Mostafa KHALEGHIPOUR
Department of Anesthesia and Operating Room Nursing, Neyshabur University of Medical Sciences, Neyshabur, Iran

Fatemeh AMINI
Department of Anesthesia and Operating Room Nursing, Neyshabur University of Medical Sciences, Neyshabur, Iran

Fatma AY
Faculty of Health Sciences, Department of Midwifery, Istanbul University-Cerrahpaşa, Turkey

Şehrinaz POLAT
Directorate of Nursing Services, Hospital of Faculty of Medicine, Istanbul University, Turkey

Tennur KASHIMI
Operating Room, Hospital of Faculty of Medicine, Istanbul University, Turkey

Gonul KURT
Faculty of Health Sciences, Department of Midwifery, Sakarya University, Sakarya, Turkey

Aygul AKYUZ
Department of Obstetrics and Gynecology Nursing, Florence Nightingale Hospital School of Nursing, Demiroglu Bilim University, Istanbul, Turkey

Index

Printed in the USA
CPSIA information can be obtained
at www.ICGtesting.com
LVHW080735221023
761596LV00011B/2134